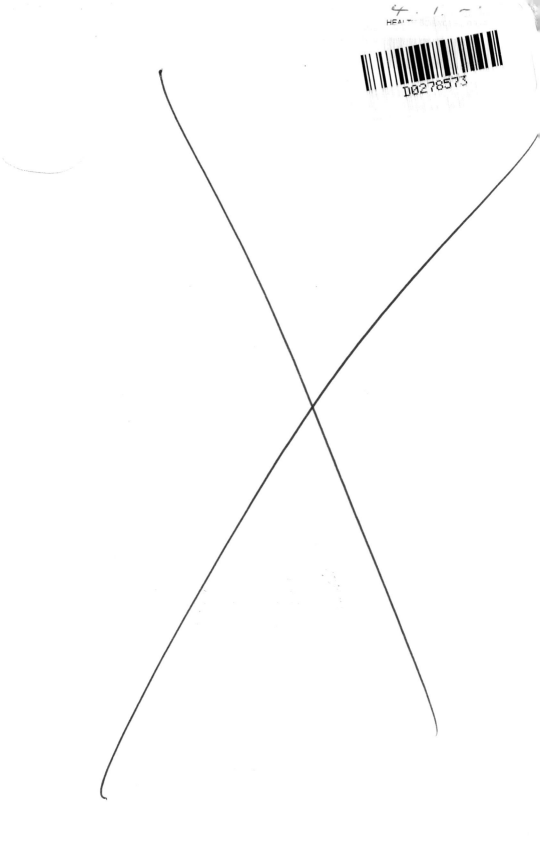

Mechanism and Management of Headache

Mechanism and Management of Headache

Seventh Edition

James W. Lance, AO, CBE, MD, Hon DSc, FRCP (London), FRACP, FAA
Consultant Neurologist, Institute of Neurological Sciences, The Prince of Wales Hospital and Emeritus Professor of Neurology, University of New South Wales, Sydney, Australia

Peter J. Goadsby, BMedSc, MB, BS, MD, PhD, DSc, FRACP
Wellcome Senior Research Fellow and Reader in Clinical Neurology, Institute of Neurology, University College London, and Consultant Neurologist, The National Hospital for Neurology and Neurosurgery, Queen Square, London, UK

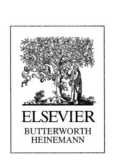

ELSEVIER
BUTTERWORTH
HEINEMANN

ELSEVIER
BUTTERWORTH
HEINEMANN

The Curtis Center
170 S Independence Mall W 300E
Philadelphia, Pennsylvania 19106

NOTICE

Medicine is an ever-changing field. Standard safety precautions must be followed, but as new research and clinical experience broaden our knowledge, changes in treatment and drug therapy may become necessary or appropriate. Readers are advised to check the most current product information provided by the manufacturer of each drug to be administered to verify the recommended dose, the method and duration of administration, and contraindications. It is the responsibility of the licensed prescriber, relying on experience and knowledge of the patient, to determine dosages and the best treatment for each individual patient. Neither the publisher nor the author assumes any liability for any injury and/or damage to persons or property arising from this publication.

Previous editions copyrighted 1998, 1993, 1982, 1978, 1973, 1969 by Judith J. Lance

International Standard Book Number: 0-7506-7530-6

Acquisitions Editor: Susan F. Pioli
Developmental Editor: Joan Ryan

Printed in the United States of America

Last digit is the print number: 9   8   7   6   5   4   3   2   1

Contents

Preface to the Seventh Edition

It is now 35 years since the first edition of this book appeared. In the 6 years since the last edition new headache entities have been described, new treatments have appeared, and research into the pathophysiology of migraine and cluster headache has intensified.

Our aim is to retain the most important findings in the older literature as a background for the presentation of new developments and to combine the practical approach to managment of previous editions with a critical analysis of the most recent information available. The format broadly follows the guidelines provided by the revised classification of the International Headache Society published in 2004. This classification introduced a new section on "Headaches attributable to psychiatric disorder." Professor Jes Olesen pointed out in his introduction to the new classification, "research illuminating this field is extremely scarce, so the chapter is very brief." For this reason we have not devoted a separate chapter to it. The important role of psychological factors in many forms of headache is considered in other chapters.

Chronic daily headache has been given a chapter to itself because it presents a common therapeutic challenge.

We trust that this new edition will prove to be a good companion for all those who suffer from headaches or treat them.

J.W.L.
P.J.G.

Preface to the First Edition

About once a month, until the age of 70 years, George Bernard Shaw suffered a devastating headache which lasted for a day. One afternoon, after recovering from an attack, he was introduced to Nansen and asked the famous Arctic explorer whether he had ever discovered a headache cure.

"No," said Nansen with a look of amazement.

"Have you ever tried to find a cure for headaches?"

"No."

"Well, that is a most astonishing thing!" exclaimed Shaw. "You have spent your life in trying to discover the North Pole, which nobody on earth cares tuppence about, and you have never attempted to discover a cure for the headache, which every living person is crying aloud for."[*]

It is easy for a person who has never been troubled with headaches to lose patience with those who are plagued by them. The reaction of the virtuous observer may pass through a phase of sympathetic concern to one of frustrated tolerance and, finally, to a mood of irritation and resentment in which the recurrence of headaches is attributed to a defective personality or escape from unpleasant life situations. The sound sleeper is traditionally intolerant of the insomniac and the speedy of bowel is just a little contemptuous of the constipated. In short, we tend to consider ourselves as the norm and to look quizzically at those whose physiological or psychological processes are at variance with our own. Such an attitude often persists in spite of years of advanced education and scientific training. To make it clear that I am not numbering myself among the righteous, I must state that I am not subject to headache and that my spirits often sink when confronted with a succession of patients whose contorted expressions testify to a lifetime of headache misery. This is about the only circumstance which I find likely to provoke headache in myself—I suppose on the principle that if you can't beat them, join them!

It would be foolish to deny that the workings of the mind are of great importance in the production of headache, but they are only part of the story.

My interest in migraine was first aroused when working at the Northcott Neurological Centre in Sydney. Each patient with migraine gave a history that was a little different from the others, but all were variations on a clearly

---

[*]Pearson, H. (1942). *Bernard Shaw*. pp. 242-243. London, Collins.

recognizable theme. It seemed that all the clues were there to point the way to the understanding of the mechanism of migraine. These thoughts led to studies of the clinical features and natural history of migraine and, later, to laboratory work which now suggests that migraine is an hereditary recurrent metabolic disturbance. If this be the case, a patient cannot be held responsible for having migraine attacks any more than a woman for having menstrual periods. The treatment of migraine has improved with better understanding of the syndrome, but knowledge of the migraine mechanism and its treatment still leave much to be desired.

Mysteries remain in the problem of tension headache, although the place of psychological factors is much more obvious in this group than in migraine and an association with chronic over-contraction of muscle is almost universal. However, many tense, frowning people do not get headaches, and the explanation for those that do must go beyond a catalogue of undesirable personality traits and bad luck in cards or love. Migraine and tension headache are given most space in this small book because they are common complaints, not always easy to diagnose and treat, and worry patients and their medical attendants. Other common forms of headache such as those arising from eye-strain or sinusitis are not emphasized as much, because their mechanism and management are more straightforward. Serious acute headaches which betoken some hazardous intracranial condition are described sufficiently to assist in diagnosis, but not dealt with at length since their management usually becomes the prerogative of the specialist neurological unit.

This book is designed to be relatively easy armchair reading for the general practitioner, senior medical student, or others who may be interested in the mechanism of headache or concerned with the practical management of headache problems. The neurologist may find something of interest in the chapters on tension headache and migraine. References are listed for those who wish to read in greater depth.

The present concept of headache mechanisms depends to a great extent on the work of the late Harold G. Wolff and his colleagues, which is described in Wolff's monograph *Headache and Other Head Pain*. The reader is referred to this work for aspects of headache which are passed over lightly here. The subject may not have all the excitement of a detective story but the talents of the great detectives of fiction would not be lost in trying to unravel some of the complexities of headache.

J.W.L.

Acknowledgments

Studies of clinical aspects, pathophysiology and treatment of headache have been conducted at The Prince Henry and Prince of Wales Hospitals, Sydney, and more recently at the National Hospital for Neurology and Neurosurgery, London, for over forty years. Those who have been or are presently engaged in the research programme include:

R. D. Adams	A. Gantenbein	M. Matharu
S. Afridi	N. Giffin	J. Michalicek
S. Akerman	V. Gordon	J. Misbach
H. Angus-Leppan	C. Hadini	D. Mitsikostas
M. Anthony	P. Hammond	E. Mylecharane
A. Bahra	M. Hellier	B. Olausson
A. Bergerot	H. Hinterberger	J. Peralta
R. Bhola	P. Holland	R. D. Piper
P. Boers	K. L. Hoskin	F. Ragaglia
C. Boes	H. Kaube	K. Shields
N. Bogduk	Y. E. Knight	T. Shimomura
E. Cittadini	G. A. Lambert	B. W. Somerville
J. Classey	M. Lasalandra	P. J. Spira
D. A. Curran	G. D. A. Lord	R. J. Storer
B. Daher	A. Lowy	A. Srikiatkhachorn
P. D. Drummond	J. Marin	K. M. A. Welch
J. W. Duckworth	N. Marlowe	A. S. Zagami
S. Evers	A. May	

We are most grateful to this happy blend of neurologists, pharmacologists, anatomists, physiologists, biochemists and psychologists for many years of stimulating association, and to our neurosurgical colleagues for their friendly collaboration in managing headache and other problems.

The research programme has been supported by the National Health and Medical Research Council of Australia and has been generously assisted by grants from the J. A. Perini Family Trust, the Adolph Basser Trust, The Australian Brain Foundation, The Migraine Trust, Sandoz AG, Basel (now Novartis), Glaxo-Wellcome (now GlaxoSmithKline) and Warren and Cheryl Anderson. Peter J. Goadsby particularly wishes to acknowledge the generous support of the Wellcome Trust, and the privilege of contributing to this book.

The manuscript has been prepared by Patricia Miller, Carol Flecknoe and Sophie Ryan. The anatomical diagrams were drawn by Dr. N. Bogduk and Mr. Marcus Cremonese. All photographs were prepared by the Department of Medical Illustration, University of New South Wales.

We are grateful to the editors of the following publications for permission to reproduce tables and figures from papers by our colleagues and ourselves: Annals of Neurology; Archives of Neurology; Brain; Cephalagia; Clinical and Experimental Neurology (Sydney, Adis Press); Headache; Journal of Neurological Sciences; Journal of Neurology, Neurosurgery and Psychiatry; Neurology; Migraine and Other Headaches (New York, Charles Scribner's Sons); Migraine: a Spectrum of Ideas (Oxford, Oxford University Press); Medical Journal of Australia; Research and Clinical Studies in Headache (Karger of Basel and New York); Wolff/Wolff's Headache and Other Head Pain (5th Edn, New York, Oxford University Press).

Chapter 1
The History of Headache

Among the beautiful frescoes in the Brancacci chapel in Florence, Italy, painted by Masaccio in the 15th century is the Expulsion from the Garden of Eden. Adam and Eve are shown with expressions of agony, Adam clasping his head with both hands, as the sad couple walk away. Was this Masaccio's idea of the First Headache?

To adopt an evolutionary approach, one might speculate that human susceptibility to headache developed when we assumed an upright posture. The discovery of trepanned skulls with bone regrowth shows that some Stone Age patients survived the trepanning procedure but does not tell us whether headache was the indication for operation. We have heard reports of a gorilla in the Toronto Zoo who sometimes curls up into a ball, shielding her eyes from the light and refusing to eat normally.

Written accounts date from about 3000 BC: Alverez (1945) quotes a couplet from a Sumerian poem in which, in some sort of heaven or Abode of the Blessed,

The sick-eyed says not "I am sick-eyed."
The sick-headed (says) not "I am sick-headed."

Also poetic, and more specific, is a reference to headache from Babylonian literature of about the same period (Sigerist, 1955; McHenry, 1969).

Headache roameth over the desert, blowing like the wind,
Flashing like lightning, it is loosed above and below;
It cutteth off him who feareth not his god like a reed,
Like a stalk of henna it slitteth his thews.
It wasteth the flesh of him who hath no protecting goddess,
Flashing like a heavenly star, it cometh like the dew;
It standeth hostile against the wayfarer, scorching him like the day,
This man it hath struck and
Like one with heart disease he staggereth,
Like one bereft of reason he is broken,

Like that which has been cast into the fire he is shrivelled,
Like a wild ass . . . his eyes are full of cloud,
On himself he feedeth, bound in death;
Headache whose course like the dread windstorm none knoweth,
None knoweth its full time or its bond.

The Atharvaveda, one of the four sacred Vedas of the Hindus, was written some time around the 10th century BC. One hymn reads,

O physician, do thou release this man from headache, free him from cough which has entered into all his limbs and joints. One should resort to forests and hills for relief from diseases resulting from excessive rains, severe wind and intense heat (Chand, 1982).

The main source of information about ancient Egyptian medicine is the Ebers Papyrus, said to have been found between the legs of a mummy in the necropolis of Thebes. The purchase and translation of this momentous and lengthy document (30 cm wide and 20.23 meters long) was arranged by George Ebers, professor of Egyptology in Leipzig, after whom the papyrus was named (Von Klein, 1905). Experts estimate that the Ebers Papyrus, which mentions migraine, neuralgia, and shooting head pains, was written or transcribed from earlier medical documents in approximately 1550 BC. The papyrus is obviously based on earlier writings, because one prescription was written for King Usaphais who reigned in 2700 BC (Major, 1930). Another six papyri on medical matters are in existence. I am indebted to Dr. John Edmeads for an artist's impression of the advice given to headache sufferers in those days (Figure 1.1). A clay crocodile was firmly bound to the head of the patient, with herbs being placed in the mouth of the crocodile. Nowadays we dispense with the clay crocodile and put the magic herbs directly into the patient's mouth.

Greek medicine may be said to have started with Aesculapius, who probably lived about 1250 BC and became so successful in his practice as a physician that the supply of souls to the underworld was imperiled. For this reason, at the request of Hades, Zeus destroyed Aesculapius with a thunderbolt. After his death, he became revered as a god and temples dedicated to healing of the sick were known throughout Greece as *asklepia*. Guthrie (1947) mentions that one of the cures recorded on stone tablets at Epidaurus was Case Number 29, a young man named Agestratos, who suffered from insomnia on account of headaches. He fell asleep in the temple and dreamed that Aesculapius cured him of his headache and then taught him to wrestle. The next day he departed cured and, shortly afterward, was crowned victor in wrestling at the Nemean games.

Egyptian medicine was probably known to Hippocrates (460 BC), who first described visual symptoms associated with migraine (Critchley, 1967):

Most of the time he seemed to see something shining before him like a light, usually in part of the right eye; at the end of a moment, a violent pain supervened in the right temple, then in all the head and neck, where the neck is attached to the spine. . . . Vomiting, when it became possible, was able to divert the pain and render it more moderate.

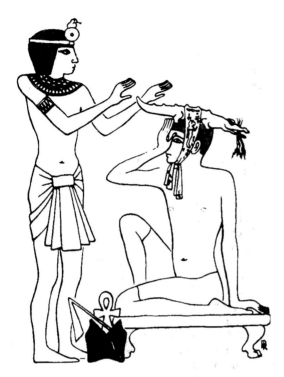

FIGURE 1.1 An interpretation of the treatment of migraine in 1200 BC. A clay crocodile with magic herbs in its mouth was bound to the patient's head. (Drawing by P. Cunningham, reproduced by permission of J. Edmeads.)

Other forms of headache, such as those caused by exercise and sexual intercourse, were noted by Hippocrates (Adams, 1939) and are discussed later in this text.

The story of migraine was elaborated by Roman authors. Cornelius Celsus, a friend of the Emperor Tiberius, described how headache could be induced by drinking wine or by the heat of a fire or the sun (Critchley, 1967). Aretaeus, born in Cappadocia (now a region of Turkey) in about AD 80, enlarged on previous descriptions of migraine by commenting that pain is often restricted to one half of the head and that afflicted patients

> . . . flee the light; the darkness soothes their disease; nor can they bear readily to look upon or hear anything agreeable; their sense of smell is vitiated, neither does anything agreeable to smell delight them, and they have also an aversion to fetid things; the patients, moreover, are weary of life and wish to die (Adams, 1841).

Galen (AD 131–201) introduced the term "hemicrania" for unilateral headache, attributing it to "the ascent of vapours, either . . . too hot or too cold." "Hemicrania" was later transformed to the Old English "megrim" and French "migraine." Galen's view of four humors that govern health and disease persisted for many centuries. It was expressed, in terms that could be given a modern interpretation, by Paul of Aegina, a Greek physician at the medical school of

Alexandria, who wrote in AD 600: "Headache, which is one of the most serious complaints, is sometimes occasioned by an intemperament solely; sometimes by redundance of humors, and sometimes by both" (Adams, 1844).

Treating headache by applying hot iron or by applying garlic to an incision in the temple was advocated by the Arab physician Abu'l Oasim (Abulcasis), born in Spain in AD 936 (Critchley, 1967). Critchley also quotes the Persian Avicenna (AD 980–1037) as saying, "Little does it concern the patient that there is an underlying cause to be treated if the practitioner proves unable to relieve his pain."

An illuminated manuscript of the 12th century by the Abbess Hildegard of Bingen describes recurrent visual phenomena that may well have been migraine equivalents: "I saw a great star, most splendid and beautiful, and with it an exceeding multitude of falling sparks with which the star followed south-ward . . . and suddenly they were all annihilated, being turned into black coals . . . and cast into the abyss so that I could see them no more" (Critchley, 1967). She explained that her headaches were unilateral, because nobody could stand it if they were on both sides of the head (Isler, 1993).

Transient sensory loss and weakness on the left side of the body accompa-nying severe headache was described by Charles Le Pois in 1618 (Riley, 1932). In 1684 Dr Willis's *Practice of Physicke,* published in London 9 years after the death of Thomas Willis (1621–1675), includes two chapters on headache (reproduced by Knapp, 1963, 1964). Headache is "a disease which falls upon . . . sober and intemperate, the empty and the full-bellied, the fat and the lean, the young and the old, yea upon men and women of every age, state or condition." Willis pointed out that the source of pain is not the brain, cere-bellum, or medulla, because "they want sensible fibres" but rather distension of the vessels, which "pulls the nervous fibres one from another and so brings to them painful corrugations or wrinklings." He described the provocation of headache by wine, overeating, lying in the sun, passion, sexual activity, long sleeping, "scirrhous tumours growing to the meninges" and "other diseases of an evil conformation." He comments on "ravenous hunger" as a premonitory symptom of migraine and on the nausea and vomiting that follows the headache.

Willis's views on therapy do not live up to the expectation aroused by his clinical observations. He starts with sage but joyless advice about avoiding wine, spiced meats, baths, sexual intercourse ("Venus"), and violent motions of the mind and body, before advocating enemas, the letting of blood, and application of leeches, and then proceeding to a bizarre polypharmacy. Although few would take umbrage at the use of vinegar, nutmeg, and rose-mary (a decoction of the dried leaves made with spring water), some would raise eyebrows at pills of amber, crab's eyes and coral, and most would draw the line at millipedes and woodlice: "We ought not to omit or postpone the use of millipedes or woodlice, for that the juice of them, wrung forth, with the dis-tilled water, also a powder of them prepared, often bring notable help, for the curing of old and pertinacious headaches." In fairness to Willis, he also administered anodynes and hypnotics to those in need.

The Swiss physician Wepfer (1620–1695) noted the alternation of migraine from one side of the head to the other in some cases, attributing migraine to relaxation of the vessels. In 1669 he observed the visual auras of migraine. Because this description was not published until 1727, long after his death, he was pre-empted by Vater, who published a dissertation on hemianopic migraine scotomas in 1723 (Isler, 1993).

Descriptions of migraine multiplied in the 18th and 19th centuries, the most comprehensive being the work of Liveing (1873), from whose treatise *On Megrim, Sick-Headache and Some Allied Disorders,* many of the following statements and quotations are borrowed, with some additions from Riley (1932), Critchley (1967), and Schiller (1975). Fordyce, in *De Hemicrania* (published 1758) observed occasional premonitory depression, polyuria during the attack, and the association with menstruation, which had been reported by Johannis Van der Linden in *De Hemicrania Menstrua* (published 1660). Fothergill in 1778 described the visual disturbances of classical migraine and was the first to use the term "fortification spectra" to describe their zigzag appearance: "After breakfast, if much toast and butter has been used, it begins with a singular kind of glimmering in the sight; objects swiftly changing their apparent position, surrounded with luminous angles like those of a fortification." Fothergill considered that "the headache proceeds from the stomach, not the reverse." He blamed certain foods, particularly "melted butter, fat meats, spices, meat pies, hot buttered toast and malt liquors when strong and hoppy." In 1796 Erasmus Darwin, the grandfather of Charles Darwin, suggested a trial of centrifugal force for the relief of headache, which, as he quaintly added, "cannot be done in private practice, and which I therefore recommend to some hospital physician. What might be the consequence of whirling a person with his head next to the centre of motion, so as to force the blood from the brain into the other parts of the body?" This challenge was taken up 150 years later by Harold G. Wolff with relief of a headache, using a centrifuge large enough for a human being.

James Ware, in 1814, described bouts of fortification spectra without a headache ensuing, later called "metastases of migraine" by Tissot (Critchley, 1967) but now known as *migraine equivalents.* Brief episodes of hemianopia without headache were described by Wollaston in 1824, and brief episodes of scintillating scotomas were described by Parry in 1825. In 1865 Sir George Airy described his visual hallucinations as "nearly resembling those of a Norman arch." A similar form of migraine manifested itself in one of Sir George's sons, Hubert Airy, who introduced the term *teichopsia* for fortification spectra and illustrated his own experience in colored plates, which were reproduced by Liveing (1873). Dysphasia with migraine was reported by Tissot, Parry, G. B. Airy, and others (Schiller, 1975).

In 1837, Labarraque implicated noise as a cause of migraine in the following words:

We all know that it is not everyone who can, with impunity, do himself the pleasure of assisting at certain theatrical representations where the glory of France is daily celebrated with noise and smoke. And how many good citizens are there not, tried patriots, whom the threatening of a migraine infallibly brought on by the unaccustomed din of drums and military music, forcibly hinders from taking part in our civic fêtes, and joining their companies on grand review days.

Marshall Hall wrote in 1849 that "Nothing is so common, nothing is viewed as of such trifling import, as the seizure termed 'sick-headache.' Yet I have known 'sick-headache' issue in paroxysmal attacks of a very severe nature, both apoplectic and epileptic" (Schiller, 1975).

The fact that the pain of migraine "mounts synchronously with the pulse of the temporal artery" was noted by Dubois-Reymond in 1859. His artery on the affected side was "like a firm cord to the touch," his eye was "small and reddened with a dilated pupil and his face became pale and warm, although his ear on the side of headache became red and hot toward the end of the attack." When he indulged "in vast and uninterrupted mental exertions," his headaches were worse, but they ceased completely on hiking trips. Parry in 1825 and later Mollendorf in 1867 observed that compressing the carotid artery made the headache disappear (Schiller, 1975). The concept of the pathophysiology of migraine was thus swinging to a vascular rather than a neural cause, although Liveing (1873) drew the analogy with epilepsy and regarded disorders of the local circulation as "among the least constant and regular of the phenomena." He was supported later by Hughlings Jackson (1890), who believed migraine to be a form of sensory epilepsy, with the headache and vomiting as an epiphenomenon (Schiller, 1975). Liveing's classic monograph *On Megrim, Sick Headache and Some Allied Disorders* was reprinted in 1997 (with an introduction by Oliver Sacks) by Arts and Boeve, Nijmegen, to commemorate the Eighth Congress of the International Headache Society, held in Amsterdam.

At about the same time as Liveing, P. W. Latham (1872) expressed the view that the disturbance of vision was due to a defective supply of blood to one side of the brain from the contraction of the cerebral arteries, after which "the action of the sympathetic is exhausted . . . the vessels become distended, the head throbs" (Schiller, 1975).

Sir Samuel Wilks (1872) gave an admirable dissertation on migraine that "runs in families, and is due to a particular nervous temperament." He states that "whatever produces a strong impression on the nervous system of such a one predisposed will cause an attack, and it may thus be induced in a hundred different ways." He lists as provocative factors a visit to the theater, a dinner party, a loud noise, an hour's visit to a picture gallery, looking through a microscope, odors of various kinds (such as of spring flowers), exposure of the body to the sun or a strong wind, and various moral causes and worry—"moving a single step out of the even tenor of their way." The various influences "alter the current of blood through the head: thus, while the face is pale, the larger vessels are throbbing, the head is hot, and the remedies which instinct suggests are cold and pressure to the part." He recommends a wet bandage around the head, profound quiet, and, if possible, sleep. He discounts the use of drugs in discussing a powder sent to him by a friend from Vancouver Island: "Alas! It must be catalogued with all the other remedies for sick-headache—it was useless."

But help was at hand. An article by Edward Woakers appeared in the *British Medical Journal* of 1868: "On ergot of rye in the treatment of neuralgia," which included hemicrania. A derivative of ergot (ergotin) was isolated in 1875 and was used by Eulenburg, who regarded migraine as being of two types: "pale" or sympatheticotonic and "red" or sympatheticoparalytic (Schiller, 1975). Gowers (1893) considered that ergot was of use, combined with bromide, in patients whose face flushed or did not change color during an attack, but he preferred the vasodilator nitroglycerin for those who became pale. He also advocated prophylactic therapy using a solution of nitroglycerin (1%) in alcohol combined with other agents, subsequently known as *Gowers mixture.* He recognized that "a hypodermic injection of morphia often acts no better than other sedatives" and employed bromide and Indian hemp, a source of cannabis, to relieve the acute attack of headache. Gowers disparaged the use of ergotin, which did no more than "lessen the throbbing intensification of the pain," commenting that "drugs that cause contraction of the arteries are almost powerless." He discussed the use of caffeine, local applications to the head and neck, hot baths of mustard and water to the feet, and, finally, electrical stimulation of the sympathetic chain ("the value of the treatment is, to say the least, seldom perceptible").

In 1925, the Swiss chemist Rothlin isolated ergotamine, which was introduced into clinical practice by Maier (1926). After the report by Graham and Wolff (1938) and the subsequent studies of Wolff and his colleagues (Wolff, 1963), ergotamine tartrate became established as the preferred treatment for acute migraine headache.

From that time on, the history of migraine, and of headache in general, blends with the present in this book. The International Headache Society was formed in 1983 to foster a systematic approach to the causes and treatment of headaches and has been responsible for a comprehensive classification of headaches, guidelines for clinical trials, and biennial scientific congresses. The history of headache is still being written; in the words of Gowers, "When all has been said that can be, mystery still envelops the mechanism of migraine."

References

Adams, F. (1841). *The extant works of Aretaeus, the Cappadocian* (p. 294). London: Sydenham Society.

Adams, F. (1844). *The seven books of Paulus Aeginata* (p. 350). London: Sydenham Society.

Adams, F. (1939). *The genuine works of Hippocrates.* Baltimore: Williams and Wilkins.

Alverez, W. C. (1945). Was there sick headache in 3000 B.C.? *Gastroenterology, 5,* 524.

Chand, D. (1982). *The Atharvaveda (Sanskrit text with English translation)* (p. 10). New Delhi: Munshiram Manoharlal.

Critchley, M. (1967). Migraine from Cappadocia to Queen Square. In *Background to migraine* (Vol. 1) (pp. 28–38). London: Heinemann.

Gowers, W. (1893). *Diseases of the nervous system* (Vol. 2) (pp. 836 & 866). Philadelphia: P. Blakiston.

Graham, J. R., & Wolff, H. G. (1938). Mechanism of migraine headache and action of ergotamine tartrate. *Arch Neurol Psychiat, 39,* 737–763.

Guthrie, D. (1947). *A history of medicine.* New York: Thomas Nelson.

Isler, H. (1993). Historical background. In J. Olesen, P. Tfelt-Hanson, & K. M. A. Welch (Eds.) *The headaches* (pp. 1–8). New York: Raven Press.

Knapp, R. D., Jr. (1963). Reports from the past. 2. *Headache, 3,* 112–122.

Knapp, R. D., Jr. (1964). Reports from the past. 3. *Headache, 3,* 143–155.

Living, E. (1873). *On megrim, sick-headache and some allied disorders: a contribution to the pathology of nerve-storms.* London: J. and A. Churchill.

Maier H. W. (1926). L'ergotamine inhibiteur du sympathique etudie en clinque, comme moyen d'exploration et comme agent therapeutique. *Revue Neurologie, 33,* 1104–1108.

Major, R. H. (1930). The Ebers Papyrus . *Ann Med Hist (New Series), 2,* 547–555.

McHenry, L. C., Jr. (1969). *Garrison's history of neurology* (p. 451). Springfield, IL: Charles C Thomas.

Riley, H. A. (1932). Special article: Migraine. *Bull Neurol Inst NY, 2,* 429–544.

Schiller, F. (1975). The migraine tradition. *Bull Hist Med, 49,* 1–19.
Sigerist, H. E. (1955). *A history of medicine. Vol. 1. Primitive and archaic medicine* (p. 451). New York: Oxford University Press.
Von Klein, C. H. (1905). 1928–1935. The medical features of the Papyrus Ebers. *JAMA, 45.*
Wilks, S. (1872). On sick-headache. *BMJ, 1,* 8–9.
Wolff, H. G. (1963). *Headache and other head pain* (pp. 259–265). New York: Oxford University Press.

Chapter 2
Recording the Patient's Case History

The most satisfying aspect of dealing with headache problems is that a diagnosis can often be made just by taking a systematic case history. Although a clearly recognizable pattern of illness, such as migraine, tension-type, or cluster headache, does not absolve the clinician from undertaking a physical examination, it may avoid unnecessary investigations and inappropriate treatment. However, the development of the disorder may indicate some serious local or systemic disturbance and urgent action. There are some patients whose headaches blur traditional boundaries and defy rigid classification. In such instances, the history at least sets the clinician thinking. It may not provide the whole answer, but it provides the clues from which the answer can finally be derived. This is part of the challenge to the knowledge, intellect, and art of the clinician.

Some clinicians prefer to let patients tell their story without interruption and reserve their questions until the end. Guide the patient gently so that the history unfolds neatly and is not obscured by side issues. This approach works well and saves a lot of time. A good history is taken not just given. Record the history of headache, like any pain history, under headings that show the characteristics, to enable recognition of the major diagnostic categories. If the patient has more than one type of headache, such as the combination of migraine and tension-type headache, it is helpful to record the characteristics of each separately, perhaps in parallel down the page, so that the diagnosis of each type becomes clear.

AGE OF ONSET

The length of the patient's illness separates possible cases into acute, subacute, and chronic groups, which reduces the number of diagnoses to be considered, as described in Chapters 4 and 18.

FREQUENCY AND DURATION OF HEADACHES

The frequency and duration of headaches define the temporal pattern of headache, which is important for establishing the diagnosis and setting a baseline for assessment of therapy. Make sure that responses from patients are consistent. For example, patients may state they have three headaches every week, possibly as three separate episodes each lasting for a day, or as a single attack persisting for 3 days. Again, patients often say they suffer several headaches each day, when they really mean they have a continuous tendency to headache, relieved by analgesics for some hours at a time. Often a simple headache diary will clarify the frequency and pattern of attacks, such as a menstrual relationship.

Ask about relapses and remissions. Patients may have periods of freedom for weeks, months, or years, a pattern characteristic in cluster headache but also in some types of migraine and trigeminal neuralgia. If headaches do recur in bouts, ask whether there is more than one attack of pain in 24 hours, how long each lasts, and whether it tends to appear at any particular time of the day or night.

TIME OF ONSET

It is important to determine whether headaches habitually arouse patients from sleep or are present on awakening. If so, ask about any premonitory symptoms that may have been experienced the previous day. If headaches develop during the daylight hours, inquire about any neurologic symptoms (aura) that immediately precede the onset of pain.

MODE OF ONSET

Early Warning Symptoms

Most patients at first deny any premonitory sensations, but one fourth recall them when prompted. This does require some leading questions. "The day before you wake up with headache do you ever feel elated, 'on top of the world' or as though you can fly through the day's work effortlessly?" "Do you ever feel unusually hungry or have a craving to eat sweet foods?" Patients may feel irritable or drowsy and yawn a lot and may complain of neck stiffness or passing more urine. Such warning symptoms help to confirm the diagnosis of migraine and to plan the timing of medication. In some cases ergotamine tartrate or some prophylactic agent can be taken at bedtime on days when warning signs are present to prevent headache the next day.

Aura

Migraine headache is sometimes preceded by focal neurologic symptoms, in which case it is called "migraine with aura" ("classical migraine"). The most common symptoms are visual disturbances such as flashes of light, rippling, or zigzag sensations with impairment or even loss of vision. These may affect one half or both of the visual fields simultaneously or may spread slowly across the field of vision (fortification spectra, scintillating scotomas). The aura usually develops over 5 to 10 minutes, persists for 20 to 45 minutes, then subsides as the headache begins, although such symptoms sometimes continue, or even arise, during headache. Paraesthesias, hemiparesis, or aphasia may also be symptoms of the aura. Nausea sometimes precedes headaches.

CHARACTERISTICS OF HEADACHE

Site and Radiation of Pain

The site and radiation of pain should be determined in relation to the following: Is the headache usually unilateral or bilateral? Is it localized to the orbital, frontal, temporal, or occipital region? Does it radiate to other areas? Does the pain spread to involve the shoulder and arm on the affected side? Is it ever felt in the ipsilateral lower limb as well?

Quality

The quality of the headache is also an important consideration. Does the headache seem to originate deep to the orbit or within the cranium, or is it felt superficially in the skin or scalp? Is it stabbing, constant, or throbbing? The term "throbbing" must be defined, because many patients use it loosely to describe a severe pain that waxes and wanes without any relationship to the pulse. I usually ask, "Does the pain get worse with each heartbeat?" or even tap my own temple rhythmically with a pen and ask, "Does it go boom, boom, boom with your pulse?" If the headache is consistent, does it feel like pressure inside the head, or like a weight on top of the head, or like a band around the head?

A sudden explosive onset ("thunderclap headache") is typical of subarachnoid hemorrhage and acute pressor responses but can occasionally occur in migraine. (See Chapters 13 and 19 for the differential diagnosis of thunderclap headache.)

Associated Symptoms

Gastrointestinal disturbances, such as nausea, vomiting, diarrhea, and abdominal pain, are common in migraine but sometimes accompany severe headaches from other causes.

Photophobia has two components. One is an expression of general hypersensitivity of the special senses—lights seem brighter, sounds seem louder, and smells seem stronger. The second component is ocular pain on exposure to light, felt only on the side affected by headache (Drummond, 1986).

Neurologic symptoms, associated with diminished cerebral blood flow, may originate in the cerebral cortex as described for the aura. Loss of concentration, confusion, and impairment of memory are common events and may rarely develop into stupor or coma. Hindbrain symptoms such as vertigo, dysarthria, ataxia, and lack of coordination are common. Circumoral paraesthesias can be a symptom of migraine but can also be caused by hyperventilation, which is often associated with headache (see Appendix A). Faintness on standing or fainting, as the result of postural hypotension, is also quite common (Selby & Lance, 1960).

An ipsilateral ocular Horner's syndrome (ptosis, miosis, and impaired thermoregulatory sweating in the supraorbital region) is common in cluster headache and occasionally in migraine and may persist between attacks. Ptosis is usually more prominent than miosis. On the side affected by cluster headache, the eye commonly reddens and lacrimates while the nostril blocks or runs. The ipsilateral forehead occasionally sweats excessively during attacks of cluster headache, because the skin area vacated by sympathetic nerves has been reinnervated by parasympathetic fibers originally destined for the lacrimal gland.

With their headaches, migraine patients may comment on distended arteries or veins in the temple, pallor (rarely flushing), dark coloration under the eyes, and swelling of the face. The hands, feet, or whole body may feel cold.

Scalp tenderness and hyperesthesia may develop during headache and persist for some days afterward, and may be reported to involve non-cranial sites.

PRECIPITATING FACTORS

Ask the patient whether it is possible to identify any trigger factor for headaches, or whether they recur regardless of circumstances. Common trigger factors include the following:

- Stress (migraine and tension-type headache)
- Relaxation after stress (migraine)
- Phases of the menstrual cycle (premenstrual and midcycle in migraine)
- Excessive afferent stimuli (glare, flickering light, noise, strong perfumes, and even having a haircut may bring on migraine and some tension-type headaches)
- The ingestion of alcohol, vasodilator drugs, or specific foods (migraine)
- Excessive intake of tea or coffee (caffeine withdrawal headache)
- Exercise (migraine and exertional vascular headaches)
- Sexual activity ("benign sex headaches")
- Coughing (intracranial vascular headaches and "benign cough headaches")
- Posture or neck movements (upper cervical syndrome and tension-type headache)
- Talking, chewing, swallowing, touching the face (trigeminal neuralgia and SUNCT see Chapter 12)
- Change in sleep pattern, too little or sleeping in (migraine)
- Weather change (migraine)

AGGRAVATING FACTORS

Ask the patient if the headache is made worse by jolting, jarring of the head, sudden movements, coughing, or straining. A positive answer suggests an intracranial vascular origin, which is typical of raised intracranial pressure or a space-occupying lesion but can also have a more banal cause such as hangover. Postural headache, developing during the day, present on standing and eased by lying down, suggests low cerebrospinal fluid pressure.

RELIEVING FACTORS

Most patients with migraine prefer to lie down in a darkened room and try to sleep when experiencing a headache, whereas patients with cluster headache usually stand or pace about. Migraine and cluster headache may be eased temporarily by local pressure or the application of hot or cold packs. Tension-type headache may be relieved by alcohol or marijuana. In about two thirds of patients with migraine who become pregnant, migraine ceases after the first trimester of pregnancy.

PREVIOUS TREATMENT

Any form of treatment tried previously should be listed, with a note about its success or failure. This list may include psychologic counseling, relaxation training, biofeedback therapy, hypnosis, chiropractic, acupuncture, and the use of transcutaneous nerve stimulation (TENS). In recording medications used in acute treatment or prophylaxis, it is important to ascertain the dosage whenever possible. Some patients may have been prescribed subtherapeutic doses, whereas others may have been consuming vast amounts of ergotamine, triptans, or analgesics without supervision. Therapy for coexisting conditions may also be relevant, because headache can be caused by bromocriptine, cyclosporin, vasodilators, cholesterol-lowering agents, antidepressants of the specific sero-tonin reuptake inhibitor type, and various other medications.

GENERAL HEALTH

It is important to determine at the outset whether headache is one facet of a sys-temic disease or is an isolated problem. Impairment of general health with loss of weight raises the possibility of chronic infections (tuberculous or cryptococ-cal meningitis, acquired immune deficiency syndrome [AIDS]), malignancy, blood dyscrasias, vasculitis, and connective tissue and endocrine disorders. The association of headache with general malaise, night sweats, and joint and mus-cle pains (polymyalgia rheumatica) suggests temporal arteritis.

System Review

When the history of the present illness is complete, it is always helpful to ask leading questions concerning each bodily system. For a patient with headache, include the eyes, ears, nose and throat, teeth, and neck in this review. The chronic obstruction of a nostril by vasomotor rhinitis or chronic respiratory tract infec-tion may suggest the possibility of sinusitis. The eye may become proptosed with retro-orbital tumors or a mucocele projecting into the orbit from the frontal sinus. Dimness of vision and "haloes" seen around lights may mark the onset of glaucoma. Complaints of impaired eyesight may draw attention to compression of the visual pathways. Papilledema may be symptomless, or the patient may notice blurring of vision on bending the head forward. In contrast, visual loss is severe in retrobulbar neuritis associated with a central scotoma.

A space-occupying lesion or other intracranial disturbance, such as progressive hydrocephalus, becomes much more likely if the recent onset of headache is associated with any of the following symptoms:

- Drowsiness at inappropriate times.
- Vomiting without apparent cause.
- Fits.
- Sudden falling attacks, in which consciousness may be retained.
- Progressive neurologic deficit of any kind, for example, mental deterioration, impairment of senses of smell, vision, or hearing. A unilateral nerve deafness may be present for years without being complained of, or even noticed, by the patient.
- Double vision.
- Weakness or sensory impairment of the face or limbs on one or other side.
- Disturbed coordination or loss of balance, with or without vertigo.
- Polyuria and polydipsia.
- Progressive change in pituitary function. Symptoms suggesting hypopituitarism are asthenia, diminished libido, reduction of body hair, lessened shaving frequency in men, premature cessation of menstruation in women, the skin becoming soft and finely wrinkled in both sexes, and the delay of pubescence in the child. In contrast, hyperpituitarism may be responsible for excessive growth and early pubescence in the young and deepening of the voice and enlargement of the jaw and hands in adults.
- Premature puberty occurs in approximately 10% of patients with a pinealoma.

PAST HEALTH

Head and neck injuries or meningitis at any time in the past may be of relevance. Subdural hematoma may follow a blow on the head that the patient considered trivial.

A number of episodes of "encephalitis" or any severe headache with neck stiffness should arouse suspicion of bleeding from a cerebral angioma or leakage of fluid from a craniopharyngioma or other cystic lesion. A useful additional point in the diagnosis of subarachnoid hemorrhage is the development of spinal root pains in the back, buttocks, and thighs some hours or days after the onset of headache, which is caused by blood tracking down the subarachnoid space to the cauda equina.

Past infections, particularly tuberculosis, should be recorded. Old tuberculous lesions may be reactivated by immunosuppressant therapy or AIDS, and an impaired immune response makes the patient vulnerable to toxoplasmosis, cryptococcal meningitis, progressive multifocal leukoencephalopathy, and primary lymphoma of the brain. Sinusitis and recurrent ear infections are also of potential relevance, particularly in children.

Vomiting attacks and motion sickness in childhood are often precursors of migraine in later life. A past history of asthma in a migraine patient cautions against the use of beta-blockers, which cause bronchoconstriction, in management.

Episodes of depression or other psychiatric disturbance may be related to the patient's present illness.

FAMILY HISTORY

Both migraine and tension headache run in families, but there is less tendency for cluster headache to do so. Information may be gained about a familial tendency to malignancy, tuberculosis, hypertension, and other disorders, which may relate to the problem of headache.

PERSONAL BACKGROUND

Occupation

Exposure at work to toxic or vasodilator substances, such as dry-cleaning fluids, may have direct relevance to the problem of headache. Some infections, such as brucellosis, leptospirosis, and Q fever, tend to occur in slaughterhouse workers, and cryptococcosis (torulosis) may occur in people who handle birds, particularly pigeons. Noise, flickering light, small video screens, unpleasant smells, and harsh air-conditioning may contribute to an unfavorable work environment, as can the tedium of a boring job: The workplace may have lost its appeal for a number of reasons. The pressure of uninspired or heavy-handed management, the inability to see the end result of one's labor, falling behind in the race for promotion, difficulty in adapting to changing techniques, financial insecurity, and the fear of unemployment or demotion are all potential causes of occupational stress. The waning of old skills may cause anxiety in the years before retirement, and when the retirement finally comes, it may remove an important source of motivation and take much of the zest from life. Yet many people enjoy both their work and their years of retirement.

Personal or Family Problems

Every stage of development abounds in potential sources of anxiety, but stress by itself is usually not enough to cause headache. The fault lies more often in failure to adapt to a situation that would not trouble most people. It is therefore important to determine any source of worry and then assess whether the patient's reaction to it is realistic.

Problems in childhood range from physical, mental, or sexual abuse to natural concerns about relationships with parents, siblings, and peers; success or failure in schoolwork and sports activities; and the making and breaking of friendships. Unrealistic goals set by parents for their children may lead to feelings of inadequacy and frustration on both sides. The self-confidence and rate of progress of a child depends largely on the attitude of parents and teachers. Some childhood headaches can be cured by changing schools. Parental separation or divorce, or a strained marriage continuing for the sake of the children, are common causes of insecurity, tension, and behavior disturbances among children.

The miraculous transformation of the body at puberty may give rise to feelings other than joy and wonder to the transformee. Puberty may arrive too early or too late. Children may feel they have grown too much or too little.

The outward and visible signs of their sexuality may seem too large or too small. They may be inadequately prepared for the onset of menstruation or may be unnecessarily laden with guilt about masturbation. As though acne were not enough! Their increasing desire for independence often conflicts with parental guidelines and the perceived need to conform to ethnic customs as well as with the discipline of a school curriculum.

Sexual problems may be important at any age. The containment within accepted social bounds of the sexual vigor of youth and the maintenance of satisfactory sexual life in marriage during the mature middle years plus the tensions of work and child raising may each bring difficulties. The unmarried of any age may be troubled by the instability of their sexual and social relationships and with the specter of loneliness at the end of the line. A tactful inquiry about sexual preference should be made when appropriate because of possible conflicts arising from the homosexual lifestyle.

Habits

The personal history also covers intake of alcohol, tea, coffee, medications, recreational drugs, and smoking. The daily consumption of analgesics, triptans, or ergotamine tartrate can transform intermittent headaches into chronic daily headache. Drinking more than six cups of tea or coffee each day or excessive intake of cola drinks can cause rebound headache from caffeine withdrawal. Alcohol, monosodium glutamate, and vasodilator drugs induce headache in susceptible people. Certain foods, missed meals, or "sleeping in" on weekends may be identified as trigger factors for headache.

EMOTIONAL STATE

As the personal history is taken, some insight is usually gained into whether the patient's symptoms are exaggerated by loneliness and introspection, or whether they are being played down by someone who has an active and interesting life. The history is a secondhand experience, which is colored by the emotional expression of the person telling the story. While the story is being recorded, the physician may be able to see whether the patient reacts to problems with physical manifestations of tension by frowning, clenching the jaws, or holding the head and neck rigidly. Look for symptoms of depression, such as loss of interest in work, home life, or personal affairs; or staying at home and not wanting to see friends or continue with previous activities. Depressive symptoms are important to recognize, because their treatment may play a big part in restoring pleasure to life, quite apart from relieving the headache, which is often a reflection of the depressive state.

References

Drummond, P. D. (1986). Quantitative assessment of photophobia in migraine and tension headache. *Headache, 26,* 465–469.

Selby, G., & Lance, J. W. (1960). Observations on 500 cases of migraine and allied vascular headache. *J Neurol Neurosurg Psychiatry, 23,* 23–32.

Chapter 3
Types of Headache

It often comes as a surprise to the general public and even to some medical students that there are many varieties of headache. To many, a headache is a headache, and that is that. When headaches are caused by some recognizable structural change or pathologic process, they can be sorted readily into appropriate categories; the task becomes more difficult when we are dealing with symptoms but no physical signs. In such cases, no help is usually forthcoming from specialized investigations and scanning techniques. Each headache must then be classified the same way we make our clinical diagnosis, by recording and analyzing the case history, including the site, nature, pattern of recurrence, and accompanying symptoms.

The first system followed the recommendations of the Ad Hoc Committee on Classification of Headache (Friedman et al., 1962). This was a useful start, but many of the definitions were qualified by adjectives such as "commonly" or "sometimes." This is difficult to avoid when headache patterns are variable, when the characteristics of one merge into another, or when two or more types of headache coexist. Drummond and Lance (1984) compared a computer classification of headache symptoms with the clinical diagnosis in 600 patients attending their neurology clinic. They found that migraine with aura and cluster headache emerged as clearly defined syndromes but that those designated clinically as "migraine without aura" and "tension headache" differed in the number rather than the nature of supposedly migrainous symptoms, suggesting that there was a spectrum of "idiopathic headache" with episodic "migraine" at one end and frequently occurring "tension headache" at the other. For example, the headache was unilateral in almost 60% of those attacks recurring from once a month to several times each week but was still unilateral in approximately 20% of patients with daily headache. The latter group included patients who had previously suffered from migraine ("transformed migraine"). Other observers (Rasmussen et al., 1991) have found a clear distinction between the symptoms of migraine and tension headache. This controversial topic is considered in Chapter 11 on chronic daily headache.

The International Headache Society (IHS) in 1988 defined and provided diagnostic criteria for headache disorders, cranial neuralgias, and facial pain and now has revised them (Headache Classification Committee of the International

Headache Society, 2004). The following summary is based on the IHS classification, but the original publication should be consulted for details.

1. Migraine (see Chapters 6 through 9)
   1.1. Migraine without aura
   This episodic headache, which used to be called "common migraine," is typically unilateral and associated with nausea, photophobia, and sensitivity to sound.
   1.2. Migraine with aura
   Migrainous headaches preceded by neurologic symptoms were termed "classic" or "classical" migraine in the past, but the IHS Committee determined that, to avoid any possibility of confusion, "migraine with aura" was preferable. The aura is commonly a visual disturbance that may affect both visual fields simultaneously, such as blurring, rippling, spots, or flashes, but in some cases moves slowly over one or both fields of vision as a zigzag pattern, leaving areas of impaired vision. These auras, known as "fortification spectra" or "scintillating scotomas," are discussed in detail in Chapter 6.
   Varieties of "migraine with aura" included familial and sporadic hemiplegic migraine, basilar migraine (when aura symptoms arise from the brainstem and occipital lobes), and episodes consisting solely of the aura without any headache ("migraine equivalents").
   Ophthalmoplegic migraine is a rare condition in which paresis of one or more of the ocular motor nerves (third, fourth, or sixth cranial nerves) follows a migraine-like headache. Recent magnetic resonance imaging (MRI) studies suggest that the ocular palsies may be caused by a demyelinating neuropathy and the condition is therefore discussed in Chapter 18.
   1.3. Childhood periodic syndromes
   Certain recurrent symptoms in a child may be associated with migraine or be precursors of migraine in later life: cyclical vomiting, abdominal migraine (abdominal pain, often associated with nausea or vomiting, "bilious" attacks), and benign paroxysmal vertigo.
   1.4. Retinal migraine
   In this rare condition visual disturbance is confined to one eye, and the headache then develops behind that eye. Amaurosis fugax from internal carotid vascular disease and ocular or orbital lesions must be ruled out.
   1.5. Complications of migraine
      1.5.1. Chronic migraine
      This term is now applied to a migraine frequency of 15 or more days per month in the absence of medication overuse.
      1.5.2. Status migrainosus
      A debilitating attack lasting for more than 72 hours.
      1.5.3. Aura symptoms persisting for more than one week without evidence of infarction on imaging
      1.5.4. Migrainous infarction
      Aura symptoms or neurologic deficit persisting with demonstration on imaging of an ischemic brain lesion.

　　　　1.5.5.　Migraine-triggered epileptic seizure
2.　Tension-type headache (see Chapter 10)
　　2.1.　Episodic
　　　　Recurrent attacks of a tight, pressing sensation in the head, usually bilateral. The episodes are usually precipitated by physical or mental stress, and a subvariety is associated with excessive muscle contraction and muscle tenderness.
　　2.2.　Chronic
　　　　Chronic tension-type headache recurs 15 or more days in a month, commonly every day. It has the same heavy or tight quality as the episodic variety and may or may not be associated with overactivity of the jaw and facial muscles. Other forms of chronic daily headache may develop from episodic migraine attacks ("transformed migraine") or start suddenly for no apparent reason ("new daily persistent headache") (see Chapter 11).
3.　Cluster headache and paroxysmal hemicrania (see Chapter 12)
　　3.1.　Cluster headache
　　　　Attacks of unilateral pain, centered on the orbital or periorbital region, usually lasting 15 to 180 minutes and recurring up to eight times a day are characteristics of cluster headache. The pain is usually severe and is accompanied by redness and lacrimation (tearing) of the eye and nasal congestion on the affected side. The disorder characteristically recurs in bouts lasting weeks or months, separated by a period of freedom for months or years (episodic cluster headache). If attacks continue for a year or more without remission, the condition is known as "chronic cluster headache." Previous names for this disorder include "ciliary neuralgia," "migrainous neuralgia," and "Horton's histaminic cephalalgia."
　　3.2.　Paroxysmal hemicrania
　　　　Paroxysmal hemicrania refers to brief episodes of headache, lasting 5 to 20 minutes, that have the characteristics of cluster headache and recur 5 to 30 times in each 24-hour period. It may be acute or chronic and responds specifically to indomethacin.
　　3.3.　Short-lasting Unilateral Neuralgiform headache attacks with Conjunctival injection and Tearing (SUNCT)
　　　　SUNCT headache is a syndrome of clusterlike head pains lasting less than 5 minutes and recurring many times in a 24-hour period.
　　　　The whole group of trigeminal-autonomic cephalgias is considered in Chapter 12.
4.　Miscellaneous headaches unassociated with a structural lesion (see Chapter 13)
　　4.1.　Primary stabbing headache
　　　　Primary stabbing headaches consist of transient stabs of pain in the head ("icepick pains") that occur spontaneously in the absence of organic disease of underlying structures.
　　4.2.　Primary cough headache
　　　　Primary couch headachcs are precipitated by coughing in the absence of any intracranial disorder.
　　4.3.　Primary exertional headache

Primary exertional headaches are brought on by exercise. Some varieties have been given specific names such as "weightlifter's headache."
4.4. Primary headache associated with sexual activity
Primary headache associated with sexual activity typically arises during sexual intercourse or masturbation, often as a dull ache increasing with sexual excitement, and becomes intense with orgasm but sometimes manifests as an explosive headache at the time of orgasm without warning. Care must be taken to exclude an underlying organic cause such as aneurysm. A rare form of postural headache after intercourse has also been described.
4.5. Hypnic headache
Hypnic headaches are dull headaches that always awaken patients from sleep.
4.6. Primary thunderclap headache
Primary thunderclap headaches are high-intensity headaches of abrupt onset mimicking that of ruptured cerebral aneurysm.
4.7. Hemicrania continua
Hemicrania continua is a persistent strictly unilateral headache responsive to indomethacin (see Chapter 11).
4.8. New daily persistent headache (NDPH)
NDPH is a headache that recurs daily from soon after onset (see Chapter 11).
5. Headache attributed to head and/or neck trauma (see Chapter 14)
5.1. Acute post-traumatic headache
Headaches developing within 7 days after head injury or regaining consciousness after head injury and resolving within 3 months are classified as "acute post-traumatic headaches."
5.2. Chronic post-traumatic headache
Headaches persisting for more than 3 months after head injury are "chronic post-traumatic headaches."
5.3. Acute headache attributed to whiplash injury
An acute headache attributed to whiplash injury develops within 7 days after whiplash injury and resolves within 3 months after whiplash injury.
5.4. Chronic headache attributed to whiplash injury
Chronic headaches attributed to whiplash injury persist for more than 3 months after whiplash injury.
5.5. Headache attributed to traumatic intracranial hematoma (see Chapter 15)
5.5.1. Epidural (extradural) hematoma
5.5.2. Subdural hematoma
5.6. Headache attributed to other head and/or neck trauma
5.7. Postcraniotomy headache (particularly common after removal of an acoustic neuroma)
6. Headache attributed to cranial or cervical vascular disorders (see Chapter 15)
6.1. Ischemic stroke or transient ischemic attack
6.1.1. Cerebral infarction
6.1.2. Transient ischemic attacks
6.2. Nontraumatic intracranial hemorrhage
6.2.1. Intracranial hemorrhage

6.2.2. Subarachnoid hemorrhage
6.3. Unruptured vascular malformations
    6.3.1. Saccular aneurysm
    6.3.2. Arteriovenous malformation (AVM)
        AVM possibly triggers migraine with aura.
    6.3.3. Dural arteriovenous fistula
    6.3.4. Cavernous angioma
        Cavernous angioma is a dubious cause of headache unless ruptured.
    6.3.5. Sturge-Weber syndrome
        Sturge-Weber syndrome may trigger migraine with aura.
6.4. Arteritis
    6.4.1. Giant cell arteritis (temporal arteritis)
    6.4.2. Primary central nervous system angiitis
    6.4.3. Secondary central nervous system angiitis
6.5. Carotid or vertebral artery pain
    6.5.1. Arterial dissection
    6.5.2. Postendarterectomy
    6.5.3. Carotid angioplasty
    6.5.4. Endovascular procedures
    6.5.5. Angiography
6.6. Cerebral venous thrombosis
6.7. Other intracranial disorders
    6.7.1. Cerebral Autosomal Dominant Arteriopathy with Subcortical Infarcts and Leukoencephalopathy (CADASIL)
    6.7.2. Mitochondrial Encephalopathy, Lactic Acidosis, and Strokelike episodes (MELAS)
    6.7.3. Benign angiopathy of the central nervous system
    6.7.4. Pituitary apoplexy
7. Headache attributed to nonvascular intracranial disorder (Chapter 16)
7.1. High cerebrospinal fluid (CSF) pressure
    7.1.1. Idiopathic (formerly "benign") intracranial hypertension (IIH)
    7.1.2. Metabolic, toxic, or hormonal causes
        Medications such as tetracycline that can elevate CSF pressure are classified under section 8 of this list by the IHS but are considered in Chapter 16 of this book.
    7.1.3. Hydrocephalus
7.2. Low CSF pressure
    7.2.1. Postural headache commonly following lumbar puncture
    7.2.2. CSF fistula
    7.2.3. Spontaneous (idiopathic) low CSF pressure (spontaneous hypoliquorrhea
7.3. Inflammatory disease (noninfectious)
    7.3.1. Neurosarcoidosis
    7.3.2. Aseptic meningitis
    7.3.3. Other noninfectious inflammatory disease
        Headache may be associated with the following:
            Acute demyelinating encephalomyelitis (ADEM)

Systemic lupus erythematosus (SLE)
Antiphospholipid antibody syndrome
Behçet's syndrome
Vogt-Koyanagi-Harada syndrome (an autoimmune disorder affecting eyes, internal ear, hair, and meninges)
7.3.4. Lymphocytic hypophysitis
Lymphocytic hypophysitis is a cause of hypopituitarism associated with pituitary enlargement, enhancing on MRI, with biopsy confirmation. It is an uncommon disorder that usually develops at the end of pregnancy or postpartum.
7.4. Intracranial neoplasm
7.4.1. Raised CSF pressure caused by neoplasm
7.4.2. Headache directly related to neoplasm
7.4.3. Carcinomatous meningitis
7.4.4. Hypothalamic or pituitary disorder causing hyper- or hyposecretion
7.5. Intrathecal injection
Headache associated with intrathecal injection develops within 4 hours after injection and resolves within 14 days.
7.6. Epileptic seizure (see Chapter 13)
7.6.1. Hemicrania epileptica
7.6.2. Postictal headache
7.7. Chiari type 1 malformation (see Chapter 13)
7.8. Syndrome of transient Headache and Neurological Deficits with CSF Lymphocytosis (HaNDL) (see Chapter 7)
7.9. Other nonvascular intracranial disorder
8. Headache associated with substances or their withdrawal (see Chapter 13)
8.1. Headache induced by acute substance use or exposure
Examples are the headaches induced by vasodilator agents, such as nitrates, nitrites, phosphodiesterase (PDE) inhibitors such as sildenafil (Viagra), or calcium channel blockers, and the inhalation of volatile hydrocarbons used in dry-cleaning and similar processes.
8.2. Medication overuse headache
8.3. Headache as an adverse event attributed to chronic medication, such as oral contraceptive pill
8.4. Headache from substance withdrawal
Substance withdrawal headaches are "rebound" headaches following the withdrawal of caffeine, narcotics, or estrogens.
9. Headache attributed to infection (see Chapter 16)
9.1. Intracranial infection
9.1.1. Bacterial meningitis
9.1.2. Viral meningitis
9.1.3. Encephalitis
9.1.4. Brain abscess
9.1.5. Subdural empyema
9.2. Systemic infection
9.3. HIV/AIDS
9.4. Chronic postinfection headache
10. Disorder of homeostasis (see Chapter 13)

10.1. Hypoxia, hypocapnia
10.2. Dialysis headache
10.3. Hypertension
10.4. Hypothyroidism
10.5. Fasting
10.6. Cardiac cephalgia
10.7. Other disorders of homeostasis
11. Headache or facial pain attributed to disorder of cranium, neck, eyes, ears, nose, sinuses, teeth, mouth, or other facial or cranial structures (see Chapter 17)
    11.1. Cranial bones
    11.2. Neck
        11.2.1. Cervicogenic headache
        11.2.2. Retropharyngeal tendonitis
        11.2.3. Craniocervical dystonia
    11.3. Eyes
        11.3.1. Acute glaucoma
        11.3.2. Refractive errors
        11.3.3. Strabismus (squint)
        11.3.4. Inflammation
    11.4. Ears
    11.5. Rhinosinusitis
    11.6. Teeth, jaws, and related structures
    11.7. Temporomandibular joint (TMJ) dysfunction (Costen's syndrome)
    11.8. Other
12. Headache attributed to psychiatric disorders
    12.1. Somatization disorder
    12.2. Psychotic disorder
13. Cranial neuralgias and central causes of facial pain (see Chapter 18)
    13.1. Trigeminal neuralgia
    13.2. Glossopharyngeal neuralgia
    13.3. Nervus intermedius neuralgia
    13.5. Nasociliary neuralgia
    13.6. Supraorbital neuralgia
    13.7. Other terminal branch neuralgias
    13.8. Occipital neuralgia
    13.9. Neck-tongue syndrome
    13.10. External compression headache
    13.11. Cold stimulus headache
    13.12. Constant pain caused by compression, irritation, or distortion of cranial nerves or upper cervical roots by structural lesions
    13.13. Optic neuritis
    13.14. Ocular diabetic neuropathy
    13.15. Head or facial pain attributed to herpes zoster
    13.16. Tolosa-Hunt syndrome
    13.17. Ophthalmoplegic "migraine"
    13.18. Central causes of facial pain
        13.18.1. Anesthesia dolorosa
        13.18.2. Central poststroke pain

13.18.3. Multiple sclerosis
13.18.4. Persistent idiopathic facial pain (formerly atypical facial pain)
13.18.5. Burning mouth syndrome
13.19. Other cranial neuralgia or other centrally mediated facial pain

The list of possible causes of headache appears formidable, but following the principles put forward in this book can usually lead to a clinical diagnosis that is satisfactory for both doctor and patient.

References

Drummond, P. D., & Lance, J. W. (1984). Clinical diagnosis and computer analysis of headache symptoms. *J Neurol Neurosurg Psychiatry, 47,* 128–133.

Friedman, A. P., Finley, K. M., Graham, J. R., Kunkle, E. C., Ostfeld, A. M., & Wolff, H. G. (1962). Classification of headache. The Ad Hoc Committee on the Classification of Headache. *Arch Neurol, 6,* 173–176.

Headache Classification Subcommittee of the International Headache Society. (2004). The international classification of headache disorders (2nd ed.). *Cephalalgia, 24*(Suppl 1), 1–160.

Rasmussen, B. K., Jensen, R., & Olesen, J. (1991). A population-based analysis of the diagnostic criteria of the International Headache Society. *Cephalalgia, 11,* 129–134.

Chapter 4
Diagnosis Based on the History

The case history and its interpretation are the most important factors in headache diagnosis. Information about the nature of the headache, under each descriptive subheading, contributes to the differential diagnosis. Each feature is considered in turn, to evaluate its significance.

AGE OF ONSET

The length of time a patient has been troubled by headache is the first guide as to whether the symptom portends some malignant or progressive neurologic disorder that requires further investigation. At one end of the scale, the sudden onset of severe headache, possibly followed by impairment of consciousness or focal neurologic signs, suggests some serious illness, such as subarachnoid hemorrhage or meningitis. At the other end of the scale, a patient who has had headaches regularly for many years is likely to have some form of primary headache, such as migraine or chronic tension-type headache. The first attack of migraine that a patient experiences may be confusing if it is not preceded by characteristic symptoms and may suggest systemic infection, encephalitis, or meningitis.

Between the very acute and very chronic headaches lie the most difficult to interpret, those that have developed over some days, weeks, or months. The subacute headache may have a relatively simple explanation, such as sinusitis, but one must be on guard against less common but more life-threatening conditions, such as subdural hematoma, cerebral tumor, or other causes of increased intracranial pressure, and, in those older than 55 years of age, the insidious onset of temporal (giant cell) arteritis.

FREQUENCY AND DURATION OF HEADACHES

The frequency and duration of the headache establish the temporal pattern, which is important in the diagnosis of recurrent headache. In this group the main

25

conditions to consider are migraine, cluster headache, trigeminal neuralgia (tic douloureux), and tension-type headache (Figure 4.1).

Migraine may recur irregularly at intervals of months or years, but commonly a pattern has become established by the time a patient seeks medical advice. The headache may be linked to the menstrual cycle or recur one or more times each week without any obvious cause, sometimes disappearing during pregnancy, holidays, admission to hospital, or other periods of prolonged rest. The headache may last from a few hours to several days but is usually followed by a period of freedom from headache before the next attack starts.

Cluster headache, in contrast, has an intriguing periodicity. It commonly recurs in bouts lasting from 2 weeks to 3 months and then vanishes completely for 3 months to as long as 4 years. During a bout, the headache returns one, two, or more times in 24 hours and lasts from 10 minutes to several hours on each occasion. The fact that the pain persists for this length of time clearly distinguishes it from trigeminal neuralgia, which recurs as transient jabs of pain, each lasting a fraction of a second, although the jabs may be repetitive. We mention the two disorders together because they are commonly confused in general practice. Many patients with cluster headache are referred with the provisional diagnosis of trigeminal neuralgia, probably because the pattern of cluster headache is not widely known. One factor the conditions have in common is the tendency to experience spontaneous remission for months or years. The distinction between the two is important, because the mechanism and treatment of each are entirely different.

Approximately 10% to 20% of patients with cluster headache suffer from a chronic form, recurring regularly without periods of remission. In this case, the distinction from migraine depends on the rapidity of onset, relative brevity of

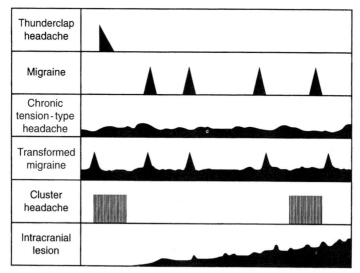

FIGURE 4.1 Temporal patterns of headache; see Chapter 11 for a discussion of primary daily headache types.

each attack, and the autonomic disturbances described in Chapters 2 and 12. Other rare headaches with similarity to cluster headache, with many brief episodes developing each day, are known as "episodic" or "chronic paroxysmal hemicrania" (CPH) and, with still shorter duration, as the SUNCT ("Short-lasting Unilateral Neuralgiform headache attacks with Conjunctival injection, Tearing, sweating, and rhinorrhea") syndrome (see Chapter 12).

Tension-type headache is set apart from those just considered by the absence of any paroxysmal quality or periodicity about its course. Although acute forms of tension-type headache may appear at the end of a stressful day in a busy office or a household of screaming children, there is usually always a headache lurking in the background. Such patients have some sort of headache all day, every day. There is a form of headache intermediate between this undulating pattern and the paroxysms of migraine, in which surges of more severe throbbing headache become superimposed every few days or weeks on an otherwise monotonous background of constant discomfort. Most of these patients have previously experienced episodic migraine and are considered to have "transformed migraine."

Time of Onset

Migraine headache commonly awakens the patient in the early hours of the morning but may come on at any time of the day. Cluster headache tends to recur punctually at certain times of the day or night, often one or two hours after the patient goes to sleep. Hypnic headaches are an unusual variety that awaken the patient, usually elderly, from sleep and are often preventable by a nocturnal cup of coffee or dose of lithium. Tension-type headache may be present on waking but more often starts on getting up and about.

The time of onset is important from the therapeutic as well as the diagnostic point of view. If headaches awaken the patient from sleep consistently, preventive medication is best taken the night before.

Mode of Onset

Early Warning Symptoms

A change of mood, such as unwarranted elation or irritability, excessive yawning, or craving sweet foods, are harbingers of migraine and should be recognized by the patient as a signal to take medication that night to prevent a headache from occurring the next day.

Aura

An aura before migraine headache is the exception rather than the rule, but when it does occur, it places the diagnosis beyond reasonable doubt. The symptoms composing the aura usually develop gradually over some minutes, persist for 10 to 45 minutes, and then subside slowly. The most common aura is a visual disturbance with positive features (flashes, zigzags, circles of light, or rippling vision) and negative features (patchy scotomas, hemianopia, bilateral blurring, or tunnel vision). One may follow the other, as in the classic fortification spectra (scintillating scotomas), in which shimmering or jittering zigzag figures pass slowly over one or both visual fields, leaving behind areas of impaired vision. Other focal neurologic symptoms, such as paresthesias, hemiparesis, and dysphasia, may develop during the aura.

Acute Onset

Headaches usually develop and increase in severity slowly, regardless of whether they are preceded by an aura. If headache strikes suddenly "like a blow to the head" (thunderclap headache), subarachnoid hemorrhage, fulminant meningitis or encephalitis, obstruction of the cerebral ventricles, or a rapid rise in blood pressure such as that which occurs in pheochromocytoma must be considered, although migraine and orgasmic headaches may present in this manner.

Site

Headache is commonly unilateral in migraine (about two thirds), cluster headache, and trigeminal neuralgia (which are almost always unilateral); as the result of local changes in the eye, sinuses, skull or scalp; and in the presence of expanding lesions of one cerebral hemisphere. An aneurysm of the internal carotid artery may cause pain behind one eye by enlarging without rupturing. Subarachnoid hemorrhage from an aneurysm or angioma may start with local pain, but headache usually becomes generalized and spreads to the back of the neck. Space-occupying lesions may cause unilateral pain by displacement of vessels, but headache becomes bilateral if cerebrospinal fluid (CSF) pathways are obstructed. The site of headache is not reliable as a means of localizing a cerebral tumor. The headache of internal carotid dissection or thrombosis is unilateral, whereas vertebrobasilar disorders may refer pain to the occipital area bilaterally. Scalp vessels may be involved separately in temporal arteritis so that pain is limited to the distribution of a specific artery.

Migraine headache often starts in one temple or occipital region (Figure 4.2), then coalesces between these areas as a bar of pain before radiating over that half of the head or becoming generalized. It may spread to involve the neck and shoulder or, rarely, the entire half of the body on the affected side. Sometimes pain may be felt more below the eye, in which case it is termed *lower-half headache* or *facial migraine*.

The pain of cluster headache characteristically involves the eye and frontal region on one side and may radiate to the occiput and the nostril, cheek, and teeth on the same side (see Figure 4.2), overlapping the distribution of lower-half headache. The stabbing pains of trigeminal neuralgia are usually felt in the cheek or chin (second and third divisions) but start in the eye or forehead (first division) in about 5% of cases. Tension-type headache is commonly bilateral but is unilateral in some 20% of patients, particularly in those who are also subject to migraine. The pain arising from a temporomandibular joint may radiate up to the temple and down over the face on that side.

"Ice-cream headache" is usually felt in the midline but may be referred to one temple, particularly when the subject is prone to experience migraine in that site (see Chapter 18). The pain of sinusitis commonly overlies the affected areas.

QUALITY

Headache may be constant, pulsatile, or stabbing. Migraine usually starts as a dull ache but may become pulsatile ("throbbing") as the intensity increases. The pain of cluster headache is described as deep, boring (drilling), and intense. Trigeminal neuralgia is a shocklike stab or series of stabs. Tension-type headache is dull, constant, and tight and presses like a band around the head or a weight on the head (Figure 4.2). Patients with tension-type headache and migraine may also be subject to sudden jabs of pain in the head ("ice-pick pains," often felt in the site of their habitual headache).

Associated Phenomena

The usual accompaniments of migraine and cluster headache are mentioned in Chapter 2 and are described in more detail in Chapters 7 and 11. Tension-type headache is notable for the absence of these distinctive features, although most patients do complain of a constant mild photophobia.

The meningeal irritation of subarachnoid hemorrhage, meningitis, and encephalitis causes a protective reflex muscle spasm of the extensor muscles of the neck, which is manifest clinically as neck rigidity.

The sudden headache caused by a colloid cyst blocking the flow of CSF in the third ventricle may be accompanied by a "drop attack," a sudden loss of power

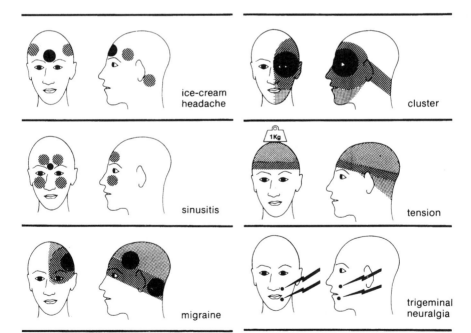

FIGURE 4.2   Sites of head and facial pain.
(From Lance, J. W. [1986]. *Migraine and other headaches.* P. H. Charles Scribner's Sons, New York. By permission of the publisher.)

in the legs caused by compression of the midline reticular formation. Consciousness is not necessarily lost during drop attacks. With any space-occupying lesion, or progressive hydrocephalus, the patient may become drowsy, yawn frequently, or vomit without preliminary nausea. Fits or other symptoms of focal cortical irritation may precede headache or appear as the headache intensifies. Diplopia may herald the onset of compression of the third cranial nerve, caused by an expanding intracranial mass forcing part of the temporal lobe downward through the tentorial opening. Dilation of the ipsilateral pupil can be a sinister sign of tentorial herniation requiring immediate action but may also be seen, occasionally, in vertebrobasilar migraine.

Rigors and sweats in any acute infectious process, nasal obstruction and bony tenderness in sinusitis, and conjunctival and circumcorneal injection in ocular conditions are all indications of the source of headache.

PRECIPITATING OR AGGRAVATING FACTORS

Any intracranial vascular headache, whether it be caused by "hangover," hypoglycemia, or intracranial tumor, will be made worse by jarring, sudden movements of the head, coughing, sneezing, or straining. "Cough headache" is not always associated with intracranial tumor but can be a benign, if unexplained, syndrome in its own right. Bending the head forward may bring on a severe paroxysmal headache in patients with a colloid cyst of the third ventricle or other forms of obstructive hydrocephalus.

Sensitivity to light is a common feature of diffuse intracranial disturbance such as meningitis or encephalitis as well as migraine. Glare, loud noises, and even strong odors are liable to initiate or worsen tension-type headache as well as migraine.

Exercise aggravates many headache types, and the occasional individual may suffer disability as a result of exercise alone. Sexual intercourse may bring on tension-type or migraines and has been known to precipitate subarachnoid hemorrhage.

Some people tend to experience a dull headache on missing a meal, and hypoglycemia or dehydration may provoke a migraine attack in susceptible patients. Certain foods are said to induce migraine, but doubt has been cast on whether fatty foods, chocolate, oranges, and other traditional migraine precipitants act specifically or by a psychologic conditioning process. Brain reactivity appears to be altered by hormonal changes, thus accounting for the association between migraine and menstruation and for the relief from migraine in some women during pregnancy.

Alcohol usually triggers cluster headache during an active bout, but not at other times. It may also bring on migraine when the patient is in a susceptible phase (not in the refractory period after an attack has recently ended). Red wines in particular have been incriminated, but in France white wines are thought to be culpable.

The lightning jabs of trigeminal neuralgia may be brought on by talking, chewing, swallowing, shaving, or even a puff of wind blowing on the face. Pain arising from the teeth is usually exacerbated by hot or cold fluids in the mouth; temporomandibular joint dysfunction is made worse by chewing or clenching the jaw. Chewing may cause pain in the temporal and masseter muscles ("claudication of the jaw muscles") when their blood supply is impaired by temporal arteritis.

The occipital headache of cervical spondylosis is understandably aggravated by neck movement. Tension-type headache may correlate with periods of turbulence caused by worry, anger, or excitement, but in the chronic form it may persist inexorably, no matter how calm the person. Migraine may occur at a time of stress, but it more commonly follows some hours after relaxation from stress or even the following day, as in "weekend migraine," when the blood supply is impaired by temporal arteritis.

Headache caused by low cerebrospinal fluid pressure develops when the patient stands and is relieved by lying down. It is often worse as the day goes on and may be absent on waking.

RELIEVING FACTORS

Pressure on the scalp and the use of hot or cold compresses are often soothing in migraine and cluster headache. The patient with migraine usually wishes to sit or lie in a darkened room, whereas a patient with the cluster headache prefers to stand or pace the floor, holding one hand over the affected eye. Rebreathing into a paper bag or inhaling carbon dioxide at 10% in air or oxygen is said to shorten the aura phase of migraine, and inhaling 100% oxygen relieves many patients with cluster headache.

The pain of sinusitis is relieved by clearing sinuses of nasal obstruction. Avoidance of chewing on one side and of excessive jaw clenching eases the pain of temporomandibular strain or arthritis.

Voluntary relaxation of forehead and jaw muscles reduces the severity of tension-type headache, and the use of alcohol may temporarily abolish it.

Acetaminophen (paracetamol) will sometimes stop the pain of migraine in childhood but usually not in adult life. Aspirin is useful in mild forms of head pain, alone or in combination with acetaminophen or caffeine, and may prevent migraine if taken in effervescent or soluble form early in the attack after a drug to promote gastric absorption, such as metoclopramide.

More specific methods of relieving headache are discussed later in the appropriate chapters.

CONCLUSION

If enough of the factors mentioned in this chapter emerge during the taking of a case history, the physician can usually form a clear clinical impression of the headache pattern and an opinion about the group to which the headache belongs and its probable cause. Well-directed inquiries may bring out important points the patient has neglected to mention. If the diagnosis is not evident after taking the case history, at least the clinician should know what to look for on physical examination and should also have formed an opinion as to whether the headache warrants further investigation.

Chapter 5
Physical Examination

The case history may direct the clinician's attention to certain aspects of the physical examination, to look for signs of meningeal irritation, raised intracranial pressure, or other signs of organic disease. Even if the story is typical of migraine, cluster headache, or tension-type headache, a general examination should be performed. This will often be completely normal, but it is important for both clinician and patient to know that it is normal. The emphasis of examination is naturally on the head, neck, and nervous system, but headache can arise in so many ways that other systems should not be neglected.

GENERAL APPEARANCE

The patient's demeanor while the history is being taken may give some indication of anxiety, depression, or hypochondriac exaggeration of symptoms. Sighing or yawning may betray a tendency to overbreathe (hyperventilate). Other manifestations of nervous tension include frowning, thrusting forward or clenching of the jaw, restless movements, and the transfer of a handkerchief from one moist palm to another. Occasionally the clinician may observe signs of an organic disorder—the large jaw and hands of acromegaly, a goiter obstructing the jugular venous outflow (see Figure 15.7), or the large head of Paget's disease or the short neck that accompanies an anomaly of the craniospinal junction, such as platybasia and Chiari malformation.

If a patient is suffering an attack of migraine at the time, the clinician may see undue pulsation of the temporal artery and its branches, whereas the skin is pale, with the area under the eyes becoming dark and puffy. The pupil on the affected side may constrict, although it dilates in rare instances of "basilar-type migraine." The changes are more striking during episodes of cluster headache, when an ocular Horner's syndrome (Figure 5.1) becomes apparent in about one third of patients, often persisting between attacks. Thickened or thrombosed scalp arteries may be visible in patients with temporal arteritis.

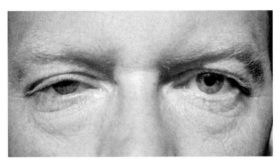

FIGURE 5.1   Ocular Horner's syndrome in cluster headache. Right ptosis and miosis is accompanied by conjunctional injection and lacrimation.

Mental State

The mental state of the patient will have been assessed superficially during history taking. Drowsiness, confusion, or disorientation may indicate a space-occupying lesion or diffuse cerebral disorder, such as meningitis or encephalitis. Focal cortical lesions can prevent normal appreciation of the body image or affect understanding of the written or spoken word, which may, therefore, give a false impression of general intellectual deterioration. Because of a lesion of the dominant hemisphere, patients may be unable to express themselves in words, mime, or writing; to calculate or perform routine tasks; or to distinguish between right and left. If cortical function is intact, the emotional tone of the patient must be assessed, because it is often altered in patients with chronic headache.

Speech

If the patient is dysphasic, always note whether the patient is right- or left-handed. The left hemisphere governs speech mechanisms in approximately 96% of right-handed individuals and in about 50% of left-handed individuals.

Skull

The skull should be examined if indicated by the case history. A search of the scalp may disclose local infection, a bone tumor, Paget's disease, or the hardened, tender arteries of temporal arteritis. The bones overlying inflamed sinuses or mastoid processes become sensitive to percussion. Bulging of the fontanels is a direct indication of increased intracranial pressure in infants. In children, measure the head circumference, because repeated recordings are of value in detecting progressive hydrocephalus. In adult life, a large head suggests hydrocephalus from aqueduct stenosis or another cause of obstruction of the cerebrospinal fluid (CSF) pathways.

Auscultation of the skull (listening over the orbits, temples, and mastoid processes) may disclose a systolic bruit in the case of angioma, vascular tumors, or stenosis of the cranial vessels. When listening over the closed eyelid, ask patients to open the other eye and hold their breath to prevent eyelid flutter and breath sounds from obscuring a bruit. Skull bruits are often normal in children under 10 years of age and may be discounted unless loud and unilateral. In patients who are unable to relax, an unexpected dividend from auscultation of the skull is that the sound of muscle contraction may be heard over the temporal and frontal muscles. The greater occipital nerve (see Figure 18.3) is tender to pressure in many patients with migraine or cluster headache as well as in those with occipital neuralgia and upper cervical syndromes.

The temporomandibular joints should be palpated while the jaw is opened and closed. Inserting a finger in each ear and pressing forward on the joint often elicits tenderness or crepitus.

Spine

The cervical spine is tested for mobility and localized tenderness. In meningeal irritation, resistance of the neck to passive flexion and Kernig's sign are usually present.

Gait and Stance

An unsteady, wide-based gait may be observed as a result of a cerebellar disturbance. It may be the only indication of a midline cerebellar lesion in the early stages and may also be the presenting symptom of hydrocephalus, because corticopontocerebellar pathways become splayed over the enlarged lateral ventricles. In some cases of posterior fossa tumor, the head may be held to one side, with the occiput tilted to the side of the lesion.

Special Senses

Smell

The nostrils are often blocked in rhinitis and sinusitis so that sense of smell cannot be adequately assessed. The sense of smell may be lost when the olfactory nerve is damaged by head injury or by a tumor in the vicinity of the olfactory groove. When a patient's intellectual ability has deteriorated, the sense of smell should always be tested, because a frontotemporal tumor may cause both anosmia and mental confusion.

Vision

Circumcorneal injection may be observed in acute angle-closure glaucoma, and increased intraocular pressure may give rise to a palpable firmness of the eye. The visual fields of those patients in whom the suspicion of an intracranial lesion has arisen should be tested to confrontation and inattention to one half-field sought if the parietal lobe is thought to be involved.

The optic discs should be examined when appropriate for signs of optic atrophy or papilloedema. Swelling of the disc occurs in about 15% of cases of retrobulbar (optic) neuritis, but in such patients, unlike patients with papilloedema from raised intracranial pressure, central vision is severely impaired.

Optic atrophy may result from interference with the blood supply to the optic nerve, long-standing papilloedema, retrobulbar neuritis, or compression of the optic nerve or the optic chiasm. Occasionally a sphenoid wing meningioma compresses one optic nerve and its surrounding subarachnoid space and then expands sufficiently to increase intracranial pressure or to impair venous return from the other eye, so that papilloedema develops on the side opposite to the origin of the lesion. This combination of optic atrophy in one eye and papilloedema in the other (Foster-Kennedy syndrome) is rarely seen now, because most tumors are detected early by computed tomography (CT) or magnetic resonance imaging (MRI).

Subhyaloid hemorrhages may be observed after subarachnoid bleeding, and perivascular nodules may rarely be seen in tuberculous meningitis or disseminated lupus erythematosus. Circumscribed areas of choroidal atrophy may be a sign of toxoplasmosis.

Hearing

The eardrums should be inspected, particularly in children, when otitis media is suspected, because infection can spread centrally to cause thrombosis of the lateral sinus (otitic hydrocephalus) or to form an abscess of the temporal lobe or cerebellum. Conduction deafness is demonstrated by tuning fork tests in the case of otitis media or Eustachian catarrh. Unilateral nerve deafness should be investigated by audiometry, loudness-balance tests, brainstem auditory evoked responses, electronystagmography, and CT scanning or MRI to ensure that an acoustic neuroma is not missed.

Other Cranial Nerves

A latent ocular imbalance may be unmasked by any infectious or debilitating illness and give rise to diplopia, which may be misinterpreted as indicating a paresis of one or other of the extraocular muscles. A sixth-nerve palsy may be found on the side of a retro-orbital lesion, and bilateral sixth-nerve palsies may develop with any case of acute hydrocephalus or cerebral edema, because the expanded brain compresses the sixth nerves in their long intracranial course.

Progressive enlargement of the pupil on one side, with or without other signs of a third-nerve palsy, is an indication for immediate action, because the third nerve may be compressed by any expanding lesion forcing the uncus and medial aspect of the temporal lobe downward through the tentorial opening into the posterior fossa (tentorial herniation). The dilated pupil is almost always on the side of the expanding lesion (such as a subdural hematoma); exceptions to this rule are rare. Inability to elevate and converge the eyes (Parinaud's syndrome) may indicate compression of the midbrain from above by a tumor such as pinealoma, but many elderly patients have difficulty in looking upward.

The sudden onset of a third-nerve palsy with pain behind the eye is most commonly caused by the sudden enlargement of an aneurysm, although this may also occur in the rare Tolosa-Hunt syndrome (Figure 5.2) and ophthalmo-plegic migraine (see Chapter 18).

Retroorbital pain, sensory impairment in the distribution of the first division of the trigeminal nerve accompanied by an ipsilateral sixth nerve palsy is known as Gradenigo's syndrome (Figure 5.3; see Chapter 18).

If the patient's consciousness becomes impaired so that voluntary eye movements are no longer possible, the integrity of the third, fourth, and sixth nerves may be tested by the "doll's-eye maneuver." When the head is rotated to one side, the eyes roll to the opposite side, producing the movements of lateral conjugate deviation. Similarly, if the chin is pushed down on the chest, the eyes elevate, and if the head is extended, the eyes roll downward.

The presence of Horner's syndrome in cluster headache has already been mentioned, and it may also be seen occasionally in migraine. The pupil of one side may remain small between paroxysms of cluster headache or after a severe attack of migraine. Both pupils may be small in a pontine lesion, and one pupil may dilate in "basilar-type migraine."

Direct compression may involve any cranial nerve. It is particularly important to test facial sensation carefully, including two-point discrimination on the lip, and to check the corneal responses in patients with trigeminal neuralgia. If there is any sensory deficit, the patient may have a lesion compressing the trigeminal nerve or a pontine plaque of multiple sclerosis.

If corticobulbar pathways are involved, weakness of the lower face is detectable, and the jaw jerk and facial reflexes may increase. A bifrontal lesion results in a pouting response to gentle tapping on the closed lips.

Motor System

Signs of an upper motor neuron or cerebellar disturbance may be detected with an expanding intracranial lesion. When the patient's arms are extended and the eyes are closed, the arm may slowly fall away on the affected side.

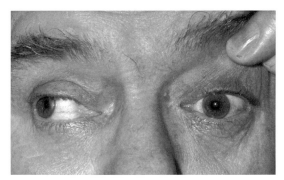

FIGURE 5.2   Left third-nerve palsy in a patient with Tolosa-Hunt syndrome. He is elevating his ptosed left eyelid with his fingers and looking to his right. The left eye fails to adduct.

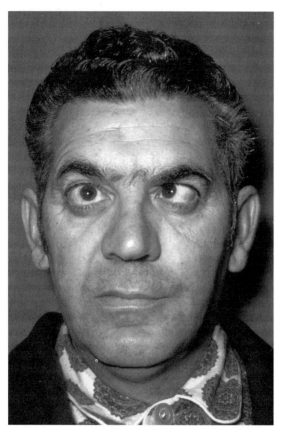

FIGURE 5.3   Gradenigo's syndrome. Pain occurs in the distribution of the first division of the trigeminal nerve, accompanied by a sixth cranial nerve palsy. The patient is unable to look to the right.

A hemiparesis is most commonly found on the side opposite to a cerebral lesion, but in a minority of patients with a rapidly expanding mass, such as subdural hematoma, the hemiparesis is found on the same side as the lesion, because the growing mass pushes the midbrain over onto the tentorial edge, compressing the cerebral peduncle. Because the pyramidal tracts cross below this level, the hemiparesis is on the same side as the causative lesion. Bilateral upper motor neuron signs may result from midbrain compression. A grasp reflex and pal-momental response indicate a lesion of the opposite frontal lobe.

With a cerebellar lesion, the affected side is hypotonic. When the elbows are resting on a table with the forearms vertical and wrist muscles relaxed, the hand hangs lower on the affected side. If the eyes are closed and the arms are lifted suddenly to a point at right angles to the body, the arm on the affected side overshoots and oscillates. The knee jerk is pendular on the affected side. Rapid and alternating movements are impaired, and finger–nose and heel–shin coordination is defective. The gait is wide based and halting, and the patient turns jerkily as if "by numbers" and tends to stumble to the side of the lesion.

Sensory System

A parietal lobe disturbance may cause subtle sensory deficit, with difficulty in discriminating two points or recognizing objects placed in the hand. Sensory inattention should be sought by touching both arms or legs simultaneously with the patient's eyes closed. Long sensory tracts may be involved with deeply placed cerebral lesions or brainstem disorders, resulting in a more clear-cut sensory disturbance.

Sphincters and Sexual Functions

Urgency of micturition may appear with upper motor neuron lesions, and a casual approach toward the time and place of relaxing the sphincters may be a feature of frontal lobe disturbance. Impotence can result from a temporal lobe lesion or from testicular atrophy secondary to hypopituitarism. In patients with impaired penile erection, it is helpful to ensure the integrity of the second and third sacral segments by testing the bulbocavernosus reflex.

GENERAL EXAMINATION

Café-au-lait patches and cutaneous nodules, seen in Von Recklinghausen's disease (neurofibromatosis type 1), indicate that there is an increased risk of pheochromocytoma (about 1%) and intracranial tumor (about 2%). Cutaneous manifestations are less obvious and may be absent in neurofibromatosis type 2, which is characterized by bilateral acoustic neuromas. The observation of cutaneous angiomas raises the possibility of an intracerebral angioma. Peutz-Jeghers syndrome is an unusual familial condition, characterized by dark pigmentation on the lips and buccal mucosa, which is associated with polyposis of the small intestine. There may be an increased tendency to intracranial tumor in this condition, as there is in polyposis coli; we have seen such a patient with multiple intracranial meningiomas.

Smoothness of the skin, paucity of body hair, and testicular atrophy or delayed development of secondary sexual characteristics in adolescents should be looked for as signs of pituitary deficiency. If the patient has noticed any lumps, examine the breasts.

Any scar in the skin warrants an inquiry about the possibility and nature of a removed lesion, because melanoma is notorious for presenting with metastases in the nervous system years after the primary tumor has been removed. Skin rashes are of importance in many infectious processes, such as meningococcemia, glandular fever, secondary syphilis, and the exanthemata associated with headache.

The association of a thin build with long fingers and toes and a high, arched palate (Marfan's syndrome) carries an increased liability to intracranial aneurysms. Other inconstant features include hypertension from coarctation of the aorta, congenital heart defects, and congenital dislocation of the lenses of the eye, which transmits a noticeable quivering movement to the iris on sudden eye movements.

Enlargement of lymph glands or spleen is relevant to the problem of headache in patients with blood dyscrasias, infectious mononucleosis, AIDS, and other infections. Ecchymoses and purpura may be observed in thrombocytopenic purpura with neurologic complications.

Urine testing does not contribute to the solution of most headache problems, but the presence of albuminuria or glycosuria may be relevant to some causes of headache. When transient cerebral episodes and headache are of recent onset, finding a cardiac valvular defect should suggest the possibility of cerebral emboli (from an atrial clot or subacute bacterial endocarditis).

Because most systemic disorders may have a neurologic component, and most cerebral disorders may have headache as a symptom, there is no need to catalog all the possible signs that careful examination could unearth that may be directly relevant to headache. However, most patients complaining of chronic headache do not have physical signs pertaining to their main symptoms, unless constant muscular overactivity and the inability to relax, which are discussed elsewhere, are included. A careful examination may disclose a number of other minor problems that require attention; many may have been a source of worry to the patient even if not mentioned in the original history. There is no better start to reassuring a patient than the knowledge that a proper physical examination has been carried out as part of a careful clinical assessment.

Chapter 6
Migraine: Varieties

The word *migraine* is of French origin and derives from the Greek *hemicrania,* like the old English term *megrim.* Although *hemicrania* literally means "only half the head," migraine involves both sides of the head from its onset in about 40% of patients. Another 40% experience strictly unilateral headaches, and approximately 20% have headaches that start on one side and later become generalized (Selby & Lance, 1960).

DEFINITION

Migraine is essentially an episodic headache, usually accompanied by nausea photophobia, and phonophobia, which may be preceded by focal neurologic symptoms (aura). The aura may be experienced without any ensuing headache; such attacks have in the past been called "migraine equivalents." Skyhøj Olsen (1990) put forward the view that migraine with and without aura may share the same pathophysiology, with the intensity of cerebral ischemia determining the presence or absence of an aura (see Chapter 8). Russell et al. (1996) consider migraine with aura and migraine without aura as distinct clinical entities, finding that the two varieties coexist in only 3.5% of males and 5.4% of females. This figure is surprisingly low, because clinical practitioners often find patients who have an aura at some stage of their lives and not at others, although the headache component retains the same characteristics (Centonze et al., 1997).

Because of the variability in migraine symptoms among patients, and even between recurrent attacks in the same patient, defining migraine has always been difficult. The problems have been tackled systematically by the Headache Classification Committee of the International Headache Society (IHS) (2004), which presented the following diagnostic criteria for migraine headache: The patient must have had five or more attacks of headache, lasting 4 to 72 hours if untreated, with at least two or four features (unilaterality, pulsating quality, moderate or severe pain intensity, and aggravation by exertion), as well as nausea, with or without vomiting, or photophobia and phonophobia. Structural abnormalities or other causative lesions should have been excluded by the history, physical examination, or, when indicated, by appropriate investigations.

These criteria have necessarily been made precise. It may be possible to make a presumptive diagnosis of migraine after one or two typical headaches, but it would be unwise to include such a patient in a clinical trial. Some headaches with migrainous characteristics last less than 4 hours, particularly in children (Maytal et al., 1995). If headaches persist for longer than 72 hours, the condition has been termed "status migrainosus." Variations in migraine symptomatology led to the allocation of attacks to subtypes of migraine under heading 1 in the IHS classification of headache (see Chapter 3).

1.1. Migraine without aura ("common migraine")
Symptoms of the headache are as just described, without any focal neurologic symptoms (Figure 6.1). The old term "common migraine" is used at times in this text for the sake of brevity.

1.2. Migraine with aura ("classical migraine")
Typical headaches preceded by neurologic symptoms such as visual, auditory, and speech disturbances, usually developing gradually over 2 to 5 minutes and lasting less than 60 minutes, are classified as migraine with aura.

1.2.1. Migraine headache with typical aura

1.2.2. Typical aura with nonmigraine headache
This term is used when the headache does not fulfill the IHS criteria for migraine.

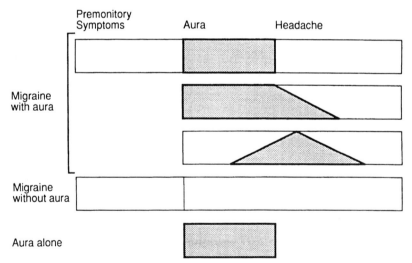

FIGURE 6.1   Classification of migraine syndromes according to the appearance of neurologic symptoms *(shaded areas)* in relation to headache. Premonitory symptoms include changes in mood, alertness, and appetite that may precede migraine by a day or so.

1.2.3. Typical aura without headache ("migraine equivalent," "transient migrainous accompaniment")

1.2.4. Familial hemiplegic migraine
Hemiparesis occurring during the attack, usually inherited as an autosomal dominant characteristic.

1.2.5. Sporadic hemiplegic migraine

1.2.6. Basilar-type migraine
Aura symptoms in basilar-type migraines arise from the brainstem (such as dysarthria, vertigo, diplopia, impaired consciousness or fainting), cerebellum, or posterior cerebral cortex.

1.3. Childhood periodic syndromes that are commonly precursors of migraine

1.3.1. Cyclical vomiting

1.3.2. Abdominal migraine

1.3.3. Benign paroxysmal vertigo of childhood

1.4. Retinal migraine
Visual symptoms are restricted to one eye.

1.5. Complications of migraine

1.5.1. Chronic migraine
Chronic migraine occurs more than 15 days each month for more than 3 months without medication abuse.

1.5.2. Status migrainosus
A debilitating migraine attack lasting for more than 72 hours is classified as status migrainosus.

1.5.3. Persistent aura without infarction

1.5.4. Migrainous infarction

1.5.5. Migraine-triggered seizures

1.6. Probable migraine

PHASES OF MIGRAINE

Premonitory Symptoms

The first indication of an impending migraine attack may be noticed 24 hours or more before headache begins (see Figure 6.1). Of 50 patients questioned by Blau (1980), 17 said that changes in mood, alertness, and appetite preceded headache by 1 to 24 hours. Drummond and Lance (1984) interviewed 530 patients with recurrent headache, ranging from typical migraine to tension-type headache, of whom 160 reported such premonitory symptoms. These patients suffered from headaches with migrainous characteristics, and about half had associated focal neurologic symptoms. Mood swings such as irritability or depression were noted by 86 patients, and a feeling of elation by 54. Of 47 who mentioned hunger, 34 craved sweet foods such as cake, cookies, and chocolate (which was specifically mentioned by 12 patients). Drowsiness and yawning were symptoms in 38 patients, and thirst in 15. These premonitory symptoms probably arise in the hypothalamus, possibly as a result of changes in monoaminergic transmission, and culminate in migraine headache, with or without aura. It could be relevant that the 5-HT$_2$ antagonist pizotyline may cause euphoria, drowsiness, and a craving to eat sweet foods. Giffin et al. (2003), using prospective collection with an electronic diary, found that the most common symptoms enabling patients to predict the onset of migraine headache were tiredness, lack of concentration, and neck stiffness. The most reliable symptom was yawning.

Aura

The aura of migraine most often arises in the visual cortex of the occipital lobe. Visual hallucinations or scotomas form part of the attack in about one third of all patients with migraine. Cluster headache with aura is rare. Silberstein et al. (2000) reported 5 patients with a visual aura and 1 with an olfactory aura out of 101 patients questioned. Fortification spectra are experienced by about 10% of patients with migraine (Lance & Anthony, 1996) and are named thus because the zigzag appearance of the hallucination resembles a medieval fortified town viewed from above. The equivalent term *teichopsia* is derived from the Greek *teichos,* meaning "wall." The fortification figures are white more often than colored and commonly shimmer or jitter as they expand across the visual field, leaving an area of impaired vision behind them, so-called scintillating scotomas. Another 25% of patients describe unformed flashes of light ("photopsia"), which usually remain in the same part of the visual field or are scattered across both visual fields. That the origin of such symptoms is the visual cortex and not the retina is clear from their distribution in the visual field and is confirmed by the fact that they occurred in a patient whose eyes had been removed (Peatfield & Rose, 1981). Some patients report that images appear split into two or more parts that may be separated from one another (Podoll & Robinson, 2000).

Symptoms that arise in areas of cortex other than the occipital lobe are much less common. Unilateral paraesthesias associated with hemiparesis or dysphasia are encountered in about 4% of all patients with migraine (Lance & Anthony, 1966). Russell and Olesen (1996) analyzed the symptoms of 163 patients experiencing migraine with aura. Almost all had visual disturbances, 31% had sensory symptoms spreading from hand and arm to the face, 18% became aphasic, and 6% developed weakness on one side. Transient temporal or parietal lobe symptoms may form part of the migraine attack. Peatfield (1991) reported a patient who experienced *déjà vu* and a dreamlike state. Olfactory hallucinations of burning, cooking, or unpleasant smells may also occur during the aura. Morrison (1990) reported that 5 of 46 patients studied had olfactory hallucinations, 3 had gustatory hallucinations, and 2 experienced distortion of self-image of their body, head, and neck with their migraine attacks. One of our patients described her fingers feeling "as long as telegraph poles" and her mouth and teeth like "a cave full of tombstones." Charles Dodgson (Lewis Carroll) suffered from migraine, and it has been suggested that the illusions of vision and body image in *Alice in Wonderland* may have been inspired by migraine. The appeal of the story is a little diminished by the knowledge that *Alice in Wonderland* was written before the author started to suffer from migraine. Oliver Sacks (1992) beautifully described and illustrated the auras of migraine.

Migraine Aura Without Headache

The waxing and waning of fortification spectra, scotomas, paresthesias, dysphasia, and other symptoms of cortical or brainstem origin over a period of 10 to 60 minutes may occur without any headache following. This has been recognized in the past as a "migraine equivalent" or acephalgic migraine (Kunkel, 1986). Focal neurologic symptoms in middle-aged and elderly patients may evolve and resolve slowly in a manner that suggests a migrainous rather than thromboembolic phenomenon. Fisher (1980) has called these episodes "transient migrainous accompaniments" (TMAs) to distinguish them from transient ischemic attacks (TIAs). Although there is no significant difference in the vascular risk factors for migraine equivalents and TIAs, TMAs carry less risk of subsequent vascular disease (Dennis & Warlow, 1992). A familial form of acephalgic migraine has been described (Shevell, 1997).

Headache

Migraine headache is primarily unilateral in two thirds of patients and is bilateral in the remainder (Selby & Lance, 1960; Lance & Anthony, 1966). It may change from one side to the other in a single attack. The pain may be felt deeply behind the eye or in the inner angle of the eye but more commonly involves the frontotemporal region. It may radiate backward to the occiput and upper neck or even to the lower neck and shoulder. In other patients it starts as a dull ache in the upper neck and radiates forward. In some patients it may remain limited to the vascular territory of frontal, temporal, or occipital arteries. In others the pain affects mainly the face (lower-half headache, facial migraine). Facial migraine is usually unilateral, and pain involves the nostril, cheek, gums, and teeth. It may spread to the neck, ear, or eye, in which case it may be confused with cluster headache. It differs from cluster headache in its pattern of recurrence, being without the remissions that usually occur between bouts of cluster headache, and with each episode lasting for 4 hours to several days. Guiloff and Fruns (1988) reported 22 patients with migraine or cluster headache who experienced pain in the upper or lower limbs on the same side as their headache, suggesting thalamic involvement in the genesis of such attacks.

It might be assumed that the headache of migraine with aura would affect the side of the head overlying the hemisphere from which the focal neurologic symptoms originated, but this is not always the case. Of 75 patients with unilateral paresthesias and unilateral headache, the headache developed on the same side as the paraesthesias in 55 and on the opposite side in only 20 (Peatfield, Gawel, & Rose, 1981). When these figures are pooled with other published reports, equal numbers of patients have headache ipsilateral and contralateral to the side of neurologic symptoms. A prospective study by Jensen et al. (1986) confirmed this important fact: Aura symptoms were ipsilateral to the headache in 19 patients and contralateral in 19.

Migraine commonly starts as a dull headache, which may become throbbing in quality (increasing with each pulse) as the headache intensifies, and reverts to a constant pain later. Many patients with migraine experience a constant headache that is never truly pulsatile. In addition, 42% of patients are subject to sudden, jabbing pains ("ice-pick pains," primary stabbing headache) in the head, whether or not they have their characteristic headache at the time, compared with only 3% of normal controls (Raskin & Schwartz, 1980).

Resolution

A feeling of exhaustion and lethargy may remain for several days after the headache stops. Blau (1987) described "postdromes" of impaired concentration, irritability, sluggishness, and diminished appetite for a day or more after the headache had gone. Less commonly, patients may experience euphoria and a craving for sweet foods, resembling the symptoms of the premonitory phase. During this "hangover phase," headache may recur briefly if patients bend forward or shake their heads.

VARIATIONS ON THE THEME OF MIGRAINE

Hemiplegic Migraine

Weakness or paralysis is an uncommon accompaniment of migraine and when it occurs is usually transient, resolving without evidence of infarction. Edema of one cerebral hemisphere has been demonstrated on computed tomography (CT) scanning during hemiplegia, and an emission CT scan using Tc^{99m} revealed a striking accumulation of isotope over the affected hemisphere, indicating a breakdown of the blood–brain barrier (Harrison, 1981), although generally this imaging is normal. Friberg et al. (1987) studied regional cerebral blood flow (rCBF) in three patients in whom hemiplegic migraine was induced by cerebral angiography. Focal hypoperfusion, preceded by hyperperfusion in two cases, developed in the frontal lobes and spread posteriorly. Rapid fluctuations in rCBF were observed, attributed to instability of cerebral vascular tone, which occasionally reached ischemic levels.

Either side of the body may be affected, sometimes alternately in successive episodes. Because the hemiplegia is often associated with dysphasia or other cortical symptoms, it is probably of hemispheric origin in most instances, and the finding that cerebral blood flow is reduced on the affected side supports this view (Staehelin Jensen et al., 1981b). Angiography demonstrated a local constriction of one internal carotid artery at the level of the skull base in one patient at the height of the attack (Staehelin Jensen et al., 1981a). Other members of this family had dysarthria, dysphagia, and drop attacks.

Reversible focal hyperperfusion of the affected part of the cerebral cortex has been demonstrated in hemiparesis persisting for 4 days (Lindahl, Allder, & Jefferson, 2002). Cerebrospinal fluid (CSF) pleocytosis has been reported at the height of hemiplegic migraine (Schraeder & Burns, 1980).

A survey of the 5.2 million inhabitants of Denmark disclosed 291 patients with hemiplegic migraine, of whom 147 were familial, coming from 44 different families, the remainder were apparently sporadic (Lykke Thomsen et al., 2002). The prevalence of hemiplegic migraine in Denmark at the end of 1999 was thus

0.01%. Familial hemiplegic migraine (FHM) is usually inherited as a dominant characteristic with mutations in the *CACNA 1A* gene on chromosome 19 in about 55% of cases (FHM$_1$) and in the *ATP1A2* gene on chromosome 1 in 15% (FHM$_2$), leaving 30% unaccounted for. The inheritance of migraine in general is discussed in Chapter 7 (page 60).

Thomsen et al. (2003) studied the characteristics of sporadic hemiplegic migraine in 105 people identified in the Danish population. As well as having weakness, 72% of these patients had become aphasic or developed visual or sensory symptoms. Weakness shifted from one side of the body to the other during an attack in 16% and was bilateral at one stage in 13%. Many met the criteria for basilar-type migraine.

Athwal and Lennox (1996) reported that FHM responds to acetazolamide, as does episodic ataxia type 2 (EA$_2$), co-localized to the same gene. We have found flunarizine (Sibelium) useful in diminishing the number and severity of attacks of hemiplegic migraine. It may take as long as 6 months to start and we have seen it work for up to 5 years in some cases with apparent tachyphylaxis.

Fitzsimons and Wolfenden (1985) reported a family in which hemiplegic migraine was associated with coma and life-threatening cerebral edema. Cerebellar ataxia followed each episode and eventually persisted. Progressive cerebellar disturbance is explicable by the discovery that the gene for FHM$_1$ on chromosome 19 overlaps the locus for episodic cerebellar ataxia type 2 (EA$_2$) and CADASIL (cerebral autosomal dominant arteriopathy with subcortical infarcts and leukoencephalopathy), which may present as familial hemiplegic migraine but usually progresses to pseudobulbar palsy associated with gross white-matter changes demonstrated by magnetic resonance imaging (MRI) (Hutchinson et al., 1995).

Hemiplegia usually clears up over a period of 24 hours, but death during an attack was reported by Guest and Woolf (1964), who found ischemic changes in the cerebrum and brainstem, and also by Neligan, Harriman, and Pearce (1977). In the case described by Neligan and colleagues, autopsy was performed 4 months after the initial episode, because life had been maintained by mechanical ventilation; microinfarcts were found in the cortex and basal ganglia, although the brainstem was apparently spared.

Alternating Hemiplegia of Childhood

Alternating hemiplegia of childhood has been proposed as an expression of migraine in children but may terminate in a dystonic state and is clearly a separate entity (Lance, 2000).

Basilar-Type Migraine

Symptoms arising from the brainstem, such as diplopia, vertigo, incoordination, ataxia, and dysarthria, are neurologic components of the migraine attack in about 25% of patients (Lance & Anthony, 1966). Bickerstaff (1961a, b) pointed out that severe brainstem symptoms in migraine were often associated with faintness, fainting, or sudden loss of consciousness, which he attributed to constriction of the basilar artery causing ischemia of the midbrain reticular formation.

Lance and Anthony (1966) found that 7% of patients with symptoms referable to the distribution of the vertebrobasilar arterial system had fainted on occasions during their attacks, whereas none of those with symptoms arising from areas supplied by the carotid artery had done so. Photopsia and fortification spectra occurred as often in association with symptoms arising from either carotid or basilar territories. The frequency of hindbrain symptoms in migraine led Klee (1968) to conclude that "the symptoms of migraine are primarily due to a dysfunction of the vertebrobasilar arterial system." Symptoms indistinguishable from those of migraine, including fortification spectra and other visual disturbances, can be precipitated by vertebral angiography (Hauge, 1954). Nevertheless, the mechanism remains obscure. Because the disturbance of cerebral metabolism extends beyond the territory supplied by the vertebrobasilar arterial system, the term *basilar-type migraine* is now preferred by the IHS.

Some children and adolescents subject to both basilar-type migraine and epilepsy have had interictal electroencephalograms (EEGs) showing slow spike-wave complexes in the occipital regions, blocking on visual attention (Camfield, Metrakos, & Andermann, 1978; Panayiotopoulos, 1980). This presumably means that the occipital cortex is in a constant state of hyperexcitability, although the relationship of this to migrainous symptoms is uncertain. The grossly abnormal EEG distinguishes this syndrome, which appears to have a good prognosis, from other forms of basilar migraine in which the EEG is usually normal between attacks.

Childhood Periodic Syndromes in the IHS Classification

Cyclical Vomiting and Abdominal Migraine

The term *cyclical vomiting* is applied to recurrent attacks of intense nausea and vomiting associated with pallor and lethargy. Episodes can last from an hour to 5 days, during which the victim may vomit four or more times an hour. Data from a single pediatric neurology practice included 1106 patients with migraine, of whom 18.5% suffered from cyclical vomiting, abdominal migraine, or both conditions (Al-Twaijri & Shevell, 2002). Typical migraine headaches occurred at other times in 70% of this group. Cyclical vomiting may be hereditary in some instances (Haan, Kars, & Ferrari, 2002).

Bille (1962) found that 20% of children with migraine were subject to paroxysmal abdominal pains compared with 4% of a control group and regarded these symptoms as a migraine equivalent. In a follow-up study only 1.5% of patients with migraine still had attacks of abdominal pain at 30 years of age or later (Bille, 1981). A history of vomiting attacks in childhood was found in 23% of patients with migraine, compared with 12% of patients subject to tension headache as studied by Lance and Anthony (1966). Lundberg (1975) reported that 12 of 100 patients with migraine suffered from recurrent abdominal pain and that some responded to antimigraine therapy.

Dignan, Abu-Arafeh, and Russell (2001) followed 54 children with abdominal migraine for 7 to 10 years and found that the condition had resolved in 31 cases (61%). Seventy percent of this group either currently (52%) or previously (18%) had migraines.

The conclusion to be drawn from the literature and from experience is that abdominal migraine is a real and important entity. There is evidence that pizotyline, cyproheptadine, and propranolol are useful in prevention (Russell, Abu-Arafeh, & Symon, 2000). Cyclical vomiting attacks may be reduced in intensity by antiemetics such as metoclopramide and domperidone (Abu-Arafeh & Hamalainer, 2000). We have found droperidol and chloropromazine useful in severe refractory cases.

Benign Paroxysmal Vertigo of Childhood (BPV)

Basser (1964) reported episodic vertigo and nystagmus in 10 girls and 4 boys, starting in the first 8 years of life and recurring on average every 6 to 8 weeks. Caloric tests demonstrated unilateral or bilateral vestibular abnormalities. The attacks ceased spontaneously after some months or years. No history of migraine headache was recorded for these children.

Abu-Arafeh and Russell (1995) estimated the prevalence of benign paroxysmal vertigo (BPV) at 2.6% and found that children with BPV had many features in common with children with migraine, considering it reasonable to regard it as a migraine equivalent. Of the 45 children, 24% were also prone to migraine headaches, compared with 10.6% of a control group. In their 19 patients Drigo, Carli, and Laverda (2001) reported a sudden onset of vertigo between the ages of 13 months and 8 years, a frequency of recurrence varying from once in 3 days to once every 4 months, and cessation of symptoms in 10 patients before the age of 10 years. Fear was experienced by nine of the children, and nystagmus was observed in seven. Migraine headache developed in three patients, and abdominal pain or cyclical vomiting in five. Six had previously suffered from benign paroxysmal torticollis.

Migrainous Vertigo in Adults

Migrainous vertigo was diagnosed in 7% of 200 patients attending a dizziness clinic and in 9% of 200 patients in a migraine clinic (Neuhauser et al., 2001). Vertigo was regularly associated with migraine headache in 15 of 33 patients and occurred with and without headache in 16 and always separately in 2.

Vertigo is a common symptom of basilar-type migraine. Kayan and Hood (1984) found abnormalities of the vestibular system in 60% of patients.

Slater (1979) used the term *benign recurrent vertigo* for attacks of spontaneous vertigo not precipitated by movement and not accompanied by cochlear or neurologic symptoms in young or middle-aged adults. This disorder has some features in common with migraine, including female preponderance, positive family history, and precipitation by alcohol, lack of sleep, and emotional stress, comparable with benign paroxysmal vertigo in children.

Behan and Carlin (1982) reported 32 patients, 7 males, and 25 females, between 8 and 65 years of age, who experienced episodes of giddiness, sometimes associated with tinnitus, deafness, ataxia, nausea, and headache, which responded to treatment with pizotifen (pizotyline) and propranolol. The paroxysmal nature of these symptoms suggests that benign recurrent vertigo may be caused by a disturbance of the internal auditory artery circulation allied to migraine. Viirre and

Baloh (1996) reported the sudden onset of deafness in 13 patients whose migraine was associated with vertigo—a less benign manifestation.

When recurrent vertigo is associated with acoustic symptoms, the diagnosis of Ménière's disease becomes more probable. Nevertheless, the link with migraine remains. In a group of 78 patients with Ménière's disease, the prevalence of migraine with and without aura was 56%, compared with 25% in a control group (Radtke et al., 2002).

Retinal Migraine and Monocular Blindness

Retinal migraine and monocular blindness are thought to be a subdivision of migraine with aura in which vision is lost in one eye (not to be confused with a homonymous hemianopia) with or without photopsia, for seconds or minutes, preceding headache or a dull ache behind the affected eye. The prevalence of retinal migraine has been estimated as 1 in 200 persons with migraine (Troost & Zagami, 2000). Compression of the optic nerve and transient ischemic attacks arising from the ipsilateral carotid artery must be excluded, particularly when monocular visual loss is not followed by headache. The mechanism is thought to involve spasm of the central retinal or ophthalmic artery. Troost and Zagami (2000) consider that "anterior visual pathway migraine" may be preferable to the term "retinal migraine," because other structures may, rarely, be involved.

Carroll (1970) presented case histories of 10 women and 5 men with retinal migraine, seven of whom had experienced typical attacks of migraine at other times. One developed a permanent visual deficit. Ischemic papillopathy has been described as a complication of migraine (McDonald & Sanders, 1971; Lee, Brazis, & Miller, 1996). Coppeto et al. (1986) summarized 12 reported cases with permanent visual impairment and added 2 of their own. Occlusion of the central retinal artery and its branches with infarction and transient retinal edema have been described most commonly, but venous obstruction has also been reported in patients with migraine.

In many cases, it is difficult to determine whether transient blindness in one eye is a migrainous variant or is thromboembolic in origin. Tomsak and Jergens (1987) reported 24 patients ranging from 19 to 61 years of age in whom cerebral angiography and cardiac investigation disclosed no source of emboli. Visual loss lasted from 30 seconds to 30 minutes, recurred from twice a year to twice a week, and was precipitated by bending over in eight patients and by strenuous exercise in four. Seven patients had suffered from migraine previously. The differential diagnosis from other forms of amaurosis remains one of exclusion.

COMPLICATIONS OF MIGRAINE

Chronic Migraine

The frequency of migraine headache may progressively increase, particularly under conditions of stress, anxiety, or depression. If the frequency exceeds 15 in a month, migraine is classified as chronic. It is included with other forms of frequent headache in Chapter 11.

Status Migrainosus

The term *status migrainosus* is applied to long-lasting, severe attacks of migraine headache; these headaches are considered in Chapter 9.

Persistent Aura Without Infarction

Some patients, many who have had migraine, report that their vision is abnormal continuously. Such patients fall into two groups. One group report a visual disturbance that is persistent and generally involves large areas, if not the entire visual field. Such patients report bright spots, sometimes colorful change or haziness, and often compare their vision to that of a poorly tuned television. The term *visual snow* is often employed. Liu and colleagues seemed to be describing such patients in their initial report (Liu et al., 1995). Case two of Rothrock's (1997) seems also to fit this description, as do cases one and two from our series (Jager et al., 2004). We have applied the term Primary Persistent Visual Disturbance (PPVD) to this clinical picture to distinguish it from more typical cases with a visual disturbance that is much more migrainous in its description. The second group of patients report a more typical aura that persists, described in Haas's original description (Haas, 1982), case one of Rothrock (1997), and Jager et al. (2004) cases three and four. The latter cases seem best classified as migraine with persistent aura, and will be subsumed by the appropriate section of the IHS classification (Headache Classification Committee of The International Headache Society, 2004). We found no changes on perfusion or diffusion weighted MRI in the four cases we studied (Jager et al., 2004). Having seen a child, aged 10, describe exactly the same disturbance of *visual snow* with blotches as adults (PJG), it is hard to believe that there is not a consistent underlying biology that distinguishes this condition in some way from more typical aura. Haan et al. (2000) reported a useful effect from acetazolamide in aura status. PPVD is often refractory to treatment.

A group of patients poorly dealt with are those with aura symptoms longer than one hour and less than seven days who would have been called prolonged aura in IHS-I (Headache Classification Committee of The International Headache Society, 1988), and have lost their classification home. This seems unfortunate.

Migrainous Infarction

Ischemic papillopathy and retinal infarction have been referred to in connection with retinal migraine. The risk of cerebral infarction in patients with migraine and the complex relationship between migraine and stroke have now been studied intensively. Welch and Levine (1990) have considered the problem under the following headings:

1. *Coexisting stroke and migraine.* The stroke occurs remote in time from a migraine attack.
2. *Stroke with clinical features of migraine.* An underlying structural lesion causes both neurologic deficit and migrainous symptoms (symptomatic migraine).
3. *Migraine-induced stroke.* The stroke occurs during the course of a migraine attack, with the neurologic deficit being in the area corresponding to the origin of aura symptoms in previous migrainous episodes. Subdivisions of this

category are those with and without risk factors, such as oral contraceptive use and cigarette smoking.

There have been many reports of strokes in the third category. It is curious that vascular occlusion demonstrated by angiography involves large arteries or their branches, the posterior cerebral more often than the middle cerebral circulation, whereas the vascular changes associated with the migrainous aura presumably affect the cortical microcirculation, because arteriography during an attack does not usually show any constriction of major vessels. Among almost 5000 patients diagnosed as having migraine or vascular headache at the Mayo Clinic over a 4-year period, 20 had migraine-associated strokes (Broderick & Swanson, 1987). Two patients had a second episode over a 7-year follow-up. The outlook for recovery was good, because 14 patients were left with only a mild deficit, and 4 had completely recovered.

Henrich and Horwitz (1989) reported that migraine with aura carried an increased risk of ischemic stroke (odds ratio 2.6). Merikangas et al. (1997) found that a history of migraine and "severe nonspecific headache" was a risk factor for stroke in general (odds ratio 1.5), whereas Carolei et al. (1996) concluded that, in the absence of other risk factors, migraine was of significance only in women younger than 35 years. Tzourio et al. (1995) studied 72 women younger than 45 years with ischemic stroke, discerning an increased risk for patients suffering from migraine without aura (odds ratio 3) as well as those with aura (odds ratio 6.2).

The risk of stroke was greatly increased for patients with migraine who smoked more than 20 cigarettes a day (odds ratio 10.2) and for those using oral contraceptives (odds ratio 13.9). They calculated that the absolute risk of young women with migraine suffering a stroke was 19 per 100,000 per year. A later publication by Tzourio et al. (2000) warns that bias in patient selection may have influenced published trials and that there is still some doubt about the risk of stroke in migraine without aura and in those patients on low-estrogen oral contraceptives.

An association between migraine and the presence of lupus anticoagulants (antiphospholipid antibodies) has been reported (Levine et al., 1987) and could be relevant to the genesis of stroke, although Hering et al. (1991) found no association between anticardiolipin antibodies and migraine. Because various antiphospholipid antibodies cross-react, it is unlikely that their presence reported in other series can be attributed to migraine alone. They may be a manifestation of some associated disorder.

Montagna et al. (1988a) found elevated blood lactate on exertion in nine patients with migraine, five of whom had suffered a migrainous stroke, and muscle biopsy disclosed ragged red fibers in one case, thus bringing up the possibility of mitochondrial disease underlying migrainous stroke. The syndrome of mitochondrial myopathy, encephalopathy, lactic acidosis, and strokelike episodes (MELAS syndrome) is a maternally inherited disorder associated with severe migraine (Montagna et al., 1988b; Goto et al., 1992), but there is no evidence for abnormalities of mitochondrial DNA in migraine with aura (Klopstock et al., 1996).

It may be concluded that prolonged cerebral oligemia in migraine predisposes to a stroke in the ischemic territory responsible for the aura (Bogousslavsky et al., 1988).

Migraine-Triggered Seizures

Marks and Ehrenberg (1993) studied the relationship between migraine and epilepsy in 395 adult patients with seizures. Seventy-nine patients (20%) also suffered from migraine, and of these, 13 stated that seizures had occurred during or after an aura. The association was particularly noticed at menstruation. EEG changes were recorded in seven patients at the time of their migraine attacks, and control of epilepsy was improved in six patients when antimigraine drugs were added to their anticonvulsant medication.

In another series of 412 adult patients with seizures, 14% had a history of migraine and 7 patients reported that migraine had induced epileptic fits (Velioglu & Ozmenoglu, 1999). There was a specific link with the menstrual cycle and migraine with aura. Four patients had fewer seizures with the addition of antimigraine therapy.

The relationship between these two paroxysmal neurologic disorders is discussed further in Chapter 7 (pages 62–63) and Chapter 13.

OTHER ENTITIES RELATED TO MIGRAINE

Recurrent Neck Pain

Episodic unilateral neck pain with tenderness of the carotid artery, responsive to ergotamine and sumatriptan, is probably a variant of migraine (De Marinis & Accornero, 1997). See also the discussion of carotidynia in Chapter 15.

Cardiac Migraine

The term *cardiac migraine* was introduced by Leon-Sotomayor (1974) to demarcate a syndrome of classical migraine, chest pain, and functional hypoglycemia. During the prodrome of an attack, patients experienced palpitations, anxiety symptoms, and chest pain that occasionally radiated to the inner aspect of the arm. This pain was reproduced in four of the patients during coronary angiography while segmental coronary spasm was demonstrated. The relationship of migraine headache to the episodes of coronary spasm is not clear from this report.

A group of 62 patients with "variant angina" (episodic angina at rest associated with transient ST segment elevation and rapidly relieved by nitroglycerin) was studied by Miller at al. (1981). Migraine was diagnosed in 26% of the patients with variant angina compared with 6% of a "coronary" control group and 10% of a "noncoronary" control group. Raynaud's phenomenon occurred in 26% of the patients with variant angina, in contrast to 5% and 3% of the two control groups. There may therefore be a tendency for spasm to occur in different vascular beds at different times in some patients. Atrial fibrillation has been reported to accompany attacks of migraine (Petersen, Scruton, & Downie, 1977), and we have observed this association in one patient who proved to have a pheochromocytoma. Hyperventilation is a common accompaniment of migraine headache (Blau & Dexter, 1980) and may give rise to symptoms such as tightness and pain in the chest, which might be misinterpreted as "cardiac migraine."

Anginal pain may be referred to the head. Headache on exertion relieved by rest may be a presenting symptom of cardiac ischemia (Lipton et al., 1997; Lance & Lambros, 1998).

Migraine Stupor

Clouding of consciousness, faintness, and syncope are not uncommon in migraine but are often associated with postural hypotension. Less often, migraine may be accompanied by stupor or coma. Lee and Lance (1977) noted cases previously reported and described seven patients from 10 to 52 years of age who had become stuporous for periods varying from 12 hours to 5 days during attacks of migraine. The diagnosis of basilar migraine was suggested by the symptoms and signs that preceded or arose during the headache: dysarthria, ataxia, incoordination, paraesthesias, dilation of one pupil, and homonymous hemianopia. However, it is not limited to the vertebrobasilar circulation. Measurement of cerebral blood flow in an episode of migraine stupor demonstrated a severe, global reduction in cerebral blood flow (Hachinski et al., 1977).

Acute Confusional Migraine

Selby and Lance (1960) reported that 3.5% of their 500 patients had experienced a confusional state as part of their migraine attacks. One woman walked out of her house, forgetting all about her children. The condition was described in children by Gascon and Barlow (1970) and is probably not uncommon, because Ehyai and Fenichel (1978) encountered five such instances in 100 successive children with migraine. Confusion lasts from 10 minutes to 20 hours, usually terminating in deep sleep. Disorientation and agitation may be thought at first to be hysterical phenomena if the headache is not a prominent feature. Attacks may be triggered by relatively minor blows to the head, particularly in children (Haas, Pineda, & Lourie, 1975), in a manner comparable with footballer's migraine (Matthews, 1972; Bennett et al., 1980). Confusion is probably the result of diffuse cerebral ischemia, like a milder form of migraine stupor.

Transient Global Amnesia

The sudden loss of short-term memory and the inability to register memory for a period of hours, known as *transient global amnesia* (TGA), was described by Fisher and Adams (1964) and may occur in epilepsy, vertebrobasilar insufficiency, and migraine. In the two latter cases, the probable cause is ischemia of the entry portals for memory, comprising the hippocampus and temporal stem situated in the medial aspect of each temporal lobe, in territory supplied by the posterior cerebral artery. For memory loss to be complete, ischemia would have to involve both sides together, suggesting that flow is reduced in the basilar artery and hence its posterior cerebral branches. Migraine was almost nine times as common as in a control population in the study presented by Melo, Ferro, and Ferro (1992) and significantly more common than a comparative group of patients with transient ischemic attacks (Hodges & Warlow, 1990). The proposition that migrainous vasospasm may be responsible for some cases of TGA is strengthened by reports of both migraine and transient global amnesia occurring in siblings (Stracciari and Rebucci, 1986; Dupuis, Pierre, & Gonsette, 1987) and by the finding of abnormalities in cerebral blood flow 1 to 5 days after an episode (Crowell et al., 1984). TGA is a frightening symptom but rarely recurs often and does not appear to be a risk factor for stroke (Hodges & Warlow, 1990).

References

Abu-Arafeh, I., & Hämäläinen, M. (2000). Childhood syndromes related to migraine. In J. Olesen, P. Tfelt-Hansen, & K. M. A. Welch (Eds.), *The headaches* (2nd ed.). (pp. 519–521). Philadelphia: Lippincott, Williams and Wilkins.

Abu-Arafeh, I., & Russell, J. (1995). Paroxysmal vertigo as a migraine equivalent in children: A population-based study. *Cephalalgia, 15,* 22–25.

Al-Twaijri, W. A., & Shevell, M. I. (2002). Paediatric migraine equivalents: Occurrence and clinical features in practice. *Paediatr Neurol, 26,* 365–368.

Athwal, B. S., & Lennox, G. G. (1996). Acetazolamide responsiveness in familial hemiplegic migraine. *Ann Neurol, 40,* 820–821.

Basser, L. S. (1964). Benign paroxysmal vertigo of childhood. A variety of vestibular neuronitis. *Brain, 87,* 141–152.

Behan, P. O., & Carlin, J. (1982). Benign recurrent vertigo. In F. Clifford Rose (Ed.), *Advances in migraine* (pp. 19–55). New York: Raven.

Bennett, D. R., Fuenning, S. I., Sullivan, G., & Weber, J. (1980). Migraine precipitated by head trauma in athletes. *Am J Sports Med, 8,* 202–205.

Bickerstaff, E. R. (1961a). Basilar artery migraine. *Lancet, 1,* 15–17.

Bickerstaff, E. R. (1961b). Impairment of consciousness in migraine. *Lancet, 2,* 1057–1059.

Bille, B. (1962). Migraine in school children. *Acta Paediat Scand, 51*(Suppl 136), 1–151.

Bille, B. (1981). Migraine in childhood and its prognosis. *Cephalalgia, 1,* 71–75.

Blau, J. N. (1980). Migraine prodromes separated from the aura; complete migraine. *BMJ, 281,* 658–660.

Blau, J. N. (1987). Adult migraine; the patient observed. In J. N. Blau (Ed.), *Migraine: Clinical and research aspects* (pp. 3–30). Baltimore: Johns Hopkins University Press.

Blau, J. N., & Dexter, S. L. (1980). Hyperventilation during migraine attacks. *BMJ, 280,* 1254.

Bogousslavsky, J., Regli, F., Van Melle, G., Payot, M., & Uske, A. (1988). Migraine stroke. *Neurology, 28,* 223–227.

Broderick, J. P., & Swanson, J. W. (1987). Migraine-related strokes. Clinical profile and prognosis in 20 patients. *Arch Neurol, 44,* 868–871.

Camfield, P. R., Metrakos, K., & Andermann, F. (1978). Basilar migraine, seizures and severe epileptiform EEG abnormalities. A relatively benign syndrome in adolescents. *Neurology, 28,* 584–588.

Carolei, A., Marini, C., De Matteis, G., & the Italian National Research Council Study Group on Stroke in the Young. (1996). History of migraine and risk of cerebral ischaemia in young adults. *Lancet, 347,* 1503–1506.

Carroll, D. (1970). Retinal migraine. *Headache, 10,* 9–13.

Centonze, V., Polito, B. M., Valerio, A., Cassiano, M. A., Amato, R., Ricchetti, G., Bassi, A., Valente, A., & Albano, O. (1997). Migraine with and without aura in the same patient: Expression of a single clinical entity. *Cephalalgia, 17,* 585–587.

Chronicle, E. P., & Mulleners, W. M. (1996). Visual system dysfunction in migraine: A review of clinical and psychophysical findings. *Cephalalgia, 16,* 525–535.

Coppeto, J. R., Lessell, S., Sciarra, R., & Bear, L. (1986). Vascular retinopathy in migraine. *Neurology, 36,* 267–270.

Crowell, G. F., Stump, D. A., Biller, J., McHenry, C. J., Jr., & Toole, J. F. (1984). The transient global amnesia-migraine syndrome. *Arch Neurol, 41,* 75–79.

De Marinis, M., & Accornero, N. (1997). Recurrent neck pain as a variant of migraine. *J Neurol Neurosurg Psychiatry, 62,* 669–670.

Dennis, M., & Warlow, C. (1992). Migraine aura without headache: Transient ischaemic attack or not? *J Neurol Neurosurg Psychiatry, 55,* 437–440.

Dignan, F., Abu-Arafeh, I., & Russell, G. (2001). The prognosis of childhood abdominal migraine. *Arch Dis Child, 84,* 415–418.

Drigo, P., Carli, G., & Laverda, A. M. (2001). Benign paroxysmal vertigo of childhood. *Brain Dev, 23,* 38–41.

Drummond, P. D., & Lance, J. W. (1984). Neurovascular disturbances in headache patients. *Clin Exp Neurol, 20,* 93–99.

Dupuis, M. J. M., Pierre, P. H., & Gonsette, R. E. (1987). Transient global amnesia and migraine in twin sisters. *J Neurol Neurosurg Psychiatry, 50,* 816–824.

Ehyai, A., & Fenichel, G. M. (1978). The natural history of acute confusional migraine. *Arch Neurol, 35,* 368–369.

Fisher, C. M. (1980). Late-life migraine accompaniments as a cause of unexplained transient ischaemic attacks. *Can J Neurol Sci, 7,* 9–17.

Fisher, C. M., & Adams, R. D. (1964). Transient global amnesia. *Acta Neurol Scand, 40*(Suppl. 9), 1–83.

Fitzsimons, R. B., & Wolfenden, W. H. (1985). Migraine coma. Meningitic migraine with cerebral oedema associated with a new form of autosomal dominant cerebellar ataxia. *Brain, 108,* 555–577.

Friberg, L., Olsen, T. S., Roland, P. E., & Lassen, N. A. (1987). Focal ischaemia caused by instability of cerebro-vascular tone during attacks of hemiplegic migraine. A regional cerebral blood flow study. *Brain, 110,* 917–931.

Gascon, G., & Barlow, C. (1970). Juvenile migraine presenting as acute confusional state. *Pediatrics, 45,* 628–635.

Giffin, N. J., Ruggiero, L., Lipton, R. B., Silberstein, S. D., Tvedskov, J. F., Olesen, J., et al. (2003). Premonitory symptoms in migraine. An electronic diary study. *Neurology, 60,* 935–940.

Goto, Y., Horai, S., Matsuoka, T., Koga, Y., Nihei, K., Kobayashi, M., & Nonaka, I. (1992). Mitochondrial myopathy, encephalopathy, lactic acidosis and stroke-like episodes (MELAS). A correlative study of the clinical features and mitochondrial DNA mutation. *Neurology, 42,* 545–550.

Guest, I. A., & Woolf, A. L. (1964). Fatal infarction of brain in migraine. *BMJ, 1,* 225–226.

Guiloff, R. J., & Fruns, M. (1988). Limb pain in migraine and cluster headache. *J Neurol Neurosurg Psychiatry, 51,* 1022–1031.

Haan, J., Kors, E. E., & Ferrari, M. D. (2002). Familial cyclic vomiting syndrome. *Cephalalgia, 22,* 552–554.

Haan, J., Sluis, P., Sluis, L. H., & Ferrari, M. D. (2000). Acetazolamide for migraine aura status. *Neurology, 55,* 1588–1589.

Haas, D. C., Pineda, G. S., & Lourie, H. (1975). Juvenile head trauma symptoms and their relationship to migraine. *Arch Neurol, 32,* 727–730.

Haas, D. C. (1982). Prolonged migraine aura status. *Annals of Neurology, 11,* 197–199.

Hachinski, V. C., Olesen, J., Norris, J. W., Larsen, B., Enevoldsen, E., & Lassen, N. A. (1977). Cerebral haemodynamics in migraine. *Can J Neurol Sci, 4,* 245–249.

Harrison, M. J. G. (1981). Hemiplegic migraine. *J Neurol Neurosurg Psychiatry, 44,* 652–653.

Hauge, T. (1954). Catheter vertebral angiography. *Acta Radiol Suppl, 109,* 1–219.

Headache Classification Committee of the International Headache Society. (1988). Classification and diagnostic criteria for headache disorders, cranial neuralgias and facial pain. *Cephalalgia, 8,* 1–96.

Headache Classification Committee, the International Headache Society. (2004). The international classification of headache disorders (2nd ed.). *Cephalalgia, 24*(Suppl 1), 24–36.

Henrich, J. B., & Horwitz, R. I. (1989). A controlled study of ischemic stroke risk in migraine patients. *J Clin Epidemiol, 42,* 773–780.

Hering, R., Couturier, G. M., Steiner, T. J., Asherson, R. A., & Clifford Rose, F. (1991). Anticardiolipin antibodies in migraine. *Cephalalgia, 11,* 19–21.

Hodges, J. R., & Warlow, C. P. (1990). The aetiology of transient global amnesia. *Brain, 113,* 639–657.

Hutchinson, M., O'Riordan, J., Javed, M., Quin, E., Macerlaine, D., Wilcox, T., Parfrey, N., Nagy, T. G., & Tournier-Lasserve, E. (1995). Familial hemiplegic migraine and autosomal dominant arteriopathy with leukoencephalopathy (CADASIL). *Ann Neurol, 38,* 817–824.

Jager H. R., Griffin N. J., & Goadsby P. J. (2004). Diffusion- and perfusion-weighted MR imaging in persistent migrainous visual disturbances. *Cephalalgia, 24,* in press.

Jensen, K., Tfelt-Hansen, P., Lauritzen, M., & Olesen, J. (1986). Classic migraine. A prospective reporting of symptoms. *Acta Neurol Scand, 73,* 359–362.

Kayan, A., & Hood, J. D. (1984). Neuro-otological manifestations of migraine. *Brain, 107,* 1123–1142.

Klee, A. (1968). *A clinical study of migraine with particular reference to the most severe cases.* Copenhagen: Munksgaard.

Klopstock, T., May, A., Seibel, P., Papagiannuli, E., Diene, H. C., & Reichmann, H. (1996). Mitochondrial DNA in migraine with aura. *Neurology, 46,* 1735–1738.

Kunkel, R. S. (1986). Acephalgic migraine. *Headache, 26,* 198–201.

Lance, J. W. (2000). Is alternating hemiplegia of childhood (AHC) a variant of migraine? *Cephalalgia, 20,* 685.

Lance, J. W., & Anthony, M. (1966). Some clinical aspects of migraine. *Arch Neurol, 15,* 356–361.

Lance, J. W., & Lambros, J. (1998). Headache associated with cardiac ischaemia. *Headache, 38,* 315–316.

Lee, A. G., Brazis, P. W., & Miller, N. R. (1996). Posterior ischemic optic neuropathy associated with migraine. *Headache, 36,* 506–509.

Lee, C. H., & Lance, J. W. (1977). Migraine stupor. *Headache, 17,* 32–38.

Leon-Sotomayor, L. A. (1974). Cardiac migraine-report of twelve cases. *Angiology, 25,* 161–171.

Levine, S. R., Joseph, R., D'Andrea, G., & Welch, K. M. A. (1987). Migraine and the lupus anticoagulant. Case reports and review of the literature. *Cephalalgia, 7,* 93–99.

Lindahl, A. J., Allder, S., & Jefferson, D. (2002). Prolonged hemiplegic migraine associated with unilateral hyperperfusion of perfusion-weighted magnetic resonance imaging. *J Neurol Neurosurg Psychiatry, 73,* 202–209.

Lipton, T. B., Lowenkopf, T., Bajwa, Z. H., Leekie, R. S., Ribeiro, S., Newman, L. C., & Greenberg, M. A. (1997). Cardiac cephalgia: A treatable form of exertional headache. *Neurology, 49,* 813–816.

Liu, G. T., Schatz, N. J., Galetta, S. L., Volpe, N. J., Skobieranda, F., & Kosmorsky, G. S. (1995). Persistent positive visual phenomena in migraine. *Neurology, 45,* 664–668.

Lundberg, P. O. (1975). Abdominal migraine-diagnosis and therapy. *Headache, 15,* 122–125.

Lykke Thomsen, L., Eriksen, M. K., Romer, S. F., Andersen, I., Ostergaard, E., Keiding, N., Olesen, J., & Russell, M. B. (2002). An epidemiological survey of hemiplegic migraine. *Cephalalgia, 22,* 361–375.

Marks, D. A., & Ehrenberg, B. L. (1993). Migraine-related seizures in adults with epilepsy, with EEG correlation. *Neurology, 43,* 2476–2483.

Mathew, N. T., Reuveni, U., & Perez, F. (1987). Transformed or evolutive migraine. *Headache, 27,* 102–106.

Matthews, W. B. (1972). Footballer's migraine. *BMJ, 3,* 326–327.

Maytal, J., Lipton, R., Young, M., & Schechter, A. (1995). International Headache Society criteria and childhood migraines. *Ann Neurol, 38,* 529–530.

McDonald, W. I., & Sanders, M. D. (1971). Migraine complicated by ischaemic papillopathy. *Lancet, ii,* 521–523.

Melo, T. P., Ferro, J. M., & Ferro, H. (1992). Transient global amnesia, a case control study. *Brain, 115,* 261–270.

Merikangas, K. R., Fenton, B. T., Cheng, S. H., Stolar, M. J., & Risch, N. (1997). Association between migraine and stroke in a large-scale epidemiological study in the United States. *Arch Neurol, 54,* 362–368.

Miller, D., Waters, D. D., Warnica, W., Szlachcic, J., Kreeft, J., & Therous, P. (1981). Is variant angina the coronary manifestation of a generalized vasospastic disorder? *N Engl J Med, 304,* 763–766.

Montagna, P., Gallassi, R., Medori, R., Govoni, E., Zeviani, M., Di Mauro, S., Lugaresi, E., & Andermann, F. (1988a). MELAS syndrome: Characteristic migrainous and epileptic features and maternal transmission. *Neurology, 38,* 751–754.

Montagna, P., Sacquegna, T., Martinelli, P., Cortelli, P., Bresolin, N., Maggio, M., Baldrati, A., Riva, R., & Lugaresi, E. (1988b). Mitochondrial abnormalities in migraine. Preliminary findings. *Headache, 28,* 477–480.

Morrison, D. P. (1990). Abnormal perceptual experiences in migraine. *Cephalalgia, 10,* 273–277.

Neligan, P., Harriman, D. G. F., & Pearce, J. (1977). Respiratory arrest in familial hemiplegic migraine: A clinical and neuropathological study. *BMJ, 2,* 732–734.

Neuhauser, H., Leopold, M., von Brevern, M., Arnold, G., & Lempert, T. (2001). The interrelations of migraine, vertigo and migrainous vertigo. *Neurology, 56,* 436–441.

Panayiotopoulos, C. P. (1980). Basilar migraine? Seizures and severe epileptic EEG abnormalities, *Neurology, 30,* 1122–1125.

Peatfield, R. C. (1991). Temporal lobe phenomena during the aura phase of migraine. *J Neurol Neurosurg Psychiatry, 54,* 371–372.

Peatfield, R. C., Gawel, M. J., & Rose, F. C. (1981). Asymmetry of the aura and pain in migraine. *J Neurol Neurosurg Psychiatry, 44,* 846–848.

Peatfield, R. C., & Rose, F. C. (1981). Migrainous visual symptoms in a woman without eyes. *Arch Neurol, 38,* 466.

Petersen, J., Scruton, D., & Downie, A. W. (1977). Basilar artery migraine with transient atrial fibrillation. *BMJ, 4,* 1125–1126.

Podoll, K., & Robinson, D. (2000). Illusory splitting as visual aura symptom in migraine. *Cephalalgia, 20,* 228–232.

Radtke, A., Lempert, T., Gresty, M. A., Brookes, G. B., Bronstein, A. M., & Neuhauser, H. (2002). Migraine and Ménière's disease. Is there a link? *Neurology, 59,* 1700–1704.

Raskin, N. H., & Schwartz, R. K. (1980). Icepick-like pain. *Neurology, 30,* 203–205.

Rothrock, J. F. (1997). Successful treatment of persistent migraine aura with divalproex sodium. *Neurology, 48,* 261–262.

Russell, G., Abu-Arafeh, I., & Symon, D. N. (2002). Abdominal migraine: Evidence for existence and treatment options. *Paediatr Drugs, 4,* 1–8.

Russell, M. B., & Olesen, J. (1996). A nosographic analysis of the migraine aura in a general population. *Brain, 119,* 355–361.

Russell, M. B., Rasmussen, B. K., Fenger, K., & Olesen, J. (1996). Migraine without aura and migraine with aura are distinct clinical entities: A study of four hundred and eighty four male and female migraineurs from the general population. *Cephalalgia, 16,* 239–245.

Sacks, O. (1992). *Migraine.* Berkeley: University of California Press.

Schraeder, P. L., & Burns, R. A. (1980). Hemiplegic migraine associated with an aseptic meningeal reaction. *Arch Neurol, 37,* 377–379.

Selby, G., & Lance, J. W. (1960). Observations on 500 cases of migraine and allied vascular headache. *J Neurol Neurosurg Psychiatry, 23,* 23–32.

Shevell, M. I. (1997). Familial acephalgic migraines. *Neurology, 48,* 776–777.

Silberstein, S. D., Niknam, R., Rozen, T. D., & Young, W. B. (2000). Cluster headache with aura. *Neurology, 54,* 201–221.

Skyhøj Olsen, T. (1990). Migraine with and without aura: the same disease due to cerebral vasospasm of different intensity. A hypothesis based on CBF studies during migraine. *Headache, 30,* 269–272.

Slater, R. (1979). Benign recurrent vertigo. *J Neurol Neurosurg Psychiatry, 42,* 363–367.

Staehelin Jensen, T., de Fine Olivarius, B., Kraft, M., & Hensen, H. J. (1981a). Familial hemiplegic migraine—A reappraisal and a long-term follow-up study. *Cephalalgia, 1,* 33–39.

Stahelin Jensen, T., Voldby, B., de Fine Olivarius, B., Tågehøj Jensen, F. (1981b). Cerebral haemodynamics in familial hemiplegic migraine. *Cephalalgia, 1,* 121–125.

Stracciari, A., & Rebucci, G. G. (1986). Transient global amnesia and migraine: Familial incidence. *J Neurol Neurosurg Psychiatry, 49,* 716–719.

Swanson, J. W., & Vick, N. A. (1978). Basilar artery migraine. Twelve patients, with an attack recorded electroencephalographically. *Neurology, 28,* 782–786.

Thomsen, L. L., Ostergaard, E., Olesen, J., & Russell, M. B. (2003). Evidence for a separate type of migraine with aura. Sporadic hemiplegic migraine. *Neurology, 60,* 595–601.

Tomsak, R. L., & Jergens, P. B. (1987). Benign recurrent transient monocular blindness: A possible variant of acephalgic migraine. *Headache, 27,* 66–69.

Troost, B. T., & Zagami, A. S. (2000). Ophthalmoplegic migraine and retinal migraine. In J. Olesen, P. Tfelt-Hensen, & K. M. Welch (Eds.), *The headaches* (pp. 513–515). Philadelphia: Lippincott, Williams and Wilkins.

Tzourio, C., Kittner, S. G., Bousser, M.-G., & Alpérovitch, A. (2000). Migraine and stroke in young women. *Cephalalgia, 20,* 190–199.

Tzourio, C., Tehindrazenarivelo, A., Iglesias, S., Alperovitch, A., Chedru, R., d'Anglejan-Chatillon, J., & Bousser, M.-G. (1995). Case-control study of migraine and risk of ischaemic stroke in young women. *BMJ, 310,* 830–833.

Velioglu, S. K., & Ozmenoglu, M. (1999). Migraine-related seizures in an epileptic population. *Cephalalgia, 19,* 797–801.

Viire, E. S., & Baloh, R. W. (1996). Migraine as a cause of sudden hearing loss. *Headache, 36,* 24–28.

Welch, K. M. A., & Levine, S. R. (1990). Migraine-related stroke in the context of the International Headache Society classification of head pain. *Arch Neurol, 47,* 458–462.

Chapter 7
Migraine: Clinical Aspects

THE EXTENT OF THE PROBLEM

Prevalence

The difficulty in defining and classifying migraine obviously extends to any survey of its prevalence, whether conducted by questionnaire or personal interview, because of the wide variation in nature, frequency, and severity of attacks. It is not uncommon to find patients who have had fewer than three migrainous attacks in their lives. The frequency of attacks may therefore range from one in a lifetime to one almost every day.

Bille (1962) studied a group of nearly 9000 Swedish children and found that the prevalence of migraine increased during childhood from 1% at 6 years of age to 5% at 11 years. Dalsgaard-Nielsen (1970) reported a higher prevalence than had Bille for each age group in Danish children, increasing from 3% at 7 years of age to 9% at 15 years of age. He found the prevalence for males remained at 11% during adult life, and prevalence for women reached 19% by 40 years of age.

A survey of almost 15,000 people conducted in 1975 by the British Migraine Trust (Green, 1977) disclosed that 10% of males and 16% of females suffered from unilateral headache with migrainous characteristics. If bilateral headaches were included, the figures rose to 20% and 26%, respectively. In a telephone interview of some 10,000 people between 12 and 29 years of age in the United States, Linet et al. (1989) found that 3% of males and 7.4% of females had suffered from a migraine headache in the month before the interview.

A national migraine study of more than 20,000 people in the United States showed that 17.6% of women and 5.7% of men experience severe migraine headaches (Stewart et al., 1992); the prevalence in lower income groups is more than 60% higher than those with an annual income of more than $30,000. This has remained constant over the past 10 years (Lipton et al., 2002).

Using the International Headache Society diagnostic criteria for migraine, Rasmussen (1995) reported that the prevalence of migraine in the Danish population was 6% for men and 15% for women. Comparable figures for France were 4% and 11.2%, respectively.

The prevalence of migraine in Japan was found to be 3.6% for men and 13.6% for women (Sakai & Igarashi, 1997). Arregui et al. (1991) assessed the prevalence of migraine in Peru, which varied from 3.6% at sea level to 12.4% in the Andes, 14,200 feet above sea level, whereas tension headache was equally common at 9.5% in both sites.

A survey of a rural community in Nigeria (Osuntokun, Bademosi, & Osuntokun, 1982) found a prevalence of 5% in males and 9% in females, increasing in females to 17% during the reproductive years of life. In Nigeria, migraine is associated with the sickle-cell trait—that is, patients with hemoglobin As (Osuntokun & Osuntokun, 1972).

A survey of citizens in the United States demonstrated striking differences in the prevalence of migraine in patients from various ethnic backgrounds. The prevalence in patients of Caucasian, African, and Asian origin was, respectively, 20.4%, 16.2%, and 9.2% for women and 8.6%, 7.2%, and 4.2% for men (Stewart, Lipton, & Liberman, 1996).

In specific groups of subjects, the prevalence is high. For example, a study of 97 narcotic addicts in a methadone treatment program found that 21% of males and 45% of females had suffered from migraine, compared with 8% and 18%, respectively, of 617 university students used as a control population (Webster et al., 1977).

Further studies are required to determine if the prevalence or severity of migraine alters when a simple village or farming existence is exchanged for life in a large city or when a subordinate job, in which the subject acts in a repetitive fashion under direction, is exchanged for one that involves frequent and difficult decision making.

Morbidity and Economic Impact

Bille (1962) found that 42% of children with migraine were subject to one or more attacks each month that were sufficiently severe to prevent the child from attending school. There was no significant difference in the hours lost from school by boys with migraine when compared with a control group, but girls with migraine lost a mean of 50 hours from school each term compared with 27 hours per term for girls who were not subject to headache.

A British Migraine Trust survey (Green, 1977) showed that patients with migraine were absent from work an average of 4 days each year because of headache. A study of 2000 patients with headache in Finland found that 13% had been absent from work in the previous year because of headache, 17% of these for more than 7 days (Nikiforow & Hokkanen, 1979). In a random sample of 514 working people in the Republic of San Marino, 255 suffered from headache, 164 reported decreased efficiency as a result, and 38 (7.4% of the population and about 15% of the group with headache) were absent from work because of headache for a total of 338 working days (Benassi et al., 1986). Of all working days lost because of illness, 8.4% were the result of headache.

Department of Social Security data from the United Kingdom for the year ending April 1989 showed 43,800 days of sickness and 276,900 days of invalid status (Blau & Drummond, 1991). The authors comment that using certified days of illness underestimates the social and economic impact of migraine, because many patients remain at work during an attack, and others, such as individuals who work in their home, would not be included. A Danish study of 119 subjects with migraine found that 43% had missed 1 to 7 days from work in the preceding year. A general practitioner had been consulted by 56% and a specialist by 16% (Rasmussen, Jensen, & Olesen, 1992). In the United States, Stewart, Lipton, and Simon (1996) examined work-related disability in 1663 patients with migraine. The average number of working days missed each year was 3.8 for men and 8.3 for women. When reduced efficiency caused by headache was considered, 51% of females and 38% of males experienced 6 or more "lost workday equivalents." Estimates of lost working days in Europe each year range from 1.8 to 7.1 days in men and from 0.9 to 10.5 days in women (Láinez, 2003).

The Migraine Disability Assessment (MIDAS) score was devised to assess the impact of migraine on the lives of sufferers. A survey of 97 patients by Stewart et al. (1999) disclosed median figures of 2 days of reduced productivity in work or school in the previous 3 months; 3 days of inability to do household tasks; 3 days of diminished efficiency in doing these tasks; and 2 days of missing family, social, or leisure activities, giving a total score of 14 compared with 4 in a control group of subjects with nonmigraine headache.

Most surveys have found that patients have difficulty in identifying their headaches as migrainous. To overcome this problem, Lipton et al. (2003) selected three of nine questions on migraine characteristics to help make the diagnosis and identify migraine. These characteristics were disability, nausea, and sensitivity to light, which discriminated migraine from other headaches with a sensitivity of 0.81 and a specificity of 0.75.

The financial impact of migraine involves the indirect costs of absence from work and reduced productivity as well as the direct costs of medical care. Láinez et al. (2003) cited the estimated annual cost to the community of disability from migraine in UK pounds from various reports (Table 7.1).

THE PATIENT WITH MIGRAINE

Sex and Age Distribution

The surveys of prevalence and morbidity show that migraine affects women more than men. In the British Migraine Trust survey of almost 15,000 people

TABLE 7.1   The cost of migraine to the community

Country	Year	Cost (million UK£)
United Kingdom	1992	950
United States	1992	4306
Spain	1996	810
Canada	1994	232
Sweden	1991	21

(Green, 1977), unilateral headaches with migrainous features were experienced by women more than men at a ratio of 3:2, and the mean age of onset was at 19 years of age. The age of migraine onset was recorded in two series, each of 500 patients attending a neurologic clinic in Sydney. Women comprised 60% of the first series (Selby & Lance, 1960) and 75% of the second (Lance & Anthony, 1966). The initial attack of migraine was experienced in the first decade of life by 25% of patients (Figure 7.1) and was uncommon after 50 years of age. It may have its onset, often unrecognized, in infancy and also in advancing years, when migrainous episodes may be confused with transient ischemic attacks (TIAs). Fisher (1980) has analyzed migraine equivalents of late onset, which may appear even in a person's 70s, and has termed them *transient migrainous accompaniments* (TMAs).

Genetic Background: The Family History

When only parents and siblings were considered, 46% of patients were found to have a family history of migraine, compared with 18% of patients with tension headache used as a control group (Lance & Anthony, 1966). If grandparents were included, 55% of patients had a positive family history (Selby & Lance, 1960). Green (1977) reported a positive family history in approximately 60% of patients with migraine and 16% of normal controls. The relative most commonly affected was the mother (53%), whereas the father was affected in 17%, a sister in 17%, and a brother in 12% of cases. Laurence (1987), in discussing the genetics of migraine, cites a risk of children developing the disorder as 70% when both parents suffer from migraine, 45% when one parent is affected, and 30%

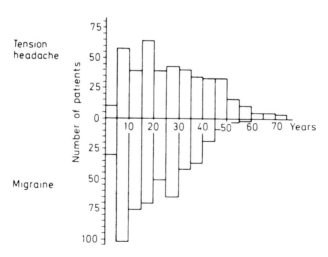

FIGURE 7.1   The age of onset of tension headache and migraine.
(From Lance, J. W., Curran, D. A., Anthony, M. (1965). Investigations into the mechanism and treatment of chronic headache. *Med J Aust, 2,* 909–914, by permission of the editor of *The Medical Journal of Australia.*)

when close relatives other than the parents have migraine. D'Amico et al. (1991) found at least one affected relative in 85% of cases and postulated a "sex-limited" transmission mode of inheritance to explain the female preponderance.

Comparisons of the prevalence of migraine in monozygotic and dizygotic twins in Australia (Merikangas, 1996) and in Sweden (Larson, Bille, & Pederson, 1995) have shown that approximately half of the susceptibility to migraine is of genetic origin and that the other half is possibly determined by environmental influences. Against the second leg of this hypothesis is the fact that twins raised separately from the age of 3 years were more similar in lifetime prevalence of migraine than twins raised together (Svennson et al., 2003).

Russell and Olesen (1995) found that the first-degree relatives of patients suffering migraine without aura (MO) had 1.9 times the risk of MO and 1.4 times the risk of migraine with aura (MA). The first-degree relatives of patients with MA had nearly four times the risk of MA but no increased risk of MO. Familial hemiplegic migraine, which is inherited as a dominant gene, is discussed further on pages 44–45 and 85–87.

"Migraine Personality"

Bille (1962) compared personality characteristics of schoolchildren who have migraine with those of their peer groups. There was no demonstrable difference in social class, intelligence, or ambition, or in such symptoms as nervous tics, nail-biting, or nocturnal enuresis. Children with migraine had a higher incidence of sleep disturbances and "night terrors," temper tantrums, recurrent abdominal pains, and motion sickness. The group with migraine performed more slowly in sensorimotor tests but with fewer errors than the control groups. The children with migraine were more fearful, tense, sensitive, and vulnerable to frustration. They were tidier and less physically enduring than their fellows without migraine. Guidetti et al. (1987) used a personality inventory to compare 40 children with migraine between 8 and 14 years of age with a control group, finding a significantly higher score for somatic concern, anxiety, and depression, but no difference in the remaining 30 scores as indices of behavior, achievement, and adjustment. Many of the traits thought characteristic of childhood migraine appear in children with other chronic pain disorders (Cunningham et al., 1987). The patient with migraine is not subject to more stress than a control group but reacts more to such stress (Henryk-Gutt & Rees, 1973).

The Minnesota Multiphasic Personality Inventory (MMPI), or variations on it, has been used repeatedly to assess patients with migraine, without evaluators being able to confirm the traditional view of the sufferer being a rigid perfectionist or indeed demonstrating any unequivocal departure from normality (Silberstein, Lipton, & Breslau, 1995).

Mental and Emotional Factors

There is a significant association among migraine, anxiety, and depression (Merikangas & Angst, 1996). Once frank psychiatric disorders have been excluded, there is still an association with neurotic traits (Breslau & Andreski, 1995). Breslau and Davis (1992) followed young adults with migraine and found they developed panic attacks 12 times as often as subjects without migraine and were four times more likely to develop major depression. The lifetime prevalence of major depression is three times higher in patients with migraine than in a control population (Breslau et al., 2000).

Academic performance from the age of 3 to 26 years was monitored in 114 patients with migraine and 109 patients with tension-type headache by Waldie et al. (2002) as part of the Dunedin Multidisciplinary Health and Development Study. Verbal ability, especially language reception, was significantly less than subjects with tension-type headache and headache-free controls. This was reflected in later examination performance. There was no correlation with time missed from school. Because the discrepancy was consistent throughout the age groups, researchers postulated that it was congenital. It is possibly relevant that people with migraine were more often ambidextrous or left-handed compared with the control group.

Migraine and Allergy

Many anecdotal reports in the past have linked migraine with allergic disorders such as asthma, hay fever, hives, and eczema. This possibility was examined prospectively in a comparative study of 500 patients with migraine and 100 patients with typical daily tension headache (Lance & Anthony, 1966). No significant difference in the family or personal history was found between the groups (Table 7.2). There is also no evidence that children with migraine are more prone to allergies than other children (Bille, 1962). Medina and Diamond (1976) were unable to demonstrate any difference in the prevalence of allergy or the plasma levels of immunoglobulin E (IgE) between groups with migraine and control groups. Merrett et al. (1983) studied the serum IgE and IgG levels in groups of patients with so-called dietary migraine, with nondietary migraine, and controls without headache but found no significant difference among the groups.

Migraine and Epilepsy

Speculation that migraine and epilepsy might share a common pathophysiology has continued for the past 100 years. Lance and Anthony (1966) undertook a prospective survey of patients referred to a headache clinic and could find no significant difference in the personal or family history of epilepsy between patients with migraine and those with tension headache (see Table 7.2). Ottman and Lipton (1996) did not find an increased risk of epilepsy in the relatives of patients with migraine, with the exception of male children of female patients, who carried a 1.8-time increased risk of epilepsy. Conversely, there was no greater risk of migraine in the relatives of epileptic patients. Because this study was carried out in adults, it does not exclude an increased risk of migraine in childhood epilepsies.

Andermann (1987), in his overview of a symposium on migraine and epilepsy, concluded that there was no genetic link between the two disorders in general but that some forms, such as benign Rolandic epilepsy; benign occipital epilepsy; and, possibly, absence attacks, were associated with a higher-than-expected prevalence of migraine. Some patients who initially

TABLE 7.2 Personal and family history of migraine, epilepsy, allergy, and vomiting attacks in migraine and tension headache in 500 patients

	Personal history			*Family history*		
	Migraine (%)	*Tension (%)*	*Significance of difference*	*Migraine (%)*	*Tension (%)*	*Significance of difference*
Migraine	100.0	0	Not applicable	46.0	18	*P < .001*
Epilepsy	1.6	2	Not significant	2.4	3	Not significant
Allergy	17.4	13	Not significant	8.2	6	Not significant
Childhood vomiting	23.2	12	*P < .02*			

have epileptic attacks only during migraine may subsequently have seizures independent of migraine. In patients with epilepsy, the characteristic postictal headache may assume migrainous characteristics.

Panayiotopoulos (1987) has suggested the term *childhood epilepsy with migrainous phenomena and occipital paroxysms* for those adolescent patients reported by him and by Campbell, Metrakos, and Andermann (1978) with migraine, seizures, and almost continuous occipital spike-wave paroxysms that were inhibited by opening the eyes and fixating on a target. The condition usually responds well to anticonvulsants, although exceptions are recorded. Panayiotopoulos (1996) has drawn attention to differences in the visual auras of migraine, which are usually linear, zigzag, arcuate, and relatively colorless, with those of occipital lobe epilepsy, which tend to be circular or of other geometric shapes and multicolored.

Benign Rolandic epilepsy is a syndrome of nocturnal epilepsy in children associated with centrotemporal spike discharges in the electroencephalogram (EEG). It was found to be associated with migraine in 21 of 30 cases reported by Bladin (1987), increasing to 24 of 30 on follow-up. The seizures responded well to anticonvulsants, but the headaches continued, even after the tendency to seizures subsided and anticonvulsants were withdrawn. Septien et al. (1991) reported that the prevalence of migraine was 63% in Rolandic epilepsy, 33% in absence epilepsy, 7% in partial epilepsy, and 9% for those whose seizures followed cranial trauma.

Features of the Migraine Attack

The varieties of migraine and the phases of migraine attacks have been considered in Chapter 6. As well as the focal neurologic symptoms and headache, which form the mainstay of migraine, the following intriguing accompaniments require explanation.

Gastrointestinal Disturbance

About 90% of patients feel nauseated with their migraine headache, and 75% vomit with some attacks. The passage of one or more loose stools at this phase of the migraine attack is noted by about 20% of patients (Lance & Anthony, 1966). These gastrointestinal symptoms are not a reaction to the pain of migraine, because they may occur with comparatively mild headaches, particularly in children, and nausea may sometimes precede headache by an hour or so. A history of migraine is common in adults as well as children with recurrent vomiting attacks (Scobie, 1983), and adults with migraine often recall periodic vomiting attacks in childhood (see Table 7.2).

The mechanism of vomiting was discussed by Baker and Bernat (1985), who reported the case of a patient presenting with nausea and projectile vomiting who was later found to have a solitary metastasis involving the lateral tegmentum of the pons. This is near the "vomiting center" in the dorsolateral reticular formation of the medulla, which receives afferents from the chemoreceptor trigger zone in the area postrema in the floor of the caudal part of the fourth ventricle as well as directly from the gastrointestinal tract. The fact that the dopamine antagonists metoclopramide, prochlorperazine, and domperidone are effective in reducing nausea and vomiting in migraine and that the intravenous infusion of the 5-HT_3 antagonist granisetron at 40 g/kg, reduced nausea more than a placebo during migraine headache (Rowat et al., 1991) implicates dopamine and 5-HT receptors, although the mechanism remains uncertain.

Migraine triggered by gastric reflux has been reported to respond to treatment of the reflux (Spierings, 2002).

Hyperacuity of the Special Senses

During migraine headache most patients are aware of an exaggeration of brightness of light (dazzle), and some feel pain on exposure to light (photophobia). Approximately 80% of patients find light unpleasant and prefer to lie down in a darkened room (Selby & Lance, 1960).

> And screened in shades from days detested glare,
> She sighs for ever on her pensive bed,
> Pain at her side, and megrim at her head.
>   (Alexander Pope, *Rape of the Lock,* Canto 4)

Moreover, about 80% of patients are subject to phonophobia. They complain that their hearing becomes more acute during migraine headache, so that the faintest sound seems louder and more disturbing (Kayan & Hood, 1984). A heightened sense of smell is also common at this time.

Drummond (1986) determined that there were two components to photophobia. The first, a general sensitivity to glare, affected both eyes and persisted to some extent between attacks in comparison with headache-free controls. The second was light-induced pain that was greater on the side of unilateral headache in 19 of 25 patients with migraine. He postulated that trigeminal and visual inputs interacted, probably in the thalamus, to produce the unilateral component, whereas the background of bilateral photophobia shared a mechanism with phonophobia and osmophobia.

Kayan and Hood (1984) suggested that a transient disturbance of cochlear function during migraine could cause phonophobia by loudness recruitment, a phenomenon common in Ménière's disease. In this condition, auditory acuity is diminished at low noise levels but improves as sound intensity increases, whereas in migraine the slightest sound appears louder than normal as one aspect of a general hyperacuity of the special senses. Auditory and visual discomfort thresholds fall substantially during attacks of migraine, suggesting a disturbance of central sensory processing mechanisms (Woodhouse & Drummond, 1993). People with migraine complained of after-images following funduscopy almost three times as often as other patients attending a neurologic clinic (de Silva, 2001). These symptoms are all consistent with a diminished gate control of afferent impulses in migraine.

Sensitivity to light has been reported as a symptom developing 3 months after infarction in the territory of one posterior cerebral artery, causing thalamic damage (Cummings & Gittinger, 1981), and the authors quote older reports in the literature that thalamic lesions cause not only hyperpathia to common sensation but also dislike of light, noise, smells, and tastes.

Hyperesthesia and Hyperalgesia

Hyperesthesia of the face and scalp may have a mechanism akin to the increased acuity of the special senses just mentioned. Tenderness of the scalp is noticed by about two thirds of patients, who may find it uncomfortable to lie on the affected side or to comb their hair (Selby & Lance, 1960). Mathew, Kailasam, and Meadors (2003) inquired about scalp symptoms in 295 patients with migraine. The scalp became sensitive to touch (allodynia) in 61 and was sore and tender in 52. Allodynia was also detected in the upper limbs in 72 patients.

Bakal and Kaganov (1977) found increased activity on electromyography (EMG) in the frontal and neck muscles of patients with migraine, during and between headaches, compared with patients who have tension headache and normal controls. During migraine headache, muscles in the areas afflicted by pain become tender to palpation (Tfelt-Hansen, Lous, & Olesen, 1981), and headache is relieved by injection of the tender areas. It remains uncertain whether hyperalgesia is the result of referred pain with reflex muscle contraction or whether muscles are a primary source of headache.

Autonomic Disturbance

Gotoh et al. (1984) investigated autonomic function in 21 patients with tension headache (10 with aura, 11 without) between headaches and compared their responses with 30 age-matched controls. Blood pressure changes with the Valsalva maneuver were diminished, postural hypotension was present, and the pupils dilated excessively after dilute (1.25%) adrenaline eye drops, more so on the habitual headache side. In accord with these indications of sympathetic hypofunction, the plasma level of noradrenaline was lower than controls and failed to rise 30 minutes after head-up tilting, unlike the normal subjects.

Fanciullacci (1979) showed that the pupils of patients with migraine dilated poorly in response to fenfluramine (which releases noradrenaline from nerve terminals), constricted more than controls after the application of guanethidine (which depletes axonal transmitter stores), and dilated excessively in response to a dilute phenylephrine (1%) eye drop. These tests indicate reduced stores of noradrenaline with receptor supersensitivity. Drummond (1987) found that the mean pupil diameter in patients with migraine was smaller during headache than that of normal controls and was significantly smaller on the affected side in patients with unilateral headache. Pupillary asymmetry was greater in darkness than in light, suggesting an acquired sympathetic deficit, similar but milder than that frequently observed in cluster headache and attributed originally by Kunkle and Anderson (1961) to involvement of the sympathetic plexus in the wall of the internal carotid artery. Autonomic disturbances have been reviewed by Schoenen and Thomsen (2000).

Because of the tendency to postural hypotension, faintness or fainting is not uncommon in migraine. In the series by Selby and Lance (1960), some 10% of patients had fainted on at least one occasion during the headache. Beware of interpreting the nonspecific symptom of "dizziness" as "faintness," because anxiety overbreathing is common during migraine headache (Blau & Dexter, 1980) and may cause lightheadedness and bilateral paraesthesias, which may incorrectly be thought to be part of the aura. Anxiety symptoms and the control of hyperventilation are discussed in Appendix A. Some patients feel cold during headache, although others sweat excessively and body temperature may increase (Sacks, 1992). Sometimes areas in the mouth or scalp may swell, resembling large hives.

Sodium and Fluid Retention

Increase in weight, with or without signs of generalized edema, is noted by about half of patients with migraine before the migraine attack. Oliguria is common before the attack, and roughly 30% of patients notice polyuria as the headache subsides. The blood sodium level has been shown to increase before and during headache, whereas serum protein concentration falls (Campbell, Hay, & Tonks, 1951). The urinary output of sodium between attacks after being given a water load of 1000 to 1500 mL is almost double in subjects with migraine compared with that of controls. There is therefore evidence that sodium and fluid retention is associated with migraine, but it is unlikely to be a cause of migraine, because the administration of diuretics, which minimizes weight fluctuations, does not prevent the regular recurrence of migraine headache. Stanford and Greene (1970) suggested that aldosterone may be responsible for the sodium and fluid retention in patients with migraine and reported the cure of premenstrual migraine by the surgical treatment of Conn's syndrome.

Precipitating Factors

Migraine headache often recurs regularly or in cycles without any obvious precipitating factors. It is probable that some internal mechanism or "biological clock" determines the pattern of the disorder in such patients.

Friedman (1970) told of one of his patients who "has an occupation that takes him through the world from the Himalayas in Tibet to Somaliland, indeed from the highest altitudes to the lowest, from the wettest to the driest—experiencing climatic, food and culture changes. But his migraine remains, for he carries his personal environment with him."

As well as the pattern of recurrence, the time of onset may depend on an internal clock or circadian rhythm, for example, those patients who are awakened from sleep by headache.

On occasions, excessive input to the nervous system may induce migraine symptoms with such rapidity that it is difficult to imagine any other than a neural mechanism being responsible. Perhaps a sudden jar to the head may also evoke a neural discharge or may initiate changes directly in the cerebral cortex ("spreading depression of Leão") or in cranial blood vessels by a vibratory stimulus to their walls, as in "footballer's migraine" (see later). The mechanism by which emotional disturbance or relaxation after a hard week's work induces migraine presumably involves both neural and humoral mechanisms, although the precise sequence of events remains obscure. Carefully listing trigger factors while taking the history is an important step in treatment, because avoiding them may lessen the frequency and severity of migraine headache.

Stress and Relaxation After Stress

A stressful event is probably the most commonly recognized precipitant of migraine (Henryk-Gutt & Rees, 1973), and the frequency of headache usually increases if the patient is worried by some protracted problem, such as an impending divorce or financial difficulties. The record diaries of 33 patients studied by Levor et al. (1986) showed a significant increase in stressful events and a decline in physical activity for the 4 days leading up to and including each headache day. At times of real emergency, when patients have to summon up all their internal resources, they usually remain free of headache, which tends to occur as soon as the crisis is resolved. The same principle underlies "weekend headache." Patients remain free while under the sustained stress of a working week but suffer from headache at the moment of "let-down" or relaxation. On some occasions, an emotional shock may be followed by the symptoms of classical migraine within seconds or minutes.

Sleep

Certain primary headache disorders such as migraine and cluster headache tend to develop during sleep, and hypnic headache occurs only during sleep. Remarkably sleep is recognized as being helpful in terminating migraine headache. Deprivation of sleep can cause headaches, whereas "sleeping in" in the morning can often trigger migraine headache. To avoid one cause of "weekend migraine," susceptible patients should make sure that they wake up and get out of bed at their regular weekday time.

Dodick, Eross, and Parish (2003) have summarized present knowledge of the physiology of sleep and its relationship to headache. Normal adult sleep consists of cycles, each lasting about 90 minutes, containing brief periods of rapid eye movement (REM) sleep during which migraine, cluster, and hypnic headache usually begin. Sleep walking is more common in migraine than control subjects, affecting 30% to 55% of patients in different reports, compared with 5% to 16% in control groups. Night terrors are also said to be common in migraine.

Trauma

A sudden jar or blow to the head may induce symptoms of migraine with aura, particularly in children. Matthews (1972) reported that soccer players who "head" the ball may experience blurring of vision within minutes, followed by headache ("footballer's migraine"). Other types of football are not exempt. Bennett et al. (1980) described three members of an American university football team who had each experienced a number of episodes of scintillating scotomas, paraesthesias, and amnesia, not always followed by headache, after a comparatively minor blow to the head. We have had as patients boys whose loss of vision after hitting their heads when tackled in rugby football gave rise to concern about serious cerebral damage but was caused by a migrainous aura. If the pupillary reaction to light is retained under these circumstances, it points to cortical blindness induced by an acute post-traumatic spreading cortical depression. Children often develop similar migrainous symptoms after bumping their head while playing, falling off a chair, or undergoing similar accidents (Haas, Pineda, & Lourie, 1975). The child may develop complete cortical blindness for 30 minutes or so, which is very worrying for one not familiar with the syndrome, and may lead to fears of serious intracranial damage.

Migraine may also be brought on by painful compression of the head, for example, by wearing tight goggles during swimming training (Pestronk & Pestronk, 1983).

Afferent Stimulation

Glare, flickering light, noise, and smells are common triggers. Marcus and Soso (1989) found that 82% of patients with migraine experienced visual discomfort while looking at a black-and-white striped pattern, compared with only 6.2% of subjects who do not have migraine. The latent period between exposure to an afferent stimulus and the development of migraine is so brief at times that it suggests a central reflex response. Psychophysical tests such as the reaction of patients with migraine to visual stimuli indicate hypersensitivity of the visual cortex (Chronicle & Mulleners, 1996). Moreover, the nature of the induced aura may resemble the precipitating stimulus. Lord (1982) cites from his personal experiences auras of central visual disturbance after exposure to a flash bulb, of visual disorientation after driving on a winding road, and of paraesthesias in one arm after using that arm vigorously to sandpaper an object. Excessive afferent stimulation may thus cause cortical depression spreading from the area of cortex subject to overload.

Food and Eating Habits

Missing a meal often induces a migraine attack, possibly as the result of hypoglycemia. About 25% of patients consider that their attacks are provoked by eating certain foods, particularly fatty foods, chocolate, and oranges (Selby & Lance, 1960). There is some doubt whether this is a delayed hypersensitivity reaction to the chemical content of these foods, or whether it depends on a conditioned reflex. Wolff (1963) quotes experiments in which incriminated foods were ingested by patients without their knowledge and without a headache ensuing.

There is contentious literature on tyramine-containing foods, described in the fourth edition of this book. It can be summarized by stating that there is no firm evidence that tyramine or abnormalities of its metabolism play any part in the genesis of migraine. Similarly, there have been contradictory reports on whether chocolate is a precipitating factor. Gibb et al. (1991) tested 20 patients who considered that their attacks followed the consumption of chocolate, by administering a 40-g chocolate bar or a placebo bar, the flavor of each being disguised by carob, in double-blind fashion. Five of the twelve patients given chocolate and none of the eight given placebo developed a migraine headache within 24 hours.

A similar trial involved patients susceptible to headache after drinking red wine being given chilled red wine or vodka, the color being concealed by a brown glass bottle from which the participants drank with a straw. A typical migraine attack developed in 9 of 11 of the red wine drinkers but in none of the 8 who drank vodka (Littlewood et al., 1988).

Whether certain foodstuffs can precipitate migraine remains controversial, because the results of elimination diets have been reported as positive (Monro et al., 1980) and negative (Medina & Diamond, 1978). In our own trial (McQueen et al., 1989) of 95 patients with migraine suffering 4 to 12 headaches each month, 36 dropped out during the first 6 weeks. The elimination diet was followed for 4 to 6 weeks by 59 patients, of whom 22 did not improve and 37 became free of headache for at least 2 weeks. Of the latter group, only 19 completed the challenge phase and were given an appropriate diet for 1 month and an inappropriate diet for 1 month in random fashion, separated by a washout period. On the appropriate diet, nine patients improved, nine were unchanged, and four were worse when compared with their period on the inappropriate diet. We may conclude that the dietary management of migraine is of little if any value, at least in adults, but it is obviously prudent for patients to avoid any food that they are convinced provokes an attack.

Vasodilators

Vasodilator agents such as alcohol, nitroglycerin (which releases nitric oxide), histamine, and prostaglandin E_1 may precipitate migraine. Applying nitroglycerin ointment to the temple of patients with migraine who usually experienced pain in that site induced headache within 30 minutes in 7 of 10 patients, whereas application of the ointment to another bodily site caused only a delayed headache, after approximately 7 hours, in 3 of 10 patients (Bonuso et al., 1989).

This was a difficult study in terms of blinding. Exposure to excessive heat or strenuous exercise sometimes triggers migraine, presumably from dilation of cerebral and extracranial vessels.

Changes in Barometric Pressure and Weather Conditions

Normal subjects have developed migrainous phenomena for the first time when subjected to rapid changes in barometric pressure in compression or decompression chambers. Appenzeller, Feldman, and Friedman (1979) considered the precipitation of migraine by flying at high altitudes and the significance of a history of migraine in air crew members.

Many patients attribute migraine attacks to changes in the weather, particularly an approaching thunderstorm. Cull (1981) correlated the incidence of migraine with changes in barometric pressure on the day of headache and for the preceding 48 hours. Curiously, the mean barometric pressure was significantly higher on migraine days than on headache-free days. A fall in barometric pressure over a 24-hour period was not associated with an increased incidence of migraine the following day, but a rise in pressure of more than 15 mbar correlated with a reduced attack rate the next day. Cull concluded that the minor changes in attack rate may be explained more easily by indirect factors, such as the lack of glare on cool, cloudy days, than by any direct effect of barometric pressure.

Sulman et al. (1970) pointed out that hot, dry winds "of ill repute" are notorious for causing irritability and headache. They include the Shirav of Israel, the Santa Ana of southern California, Arizona desert winds, the Argentine Zonda, the sirocco of the Mediterranean, the Maltese xlokk, the chamsin of Arab countries, the foehn of Switzerland, and the North Winds of Melbourne. These researchers attributed the symptoms of nervous tension and headache to the increased ionization of the air that precedes the arrival of the hot, dry wind, and correlated this with excessive urinary excretion of serotonin. Winds need not be "of ill repute" to cause headaches. The chinook is welcome in the Canadian province of Alberta, because it brings warmer weather in the cold winter. Nevertheless, there is an increased susceptibility to migraine headache, particularly when the velocity exceeds 38 km per hour (Cooke, Rose, & Becker, 2000).

Hormonal Changes

Johannis van der Linden in *De Hemicrania Menstrua* (1660) described a unilateral headache accompanied by nausea and vomiting that the Marchioness of Brandenburg suffered each month "during the menstrual flux."

The periodicity of migraine is related to the menstrual cycle in about 60% of women patients, the headaches appearing or becoming more severe just before menses. Migraine is relieved by pregnancy in about 60% of women, but this does not depend on a previous association with menstruation, although there is a positive correlation. Of women whose migraine was linked with menses, 64% lost their headache during pregnancy, compared with 48% of those in whom this relationship was absent (Lance & Anthony, 1966). There is no link between relief during pregnancy and the sex of the fetus. Some women may experience migraine for the first time during pregnancy, but the migraine may cease to be a problem after the child is born (Chancellor, Wroe, & Cull, 1990).

Clustering of migraine headaches around the menstrual period (−2 to +3 days of the cycle) was reported by 21% of women subject to migraine without aura and by only 4% of those with aura (Mattson, 2003). Improvement after menopause was not significant.

Somerville (1972b) surveyed 200 women attending an antenatal clinic during the last 4 weeks of pregnancy. He found that 31 patients had been subject to migraine headache in the 12 months before becoming pregnant, giving a prevalence of 15% of women in the reproductive years. Of the 31 patients, 24 improved during pregnancy, 7 becoming completely free of headache. Only 7 patients had developed migraine for the first time in the current pregnancy, mostly in the first trimester. Somerville found no significant difference in the plasma progesterone of those women whose migraine had improved (98.4 ng/mL), those women whose migraine continued during pregnancy (101.2 ng/mL), and the control patients without migraine (119.4 ng/mL).

Somerville (1971, 1972a) clarified the relationship of migraine to the hormonal changes of the menstrual cycle. Normal women and women with migraine had a similar fluctuation of hormone levels. Plasma estradiol rose to an early preovulatory peak, followed by a rapid fall, then a secondary rise during the luteal phase with a final fall before menstruation. Plasma progesterone remained low during menstruation and the follicular phase, then increased at or just after midcycle to a plateau during the luteal phase, before declining premenstrually. No significant differences appeared between the peak progesterone concentrations in women with and without migraine.

Premenstrual migraine occurred regularly during or after the time at which plasma estradiol and progesterone fell to their lowest levels. To determine which of these hormones was more influential in triggering migraine headache, Somerville treated six women with progesterone and six women with estradiol in the premenstrual phase while measuring their hormone levels daily. He found that administering progesterone to maintain artificially high blood levels postponed uterine bleeding, but that the migraine attack occurred in five out of the six women at the expected time in the cycle. However, injecting estradiol did not postpone menstruation but delayed the onset of migraine headache in all patients by 3 to 9 days (Figure 7.2). Migraine began after the estradiol level fell below 20 ng/100 mL and could not be postponed further if another injection of estradiol was given at this time. Two other women had consistently low levels of progesterone, indicating the absence of ovulation. One developed migraine 10 days after an injection of estradiol, followed on the 11th day by estrogen-withdrawal bleeding. The second patient, who was menopausal, suffered a typical episode of migraine as the estrogen level fell 9 days after injection, without any withdrawal bleeding.

Therefore the withdrawal of estrogen, rather than progesterone, apparently sets in motion a series of changes that culminate in the onset of migraine. This could account for the midcycle headache that afflicts some women in addition to their menstrual migraine. There is probably some intermediary between estrogen withdrawal and the sequelae of menstruation and migraine. The prostaglandins are possible contenders because of their actions on the uterus and the known effect of PGE_1 in precipitating migraine when infused into normal subjects (Carlson,

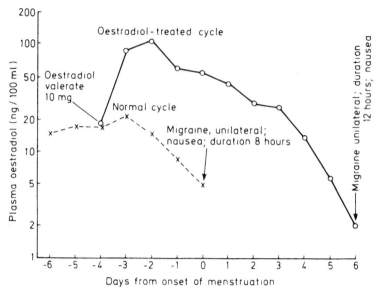

FIGURE 7.2   Estrogen-treated cycle *(continuous line)* and normal cycle *(dashed line)* in the same patient. The onset of migraine is postponed until the estrogen level falls. (From Somerville, 1972a, by permission of the editor of *Neurology*.)

Ekelund, & Oro, 1968). Alternatively, the hypothalamopituitary axis may be responsible for hormonal changes and migraine occurring together.

The use of oral contraceptive tablets containing a high dose of estrogen commonly exacerbates migraine. Pills containing 30 μg or less of ethinylestradiol reduced headache incidence to 5% or less by the sixth cycle (Massiou & MacGregor, 2000).

Radiotherapy

Migraine-like headaches with prominent aura symptoms have been reported in children after cranial irradiation and chemotherapy (Parker, Vezina, & Stacy Nicholson, 1994). We have had an adult patient who developed similar features years after cranial radiotherapy.

Possible Viral Infection and HaNDL Syndrome

The finding of lymphocytic pleocytosis in the cerebrospinal fluid (CSF) of patients suffering from severe migraine-like headache has been well documented (Gomez-Aranda et al., 1997), posing the question of whether the headache is "pseudomigraine" as a symptom of infection or whether the migrainous process can induce CSF changes resembling that of a viral meningoencephalitis.

The association of headache, neurologic deficit, and CSF lymphocytosis (HaNDL) is now recognized as a distinct benign headache syndrome. Toth

(2002) reported eight patients with HaNDL, only two of whom had suffered from migraine. The average number of episodes was 3.7, with an average duration of 17 days. Most patients had a hemiparesis or sensory deficit accompanying their headache. Half developed a homonymous hemianopia, and one had cortical blindness. Three patients had symptoms suggesting a viral infection 3 to 7 days before the headache started. CSF opening pressure, protein content, and white cell count (mainly lymphocytes) were elevated, with a normal glucose level. Some CSF abnormalities remained even after a follow-up of 56 to 196 days. No patient had a persisting neurologic deficit.

Fumal et al. (2003) carried out neurophysiologic studies in a patient with HaNDL to determine whether the findings resembled those of patients with migraine. The potentiation of pattern-reversal evoked potentials reverted to habituation after transcranial magnetic stimulation, and increased "jitter" was demonstrated in single-fiber EMG, both abnormalities previously demonstrated in migraine. This supports the concept of HaNDL being a variant of migraine with aura, possibly precipitated by infection.

Associated Diseases

1. Ménière's Disease

Radtke et al. (2002) found the lifetime prevalence of migraine in patients with Ménière's disease to be higher (56%) than in orthopedic control subjects (25%). Of 78 patients, 28% had experienced migrainous headache, and 52% photophobia with their attacks of vertigo. Scintillating scotomas or spreading sensory symptoms had been experienced by 10%.

Recurrent vertigo without acoustic symptoms as a migraine equivalent is described in Chapter 6, pages 47–48.

2. Multiple Sclerosis

Watkins and Espir (1969) found that 27% of 100 patients with multiple sclerosis (MS) suffered from migraine compared with a control group matched for age and sex. Rolak (1985) confirmed that headache was more common in patients with MS than in controls but could find no correlation with signs and symptoms of MS.

Acute demyelination of the pons can give rise to a unilateral headache associated with brainstem and cerebellar symptoms (Nager, Lanska, & Daroff, 1989). MS may present with a severe headache (Galer et al., 1990), probably caused by a plaque of demyelination in the region of the periaqueductal gray matter, as illustrated in the report by Haas, Kent, and Friedman (1993).

3. Behçet's Disease

Behçet's disease is a multisystem vasculitis characterized by recurrent oral and genital ulcerations with uveitis.

Migraine without aura was significantly more frequent in 27 patients with Behçet's disease (44%) compared with controls (11%) even when there was no neurologic involvement (Monastero et al., 2003).

4. Celiac Disease

Subclinical celiac disease has been associated with neuropathy, cerebellar ataxia, and other neurologic disorders. Gabrielli et al. (2003) screened 90 patients with migraine by estimating antiendomysium and transglutaminase antibodies, specific tests for celiac disease, and found them positive in four patients in whom the diagnosis was confirmed by endoscopy. All four improved on a gluten-free diet, and one was free of headache for the 6 months of the trial.

Brain magnetic resonance imaging (MRI) in patients with gluten sensitivity shows areas of high signal in the white matter that may become confluent (Hadjivassiliou et al., 2001) and that resemble the changes of CADASIL.

5. Strokelike Syndromes

MELAS, a syndrome of mitochondrial myopathy, encephalopathy, lactic acidosis, and strokelike episodes, is a disorder that is inherited through the mother (see Chapter 6, page 50). It starts in childhood, and focal neurologic deficits later accompany migraine-like headache. Imaging demonstrates multiple areas of infarction progressing to generalized atrophy. Muscle biopsy shows ragged red fibers and abnormal mitochondria (Koo et al., 1993).

An antiphospholipid syndrome (Hughes's syndrome) consists of transient ischemic attacks, strokes, and headaches including migraine with episodes resembling those of MS. It has been reported to respond to anticoagulation with warfarin (Hughes, 2003). The evidence for other links between migraine and antiphospholipid antibodies is weak. Intiso et al. (2002) looked for anticardiolipin antibodies in 70 patients with migraine, 40 with aura, and found that serum levels were not increased. Published studies have not demonstrated any comorbidity with systemic lupus erythematosus.

6. Prolapsed Mitral Valve and Patent Foramen Ovale

Pfaffenrath et al. (1991) could not support the proposed association of migraine with prolapsed mitral valve.

Patent foramen ovale (PFO) is quite common, being present in about 20% of normal subjects. Anzola et al. (1999) found the prevalence of PFO to be 48% (54/113) in patients who had migraine with aura and 23% in 53 patients without aura. They postulate that the increased risk of stroke in patients with migraine with aura might be explained by an increased proneness to paradoxical cerebral embolism. Reduction or abolition of migrainous auras after closure of right to left shunts, atrial septal defect or PFO, has been reported (Wilmshurst et al., 2000). There are no population-based data for this assertion and no controlled studies at the moment.

7. Angiomas

ARTERIOVENOUS MALFORMATIONS.   The relationship between AVMs and migraine is controversial. Monteiro et al. (1993) reviewed medical records to check the prevalence of headaches in 51 patients with intracranial arteriovenous malformations (AVMs), finding that 47% had migrainous headaches and that the site of the AVM strongly correlated with side of the headache. The authors considered that a prospective study was required to determine whether there was a pathophysiologic relationship between these entities.

STURGE-WEBER SYNDROME. Klapper (1994) found a prevalence of migraine of 31% in patients younger than the age of 10 years in a sample of 71 patients with Sturge-Weber syndrome, compared with the usual figure of 5% for this age group. Overall, migraine prevalence was 28% for males and females.

8. Raynaud's Phenomenon

O'Keeffe, Tsapatsaris, and Beetham (1993) found that 24 of 41 hospital employees with Raynaud's phenomenon were also subject to migraine, compared with only 10 of 41 of a control group. Nevertheless, Corbin and Martin (1985) showed the response of the digital arteries to cold to be normal.

9. Other Precipitating or Aggravating Conditions

Migraine may be aggravated by hypertension, aldosteronism (Stanford & Greene, 1970), and hyperthyroidism (Thomas et al., 1996). It has been reported as a symptom of hyper-pre-beta-lipoproteinemia, possibly because of changes in plasma viscosity or red cell aggregation, and it disappears with restoration of serum lipids to normal (Leviton & Camenga, 1969). Migraine has been recorded during episodes of thrombocytopenia (Damasio & Beck, 1978), and instances are reported of migraine with aura being precipitated or aggravated by dissection or obstruction of cerebral arteries (Welch & Levine, 1990). Migraine is the most common form of headache in patients with pituitary tumors with 76% of 84 patients presenting with typical headaches (Levy et al., 2003).

Physical Examination

No physical signs of migraine are detectable between attacks apart from subtle signs of cerebellar impairment detected by special techniques (Sandor et al., 2001). Hearing a bruit over the skull or orbits may give rise to concern and warrant carotid angiography to exclude the presence of an intracranial angioma or vascular tumor. In one series of 500 patients, 10 had an audible cranial bruit (Selby & Lance, 1960). Two were children younger than 10 years, in whom skull bruits are usually not of any significance. In four adult patients the bruit was heard over both eyes, and in four it was unilateral. Carotid angiograms in three of the latter were completely normal.

In the just-mentioned series, a blood pressure of more than 150 mm Hg systolic and 100 mm Hg diastolic was found in 13% of patients. Hypertension is significantly more common in patients older than 50 years of age with migraine than in the general population (see Chapter 15).

While a migraine headache is in progress, excessive pulsation of temporal arteries may be noted, and veins are often prominent on the forehead and temple (see Figure 7.3). The face and scalp are commonly pale and sweaty in severe attacks. The patient may be mentally confused, stuporous, or even briefly lose consciousness. Speech may be slurred (dysarthria), or the person may be unable

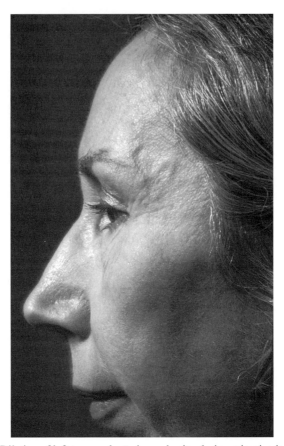

FIGURE 7.3   Dilation of left temporal arteries and veins during migraine headache.

to choose the correct word or phrase (dysphasia). A transient Horner's syndrome or dilated pupil may occur on the side of the headache and, very rarely, paresis of extraocular muscles (ophthalmoplegic migraine). Weakness of upper motor-neuron type may be observed (hemiparetic migraine) or, uncommonly, dystonic postures or involuntary movements.

Differential Diagnosis and Investigation

Because the differential diagnosis of migraine includes almost every cause of intermittent focal neurologic symptoms and every cause of recurrent headache, the list of conditions to consider could be extensive. In practice, the recurrent pattern of migraine is so characteristic that it is rarely necessary to undertake any investigations. The first attack of migraine with aura in the absence of a family history can be worrying and, if there is any doubt about the diagnosis, the appropriate tests can be carried out as outlined in Chapter 19.

Episodes of cerebral embolism, as in subacute bacterial endocarditis, can sometimes mimic migraine. The focal neurologic symptoms of migraine with aura may also suggest a viral meningoencephalitis at times, particularly if the episode is accompanied by a fever. Lumbar puncture may indeed disclose a mononuclear pleocytosis in the CSF at the height of such a migraine attack (see earlier discussion of HaNDL). We must stress that there is no indication for lumbar puncture in typical uncomplicated migraine.

Electroencephalography

The EEG is not usually helpful in diagnosing or managing migraine. Many reports of uncontrolled observations in the past have suggested that EEG abnormalities may be more common in patients with migraine. Focal slow-wave changes have been described in patients with severe and prolonged attacks, in hemiplegic migraine for example, but Lauritzen, Trojaborg, and Olesen (1981) could find no abnormality in a study of 21 patients during migraine attacks with or without aura, including 3 patients examined while they were experiencing photopsia. Bille (1962) did not find any significant difference between the EEGs of children with migraine and those of a control group. Certain patients with Basilar-type migraine, discussed earlier in this chapter, have EEG abnormalities, including some with an almost continuous pattern of occipital spike-wave discharges (Camfield, Metrakos, & Andermann, 1978; Panayiotopoulos, 1980). There is a tendency toward synchronization of the rhythms in the visual cortex of patients with migraine, and EEG abnormalities may appear in association with severe neurologic symptoms in migraine; a minority of patients do show epileptiform abnormalities, although their relationship to migraine is uncertain. There does not appear to be any basis for the concept of "dysrhythmic migraine" (Winter, 1987).

Cortical Evoked Potentials and Habituation

Visual evoked potentials (VEPs) are attenuated during a migraine attack when it is accompanied by visual symptoms. Between attacks, the positive wave, which appears at a latency of about 100 ms (P100), is not delayed with flash stimulation, but the trough between P100 and the ensuing negative wave (N120) is enhanced in subjects with migraine compared with a control group (Connolly, Gawel, & Clifford Rose, 1982). The increase in amplitude of this primary response in the visual cortex to an afferent volley, and its failure to habituate with repeated stimulation (Schoenen & Thomsen, 2000), could underlie the sensitivity of the patient with migraine to glare and flickering light.

A similar failure to habituate of brainstem auditory evoked potentials (BAEPs) and the contingent negative variation (CNV) supports the concept of defective modulatory mechanisms in migraine (Siniatchkin et al., 2003). The CNV is a potential recorded from the cortex when a subject is alerted to perform a movement.

Blink reflexes elicited by a concentric electrode designed to stimulate cutaneous pain fibers selectively ("nociceptive" blink reflexes) demonstrate enhancement and lack of habituation between migraine attacks, supporting the concept of abnormal trigeminal processing of pain (Katsarava et al., 2003).

These observations are helpful in understanding the mechanism of migraine but are not useful as clinical tools.

Brain Imaging and Cerebral Angiography

Computed tomography (CT) scanning has demonstrated cerebral edema, cortical infarction, and areas of cortical atrophy in patients with migraine (Hungerford, du Boulay, & Zilkha, 1976; Mathew et al., 1977; Dorfman, Marshall, & Enzmann, 1979). MRI showed punctate white matter abnormalities in 7 of 17 patients suffering from migraine, and in 4 of 7 patients with associated neurologic deficits a cerebral or cerebellar infarct was demonstrated (Soges et al., 1988). Ziegler et al. (1991) compared the MRI scans of 18 patients subject to migraine with aura and those of 15 headache-free controls. A cortical infarction was noted in one patient with migraine, but small white-matter lesions were found in two controls as well as in three of the patients. However, Igarashi et al. (1991) found a significant difference between 91 subjects with migraine and 98 controls. Small white-matter lesions were found in 30% of patients younger than 40 years of age, compared with 11% of age-matched controls, and the prevalence of abnormalities over the whole age range was 40%. Lesions were no more frequent in patients with than without aura, and their cause remains to be determined. A recent population-based study confirmed an excess of lesions on MRI in patients with migraine with aura (Kruit et al., 2004) emphasizing the need to understand their nature.

Cerebral angiography is indicated only if there is some doubt about the diagnosis, and aneurysm or other vascular abnormalities must be excluded. There has always been some reluctance to perform angiography in patients with migraine, but Shuaib and Hachinski (1988) found that focal cerebral events followed the procedure in only 2.6% of patients with migraine compared with 2.8% in a prospective study of 1002 patients undergoing angiography for different reasons. MR angiography, a noninvasive alternative, is often sufficient.

Electromyography

Single-fiber EMG shows a variable latency of response to nerve stimulation ("jitter") and impulse blocking in patients subject to migraine with aura (Ambrosini et al., 2001). The authors postulate an underlying calcium channelopathy.

NATURAL HISTORY AND PROGNOSIS

The prognosis of migraine may be deduced from the little we know about its natural history. A child with migraine has a 60% chance of remission in adolescence. Of the patients who remit, one third start to have attacks again, so 60% of affected children are still subject to migraine at 30 years of age (Bille, 1981). Migraine seems to run a more benign course in boys, because at 30 years of age 52% of males and only 30% of females were free of migraine. Between 37 and 43 years of age, 53% still suffered from migraine (Bille, 1989). One third of the original cohort of 73 patients had suffered from migraine ever since childhood. In half the cases, the adult attacks were less severe and less frequent than in childhood. The latest follow-up at 40 years disclosed that more than 50% of patients were still subject to migraine in the age group 47 to 53 years (Bille, 1997). A study of adolescents over a 10-year period up to a mean age of 22 years found that about 40% had remitted (Monastero, 2003). Of patients with migraine in adult life, 70% lose their headaches or improve over a period of 14 years, although 50% may still be liable to occasional attacks at 65 years of age (Whitty & Hockaday, 1968).

References

Ambrosini, A., Maertens de Noordhout, A., & Schoenen, J. (2001). Neuromuscular transmission in migraine. *Neurology, 56,* 1038–1043.

Andermann, F. (1987). Migraine and epilepsy: An overview. In F. Andermann & E. Lugaresi (Eds.), *Migraine and epilepsy* (pp. 405–422). Boston: Butterworths.

Anzola, G. P., Magoni, M., Guindani, M., Rozzini, L., & Dalla Volta, G. (1999). Potential source of cerebral embolism in migraine with aura. *Neurology, 52,* 1622–1625.

Appenzeller, O., Feldman, R. G., & Friedman, A. P. (1979). Neurological and neurosurgical conditions associated with aviation safety. Migraine, headache and related conditions. *Arch Neurol, 36,* 784–805.

Arregui, A., Cabrera, J., LeonVelarde, F., Parades, S., Viscarra, D., & Arbaiza, D. (1991). High prevalence of migraine in a high altitude population. *Neurology, 41,* 1668–1670.

Bakal, D. A., & Kaganov, I. A. (1977). Muscle contraction and migraine headache: Psychophysiologic comparison. *Headache, 17,* 208–215.

Baker, C. H. B., & Bernat, J. L. (1985). The neuroanatomy of vomiting in man: Association of projectile vomiting with a solitary metastasis in the lateral tegmentum of the pons and the middle cerebellar peduncle. *J Neurol Neurosurg Psychiatry, 48,* 1165–1168.

Benassi, G., D'Alessandro, R., Lenzi, P. L., Manzaroli, D., Baldrati, A., & Lugaresi. E. (1986). The economic burden of headache: An epidemiological study in the Republic of San Marino. *Headache, 26,* 457–459.

Bennett, D. R., Fuenning, S. I., Sullivan, G., & Weber, J. (1980). Migraine precipitated by head trauma in athletes. *Am J Sports Med, 8,* 202–205.

Bille, B. (1962). Migraine in schoolchildren. *Acta Paediat Stockh, 51*(Suppl. 136), 1–151.

Bille, B. (1981). Migraine in childhood and its prognosis. *Cephalalgia, 1,* 71–75.

Bille, B. (1989). Migraine in childhood: A 30-year follow-up. In G. Lanzi, V. Balottin, & A. Cernibori (Eds.), *Headache in children and adolescents* (pp. 19–26). Amsterdam: Elsevier.

Bille, B. (1997). A 40-year follow-up of school children with migraine. *Cephalalgia, 17,* 488–491.

Bladin, P. F. (1987). The association of benign Rolandic epilepsy with migraine. In F. Andermann & E. Lugaresi (Eds.), *Migraine and epilepsy* (pp. 145–152). Boston: Butterworths.

Blau, J. N., & Dexter, S. L. (1980). Hyperventilation during migraine attacks. *BMJ, 280,* 1254.

Blau, I. N., & Drummond, M. F. (1991). *Migraine.* London: Office of Health Economics.

Bonuso, S., Marano, E., Di Stasio, E., Sorge, F., Barbieri, F., & Ullucci, E. (1989). Source of pain and primitive dysfunction in migraine: An identical site? *J Neurol Neurosurg Psychiatry, 52,* 1351–1354.

Breslau, N., & Andreski, P. (1995). Migraine, personality and psychiatric comorbidity. *Headache, 35,* 382–386.

Breslau, N., & Davis, G. C. (1992). Migraine, major depression and panic disorder: A prospective epidemiologic study of young adults. *Cephalalgia, 12,* 85–90.

Breslau, N., Schultz, L. R., Stewart, W. F., Lipton, R. B., Lucia, V. K., & Welch, K., M. (2000). Headache and major depression. Is the association specific to migraine? *Neurology, 54,* 308–313.

Camfield, P. R., Metrakos, K., & Andermann, F. (1978). Basilar migraine, seizures and severe epileptiform EEG abnormalities. *Neurology, 28,* 584–588.

Campbell, D. A., Hay, K. M., & Tonks, E. M. (1951). An investigation of salt and water balance in migraine. *BMJ, 2,* 1424–1429.

Carlson, L. A., Ekelund, L. G., & Oro, L. (1968). Clinical and metabolic effects of different doses of prostaglandin E in man. *Acta Med Scand, 183,* 423–430.

Chancellor, A. M., Wroe, S. J., & Cull, R. E. (1990). Migraine occurring for the first time in pregnancy. *Headache, 30,* 224–227.

Chronicle, E. P., & Mulleners, W. M. (1996). Visual system dysfunction in migraine: A review of clinical and pathophysiological findings. *Cephalalgia, 16,* 525–535.

Connolly, F. J., Gawel, M., & Clifford Rose, F. (1982). Migraine patients exhibit abnormalities in the visual-evoked potential. *J Neurol Neurosurg Psychiatry, 45,* 464–467.

Cooke, L. J., Rose, M. S., & Becker, W. J. (2000). Chinook winds and migraine headache. *Neurology, 54,* 302–307.

Corbin, D., & Martyn, C. (1985). Migraine is not a manifestation of a generalized vasospastic disorder. *Cephalalgia, 5*(Suppl. 3), 458–459.

Cull, R. E. (1981). Barometric pressure and other factors in migraine. *Headache, 21,* 102–104.

Cummings, J. L., & Gittinger, J. W. (1981). Central dazzle. A thalamic syndrome? *Arch Neurol, 38,* 372–374.

Cunningham, S. J., McGrath, P. J., Ferguson., H. B., Humphreys, P., D'Astous, J., Latter, J., Goodman, J. T., & Firestone, P. (1987). Personality and behavioural characteristics in pediatric migraine. *Headache, 27,* 16–20.

Dalsgaard-Nielsen, J. (1970). Some aspects of the epidemiology of migraine in Denmark. In *Kliniske Aspekter i Migraeneforskningen* (pp. 18–30). Copenhagen: Nordlundes Bogtrykkeri.

Damasio, H., & Beck., D. (1978). Migraine, thrombocytopenia and serotonin metabolism. *Lancet,* i, 240–242.

D'Amico, D., Leone, M., Macciardi, F., Valentini, S., & Bussone, G. (1991). Genetic transmission of migraine without aura: A study of 68 families. *Ital J Neurol Sci, 12,* 581–584.

de Silva, R. N. (2001). A diagnostic sign in migraine? *J R Soc Med, 94,* 286–287.

Dodick, D. W., Eross, E. J., & Parish, J. M. (2003). Clinical, anatomical and physiologic relationship between sleep and headache. *Headache, 43,* 282–292.

Drummond, P. D. (1986). A quantitative assessment of photophobia in migraine and tension headache. *Headache, 26,* 465–469.

Drummond, P. D. (1987). Pupil diameter in migraine and tension headache. *J Neurol Neurosurg, Psychiatry, 50,* 228–230.

Essink-Bot, M. L., van Royen, L., Krabbe, P., Bonsel, G. J., & Rutten, F. F. H. (1995). The impact of migraine on health status. *Headache, 35,* 200–206.

Fanciullacci, M. (1979). Iris adrenergic impairment in idiopathic headache. *Headache, 19,* 8–13.

Fisher, C. M. (1980). Late-life migraine accompaniments as a cause of unexplained transient ischemic attacks. *Can J Neurol Sci, 7,* 917.

Friedman, A. P. (1970). The (infinite) variety of migraine. In A. L. Cochrane (Ed.), *Background to migraine. Third Migraine Symposium* (pp. 165–180). London: Heinemann.

Fumal, A., Venheede, M., DiClemente, L., Jacquart, J. Gerard, P., Maertens de Noordhout, A., et al. (2003). "Pseudomigraine" with temporary neurologic symptoms and CSF lymphocytosis (or HaNDL) is pathophysiologically similar to migraine with aura: Results from an evoked potential and single fiber EMG study. *Cephalalgia, 23,* 619.

Gabrielli, M., Cremonini, F., Fiore, G., Addolorato, C., Padalino, C., Candelli, M., et al. (2003). Association between migraine and celiac disease: Results from a preliminary case-control and therapeutic study. *Am J Gastroenterol, 98,* 625–629.

Galer, B. S., Lipton, R. B., Weinstein, S., Bello, L., & Solomon, S. (1990). Apoplectic headache and oculomotor nerve palsy: An unusual presentation of multiple sclerosis. *Neurology, 40,* 1465–1466.

Gibb, C. M., Davies, P. T. G., Glover, V., Steiner, T. J., Clifford Rose, F., & Sandler, M. (1991). Chocolate is a migraine-provoking agent. *Cephalalgia, 11,* 93–95.

Gomez-Aranda, F., Canadillas, F., Marti-Masso, J. F., Diez-Tejedor, E., Serano, P. J., Leira, R., Gracia, M., & Pascual, J. (1997). Pseudo-migraine with temporary neurological symptoms and lymphocytic pleocytosis. A report of 50 cases. *Brain, 120,* 1105–1113.

Gotoh, F., Komatsumoto, S., Araki, N., & Gomi, S. (1984). Noradrenergic nervous activity in migraine. *Arch Neurol, 41,* 951–955.

Green, J. E. (1977). A survey of migraine in England 1975–1976. *Headache, 17,* 67–68.

Guidetti, V., Fornara, R., Ottaviano, S., Petrilli, A., Seri, S., & Cortesi, F. (1987). Personality inventory for children and childhood migraine. *Cephalalgia, 7,* 225–230.

Haas, D. C., Kent, P. F., & Friedman, D. I. (1993). Headache caused by a single lesion of multiple sclerosis in the periaqueductal grey area. *Headache, 33,* 452–455.

Haas, D. C., Pineda, G. S., & Lourie, H. (1975). Juvenile head trauma syndromes and their relationship to migraine. *Arch Neurol, 32,* 727–737.

Hadjivassiliou, M., Grünewald, R. A., Lawden, M., et al., (2001). Headache and CNS white matter abnormalities associated with gluten sensitivity. *Neurology, 56,* 385–388.

Henry, P., Auray, J. P., Gaudin, A. F., Dartigues, J. F., Duru, G., Lanteri-Minet, M., et al. (2002). Prevalence and clinical characteristics of migraine in France. *Neurology, 59,* 232–237.

Henryk-Gutt, R., & Rees, W. L. (1973). Psychological aspects of migraine. *J Psychosom Res, 17,* 141–153.

Hughes, G. R. (2003). Migraine, memory loss and "multiple sclerosis." Neurological features of the antiphospholipid (Hughes") syndrome. *Postgrad Med J, 79,* 81–83.

Hungerford, G. D., du Boulay, G. H., & Zilkha, K. J. (1976). Computerized axial tomography in patients with severe migraine: A preliminary report. *J Neurol Neurosurg Psychiatry, 39,* 990–994.

Igarashi, H., Sakai, F., Kan, S., Okada, J., & Tazaki, Y. (1991). Magnetic resonance imaging of the brain in patients with migraine. *Cephalalgia, 11,* 69–74.

Intiso, D., Crociani, P., Fogli, D., et al. (2002). Occurrence of factor V Leiden mutation (Arg 506 G1n) and anticardiolipin antibodies in migraine patients. *Neurol Sci, 22,* 455–458.

Katsarava, Z., Giffin, N., Diener, H.-C., & Kaube, H. (2003). Abnormal habituation of "'nociceptive'" blink reflex in migraine. Evidence for increased excitability of trigeminal nociception. *Cephalalgia, 23,* 814–819.

Kayan, A., & Hood, J. D. (1984). Neuro-otological manifestations of migraine. *Brain, 107,* 1123–1142.

Klapper, J. (1994). Headache in Sturge-Weber syndrome. *Headache, 34,* 521–522.

Koo, B., Becker, L. E., Chuang, S., et al. (1993). Mitochondrial encephalomyopathy, lactic acidosis, stroke-like episodes (MELAS). Clinical, radiological, pathological and genetic observations. *Ann Neurol, 34,* 25–32.

Kruit, M. C., van Buchem, M. A., Hofman, P. A., Bakkers, J. T., Terwindt, G. M., et al. (2004). Migraine as a risk factor for subclinical brain lesions. *Jama, 291,* 427–434.

Kunkle, E. C., & Anderson, W. B. (1961). Significance of minor eye signs in headache of migraine type. *Arch Ophthalmol, 65,* 504–508.

Kruit, M. C., van Buchem, M. A., Hofman, P. A., Bakkers, J. T., Terwindt, G. M., et al. (2004). Migraine as a risk factor for subclinical brain lesions. *JAMA, 291,* 427–434.

Láinez, M. J. A., Monzón, & the Spanish Occupational Migraine Study Group. (2003). The socio-economic impact of migraine in Spain. In J. Olesen, T. J. Steiner, & R. B. Lipton (Eds.), *Reducing the burden of headache* (pp. 255–299). New York: Oxford University Press.

Lance, J. W., & Anthony, M. (1966). Some clinical aspects of migraine: A prospective survey of 500 patients. *Arch Neurol, 15,* 356–361.

Larsson, B., Bille, B., & Pederson, N. L. (1995). Genetic influence in headaches: A Swedish twin study. *Headache, 35,* 513–519.

Laurence, K. M. (1987). Genetics of migraine. In J. N. Blau (Ed.), *Migraine. Clinical and research aspects* (pp. 479–484). Baltimore: Johns Hopkins University Press.

Lauritzen, M., Trojaborg, W., & Olesen, J. (1981). EEG during attacks of common and classical migraine. *Cephalalgia, 1,* 63–66.

Leviton, A., & Camenga, D. (1969). Migraine associated with hyper-pre-beta-lipoproteinemia. *Neurology, 19,* 963–966.

Levor, R. M., Cohen, M. J., Naliboff, B. D., & McArthur, D. (1986). Psychosocial precursors and correlates of migraine headache. *J Consult Clin Psychol, 54,* 347–353.

Levy, M. J., Matharu, M. S., Powell, M. P., Meeran, K., & Goadsby, P. J. (2003). Phenotype characterisation of the headache associated with pituitary tumors. *Cephalagia, 23,* 621.

Linet, M. S., Stewart, W. F., Celentano, D. D., Ziegler, D., & Sprechner, M. (1989). An epidemiologic study of headache among adolescents and young adults. *JAMA, 261,* 2211–2216.

Lipton, R. B., Dodick, D., Sadovsky, R., Kolodner, K., Endicott, J., Hettiarachchi, J., et al. (2003). A self-administered screener for migraine in primary care. The ID Migraine validation study. *Neurology, 61,* 375–382.

Lipton, R. B., Scher, A. I., Kolodner, K., Liberman, J., Steiner, T. J., & Stewart, W. F. (2002). Migraine in the United States. Epidemiology and patterns of health care use. *Neurology, 58,* 885–894.

Lipton, R. B., Silberstein, D. S., & Stewart, W. F. (1994). An update on the epidemiology of migraine. *Headache, 34,* 319–328.

Litman, G. I., & Friedman, H. M. (1978). Migraine and the mitral valve prolapse syndrome. *Am Heart J, 96,* 610–614.

Littlewood, J. T., Gibb, C., Glover, V., Sandler, M., Davies, P. T. G., & Clifford Rose, F. (1988). Red wine as a cause of migraine. *Lancet,* i, 558–559.

Lord, G. D. A. (1982). A study of premonitory focal neurological symptoms in migraine. In F. Clifford Rose (Ed.), *Advances in migraine research and therapy* (pp. 45–48). New York Raven Press.

Marcus, D. A., & Soso, M. J. (1989). Migraine and stripe-induced visual discomfort. *Arch Neurol, 46,* 1129–1132.

Massiou, H., & MacGregor, E. A. (2000). Evolution and treatment of migraine with oral contraceptives. *Cephalalgia, 20,* 170–174.

Mathew, N. T., Kailasam, J., & Meadors, L. (2003). Allodynia in migraine. *Cephalalgia, 23,* 637.

Mathew, N. T., Meyer, J. S., Welch, K. M. A., & Neblett, C. R. (1977). Abnormal CT scans in migraine. *Headache, 16,* 272–279.

Matthews, W. B. (1972). Footballer's migraine. *BMJ, 1,* 326–327.

Mattson, P. (2003). Hormonal factors in migraine: A population based study of women aged 40 to 74 years. *Headache, 43,* 27–35.

McQueen, J., Loblay, R. H., Swain, A. R., Anthony, M., & Lance, J. W. (1989). A controlled trial of dietary modification in migraine. In F. Clifford Rose (Ed.), *New advances in headache research* (pp. 235–242). London: Smith-Gordon.

Medina, J. L., & Diamond, S. (1976). Migraine and atopy. *Headache, 15,* 271–274.

Medina, J. L., & Diamond, S. (1978). The role of diet in migraine. *Headache, 18,* 31–34.

Merikangas, K. R. (1996). Sources of genetic complexity in migraine. In M. Sandler, M. Ferraris, & S. Harnett (Eds.), *Migraine, pharmacology and genetics* (pp. 254–2810). London: Chapman and Hall.

Merikangas, K. R., & Angst, J. (1990). Depression and migraine. In M. Sandler & G. Collins (Eds.), *Migraine, a spectrum of ideas* (pp. 248–258). Oxford, UK: Oxford University Press.

Merrett, J., Peatfield, R. C., Clifford Rose, F., & Merrett, T. G. (1983). Food-related antibodies in headache patients. *J Neurol Neurosurg Psychiat, 46,* 738–742.

Monastero, R., Mannino, M., Lopez, G., et al. (2003). Prevalence of headache in patients with Behçets disease without overt neurological involvement. *Cephalalgia, 23,* 105–108.

Monro, J., Brostoff, J., Carini, C., & Zilkha, K. (1980). Food allergy in migraine: study of dietary exclusion and RAST. *Lancet,* ii, 1–4.

Monteiro, J. M., Rosas, M. J., Correia, A. P., & Vaz, A. R. (1993). Migraine and intracranial vascular malformations. *Headache, 33,* 563–565.

Nager, B. J., Lanska, D. J., & Daroff, R. B. (1989). Acute demyelination mimicking vascular hemicrania. *Neurology, 29,* 423–424.

Nikiforow, R., & Hokkanen, E. (1979). Effects of headache on working ability: A survey of an urban and a rural population in Northern Finland. *Headache, 19,* 214–218.

O'Keeffe, S. T., Tsapatsasis, N. P., & Beetham, W. P., Jr. (1993). Association between Raynaud's phenomenon and migraine in a random population of hospital employees. *J Rheumatol, 20,* 1187–1188.

Osuntokun, B. O., Bademosi, O., & Osuntokun, O. (1982). Migraine in Nigeria. In F. Clifford Rose (Ed.), *Advances in migraine research and therapy* (pp. 25–38). New York: Raven Press.

Osuntokun, B. O., & Osuntokun, O. (1972). Complicated migraine and haemoglobin AS in Nigerians. *BMJ, 2,* 621–622.

Ottman, R., & Lipton, R. B. (1996). Is the comorbidity of epilepsy and migraine due to a shared genetic susceptibility? *Neurology, 47,* 918–924.

Panayiotopoulos, C. P. (1987). Difficulties in differentiating migraine and epilepsy based on clinical and EEG findings. In F. Andermann & E. Lugaresi (Eds.), *Migraine and epilepsy* (pp. 31–46). Boston: Butterworths.

Panayiotopoulos, C. P. (1996). Elementary visual hallucinations in migraine and epilepsy. *J Neurol Neurosurg Psychiatry, 60,* 117.

Parker, R. J., Vezina, G., & Stacy Nicholson, H. (1994). Complicated "migraine-like" headaches in children following cranial irradiation and chemotherapy. *Ann Neurol, 36,* 509–510.

Pestronk, A., & Pestronk, S. (1983). Goggle migraine. *N Engl J Med, 308,* 226–227.

Pfaffenrath, V., Kommissari, I., Pollman, W., Kaube, H., & Rath, M. (1991). Cerebrovascular risk factors in migraine with prolonged aura and without aura. *Cephalalgia, 11,* 257–261.

Radtke, A., Lempert, T., Gresty, M. A., et al. (2002). Migraine and Ménière's disease. If there a link? *Neurology, 59,* 1700–1704.

Rasmussen, B. K., Jensen, R., & Olesen, J. (1992). Impact of headache on sickness absence and utilisation of medical services: A Danish population study. *J Epidemiol Community Health, 46,* 443–446.

Rasmussen, B. K., Jensen, R., Schroll, M., & Olesen, J. (1991). Epidemiology of headache in a general population: A prevalence study. *J Clin Epidemiol, 44,* 1147–1157.

Rasmussen B. K. (1995). Epidemiology of headache. *Cephalalgia, 15,* 45–68.

Rolak, L. A. (1985). Headache in patients with multiple sclerosis. *Neurology, 35*(Suppl. 1), 267.

Rowat, B. M. T., Merrill, C. F., Davis, A., & South, V. (1991). A double-blind comparison of granisetron and placebo for the treatment of acute migraine in the emergency department. *Cephalalgia, 11,* 207–213.

Russell, M. B., & Olesen, J. (1995). Increased familial risk and evidence of genetic factor in migraine. *BMJ, 311,* 541–544.

Sacks, O. W. (1992). Migraine (pp. 37–38). Berkeley: University of California Press.

Sakai, F., & Igarashi, H. J. (1997). Prevalence of migraine in Japan: A nationwide survey. *Cephalalgia, 17,* 15–22.

Sándor, P. S., Mascia, A., Seidel, L., et al. (2001). Subclinical cerebellar impairment in the common types of migraine: A three dimensional analysis of reaching movements. *Ann Neurol, 49,* 668–672.

Schoenen, J., & Thomsen, L. L. (2000). Neurophysiology and autonomic dysfunction in migraine. In J. Olesen, P. Tfelt-Hensen, & K. M. A. Welch (Eds.), *The headaches* (2nd ed., pp. 301–312).

Scobie, B. A. (1983). Recurrent vomiting in adults. A syndrome? *Med J Aust, 1,* 329–331.

Selby, G., & Lance, J. W. (1960). Observations on 500 cases of migraine and allied vascular headache. *J Neurol Neurosurg Psychiatry, 23,* 23–32.

Septien, L., Pelletier, J. L., Brunotte, F., Giroud, M., & Dumas, R. (1991). Migraine in patients with history of centro-temporal epilepsy in childhood. *Cephalalgia, 11,* 281–284.

Shuaib, A., & Hachinski, V. C. (1988). Migraine and the risks from angiography. *Arch Neurol, 45,* 911–912.

Silberstein, S. D., Lipton, R. B., & Breslau, N. (1995). Migraine: Association with personality characteristics and psychopathology. *Cephalalgia, 15,* 358–369.

Siniatchkin, M., Kropp, P., & Gerber, W.-D. (2003). What kind of habituation is impaired in migraine patients? *Cephalalgia, 23,* 511–518.

Soges, L. J., Cacayorin, E. D., Petro, G. R., & Ramachandran, T. S. (1988). Migraine: Evaluation by MR. *AJNR (Am J Neuroradiol), 9,* 425–429.

Somerville, B. W. (1971). The role of progesterone in menstrual migraine. *Neurology, Minneap, 21,* 853–859.

Somerville, B. W. (1972a). The role of oestradiol withdrawal in the etiology of menstrual migraine. *Neurology, Minneap, 22,* 355–365.

Somerville, B. W. (1972b). A study of migraine in pregnancy. *Neurology, Minneap, 22,* 824–828.

Spierings, E. L. H. (2002). Reflux-triggered migraine headache originating from the upper gum/teeth. *Cephalalgia, 22,* 555–556.

Stanford, E., & Green, R. (1970). A case of migraine cured by treatment of Conn's syndrome. In *Background to migraine. Third British Migraine Symposium* (pp. 53–57). London: Heinemann.

Stewart, W. F., Lipton, R. B., Celentano, D. D., & Reed, M. L. (1992). Prevalence of migraine headache in the United States. Relation to age, income, race and other sociodemographic factors. *JAMA, 267,* 64–69.

Stewart, W. F., Lipton, R. B., Kolodner, K., Liberman, J., & Sawyer, J. (1999). Reliability of the migraine disability assessment score in a population-based sample of headache sufferers. *Cephalalgia, 19,* 107–114.

Stewart, W. F., Lipton, R. B., & Liberman, J. (1996). Variation in migraine prevalence by race. *Neurology, 47,* 52–59.

Stewart, W. F., Lipton, R. B., & Simon, D. (1996). Work-related disability: Results from the American Migraine Study. *Cephalalgia, 16,* 231–238.

Sulman, F. G., Danon, A., Pfeifer, Y., Tal, E., & Weller, C. P. (1970). Urinalysis of patients suffering from climatic heat stress. *Int J Biometeorol, 14,* 45–53.

Svensson, D. A., Larsson, B., Waldenlind, E., & Pedersen, N. L. (2003). Shared rearing environment in migraine: Results from twins reared apart and twins reared together. *Headache, 43,* 235–244.

Tfelt-Hansen, P., Lous, I., & Olesen, J. (1981). Prevalence and significance of muscle tenderness during migraine attacks. *Headache, 21,* 49–54.

Thomas, D. J., Robinson, S., Robinson, A., & Johnson, D. G. (1996). Migraine threshold is altered in hyperthyroidism. *J Neurol Neurosurg Psychiatry, 61,* 222.

Toth, C. C. (2002). Persistent cerebrospinal fluid abnormalities in the syndrome of headache, neurological deficit, and cerebrospinal fluid lymphocytosis despite resolution of clinical symptomatology. *Headache, 42,* 1038–1043.

van der Linden, J. A. (1660). *De hemicrania menstrua.* Amsterdam: Elsevier.

Waldie, K. E., Hausmann, M., Milne, B. J., & Poulton, R. (2002). Migraine and cognitive function. A life-course study. *Neurology, 59,* 904–908.

Watkins, S. M., & Espir, M. (1969). Migraine and multiple sclerosis. *J Neurol Neurosurg Psychiatry, 32,* 35–37.

Webster, I. W., Waddy, N., Jenkins, L. V., & Lai, Y. C. L. (1977). Health status of a group of narcotic addicts in a methadone treatment programme. *Med J Aust, 2,* 485–491.

Welch, K. M. A., & Levine, S. R. (1990). Migraine-related stroke in the context of the International Headache Society classification of head pain. *Arch Neurol, 47,* 458–462.

Whitty, C. W. M., & Hockaday, J. M. (1968). Migraine. A follow-up study of 92 patients. *BMJ, 1,* 735–736.

Wilmshurst, P. T., Nightingale, S., Walsh, K. P., & Morrison, W. L. (2000). Effect on migraine of closure of cardiac right to left shunts to prevent recurrence of decompression illness or stroke or for haemo-dynamic reasons. *Lancet, 356,* 1648–1651.

Winter, A. L. (1987). Neurophysiology and migraine. In J. N. Blau (Ed.), *Migraine: Clinical and research aspects* (pp. 485–510). Baltimore: Johns Hopkins University Press.

Wolff, H. G. (1963). *Headache and other head pain.* New York: Oxford University Press.

Woodhouse, A., & Drummond, P. D. (1993). Mechanisms of increased sensitivity to noise and light in migraine headache. *Cephalalgia, 13,* 417–421.

Ziegler, D. K., Batnitzky, S., Barter, R., & McMillan, J. H. (1991). Magnetic resonance image abnormality in migraine with aura. *Cephalalgia, 11,* 147–150.

Chapter 8
Migraine: Pathophysiology

Migraine is a hereditary susceptibility of the brain to relax modulation of afferent impulses periodically, thus permitting and augmenting the perception of head pain; vascular pulsation; scalp tenderness; and sensitivity to light, sounds, and smells.

Migrainous headaches may be preceded by or associated with progressive cortical "shutdown," causing positive and then negative cerebral symptoms such as scintillating scotomas that we recognize as an aura but that more commonly cause lack of concentration and confusion, with other subtle signs of mental impairment. The two arms of migraine—aura and headache—are often linked sequentially, but more often headache is the dominant symptom without recognizable cortical symptoms. At other times, a classical aura may develop with little or no headache following.

The aura phase is substantially a cortical phenomenon that may be caused directly by excessive afferent input to the visual or other areas of the cerebral cortex or that may be initiated by an "upstream discharge" from hypothalamus or brainstem structures to the cortex (Figure 8.1). The headache phase results from a "downstream discharge" from cortex or hypothalamus to inhibit the endogenous pain-control pathway (Figure 8.2).

The frequency of migraine headache varies from once in a lifetime to almost daily, so no clear line may divide a migrainous and a nonmigrainous brain, although the degree of predisposition may vary. Our present concept is one of a threshold of susceptibility determined by some of the following factors. It remains unresolved as to whether this is a universal susceptibility.

THE PREDISPOSITION—A MIGRAINOUS BRAIN

What factors may play a part in setting the migrainous threshold?

Genetic Factors

A rare form of migraine that is clearly autosomal dominant, familial hemiplegic migraine, can be caused by mis-sense mutations in the α-1 subunit of the P/Q type voltage-gated calcium channel on chromosome 19 (Ophoff et al., 1996). This

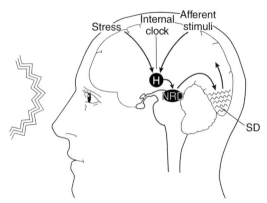

FIGURE 8.1 Aura. A simple schema of the way that internal or external trigger factors could initiate a migrainous aura via the hypothalamus (H) and serotonergic projections from the nucleus raphe dorsalis (NRD) to the occipital cortex.

mutation explains about 55% of cases, with a further 15% being recently localized to chromosome 1 (Ducros et al., 1997; de Fusco et al., 2003) and the final 30% still being unaccounted for. This finding in this rare form of migraine has an important biologic implication. Neurologic disorders caused by abnormalities in channels, so-called channelopathies (Griggs & Nutt, 1995), often have the characteristic of episodicity that is so much a part of migraine. Abnormalities on

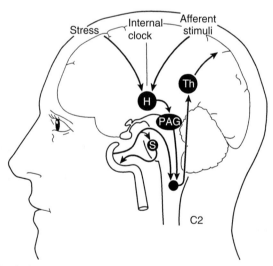

FIGURE 8.2 Headache. A possible mechanism for the hypothalamus (H) influencing the periaqueductal gray matter (PAG) to inhibit the endogenous pain-control system and excite the nucleus salivatorius (S) to dilate cerebral blood vessels via the parasympathetic outflow. Afferent input from the vessels projects to the cortex through the thalamus (Th) and augments the outflow from S.

chromosome 19 may account in part for some patients' genetic susceptibility to other types of migraine (May et al., 1995).

Magnesium Deficiency

The measurement of brain phosphates by nuclear magnetic resonance spectroscopy after the intravenous injection of 31_p has enabled the indirect assay of magnesium content by examining the chemical shift properties of the 31_p resonance signals. By using this noninvasive technique, Welch's group (Ramadan et al., 1989) found that magnesium ion concentration was lower during migraine headache. Magnesium ion concentration gates and blocks the N-methyl-d-aspartate (NMDA)-subtype glutamate receptor so that this preliminary result suggests a basis for cerebral hyperexcitability via increased activity at NMDA receptors (Welch & Ramadan, 1995). Given that NMDA-mediated activation is essential for spreading depression (Lauritzen, 1994), a relative reduction in brain magnesium may make the brain more susceptible to the triggering of spreading depression.

Excitatory Amino Acids

D'Andrea, Cananzi, and Joseph (1989a) reported that the platelet content of glutamate and aspartate was increased in patients subject to migraine with aura, during headache-free periods, compared with normal controls and patients with migraine without aura. The glutamate level rose further during headache. Ferrari et al. (1990) measured these amino acids in plasma and found the level elevated in patients with migraine between attacks, more so in those patients whose migraine was accompanied by an aura, and increased further during headache. If a similar elevation of excitatory amino acids were shown to exist in the cortex, this would also increase its excitability.

Neurophysiologic Changes

The results of electrophysiologic tests in migraine have been presented in Chapter 7, with the lack of habituation between migraine headaches being the most constant finding. The many studies of visual and auditory evoked potentials, the contingent negative variation, and the results of transcranial magnetic stimulation and electromyography are summarized by Ambrosini et al. (2003). These authors explain the normalization of habituation during migraine headache by postulating an increase in cortical excitability before the attack begins, related to enhanced activity in raphe-cortical pathways, that then reverts to normal as headache begins. They comment on observations by Evers et al. (1999) that serotonin content of blood platelets decreases as the habituation of visual evoked responses normalizes. The discharge of platelet serotonin at the onset of migraine headache, first established in our laboratory in the 1960s (Anthony, Hinterberger, & Lance, 1967), is thought to reflect depletion of serotonin at central synapses.

The use of the blink response to explore trigeminal pathway sensitivity has been refined by Kaube et al. (2000), using a concentric stimulating electrode that selectively stimulates superficial cutaneous nociceptive fibers. This "nociceptive" blink response failed to habituate outside the migraine attack (Katsarava et al., 2003). The R_2 component of the blink reflex, which is nociception specific, was augmented by 680% on the headache side and 230% on the nonheadache side during a migraine attack and was also reduced in latency (Kaube et al., 2002).

The failure of habituation before headache begins indicates increased cortical excitability that would be consistent with susceptibility to the development of migraine aura, whereas the increase in sensitivity of central trigeminal pathways in migraine headache indicates withdrawal of the normal modulating action of the endogenous pain-control system.

The Hypothalamo-Pituitary Axis and Dopaminergic Transmission

Some interesting evidence suggests a role for dopaminergic transmission in the pathophysiology of migraine (Peroutka, 1997). About 25% of patients report symptoms of elation, irritability, depression, hunger, thirst, or drowsiness during the 24 hours preceding headache. Most of these manifestations can arise in the hypothalamus (Kupfermann, 1985), and this, along with circadian functions in the region of the suprachiasmatic nucleus (Swaab et al., 1993), suggests a central site for their evolution. A substantial proportion of patients with migraine report yawning (Russell et al., 1996), which, of all the premonitory symptoms, is most distinctively dopaminergic.

Patients with "essential headache," including migraine, are more responsive to hallucinogenic agents such as LSD and psilocybin than are control subjects (Fanciullacci, Franchi, & Sicuteri, 1974). Patients with migraine are unusually sensitive to the emetic effects of apomorphine (Sicuteri, 1977) and become hypotensive more readily when given bromocriptine (Fanciullacci et al., 1980). Information presently available therefore suggests a dopamine deficiency in migraine with supersensitivity of dopamine receptors.

Opioids and the Endogenous Pain-Control System

Endogenous opioids have been implicated as inhibitory neurotransmitters liberated from interneurons in the central regulation of pain pathways. They comprise beta-endorphin, enkephalins, and dynorphins. There have been conflicting reports on plasma beta-endorphin levels in migraine. Bach et al. (1985) could not detect any difference between plasma levels in and out of attacks. Plasma methionine-metenkephalin levels are higher in patients with migraine than in normal controls and increase further during headache (Mosnaim et al., 1985; Ferrari et al., 1987). The extent to which blood and cerebrospinal fluid (CSF) levels reflect central opioid function remains uncertain. It is interesting that the intramuscular injection of naloxone 0.8 mg shortened the migrainous aura in most patients, but when the aura followed its usual course, the ensuing headache was of normal severity (Sicuteri et al., 1983).

Pain control mechanisms must be partially defective in patients with migraine, because spontaneous jabs of pain in the head ("ice-pick pains;" primary stabbing headache) and headaches induced by eating ice cream are more common in patients with migraine than in control subjects. Drummond and Lance (1984) found that both these pains were felt in the part of the head habitually affected by migraine headache in about one third of patients, indicating a latent defect in that part of the endogenous pain-control system.

Vascular Reactivity

The cerebral vasodilator response to carbon dioxide is greater in patients with migraine than in normal controls (Sakai & Meyer, 1979), and the reaction of extracranial arteries to exercise (Drummond & Lance, 1981) and stress (Drummond, 1982) is greater on the side of their usual migraine headache.

THE TRIGGER—INITIATION OF THE MIGRAINE ATTACK

Given that the brain of susceptible subjects has a low "migraine threshold," as just outlined, what triggers each episode? For many patients, no external factor can be identified. Episodes may recur regularly, as though determined by some internal clock. Probably the relevant biological clock involves the hypothalamus (Figure 8.3), because premonitory symptoms, such as elation, drowsiness, thirst, or a craving for sweet foods, may precede headache by some 24 hours (Blau, 1980; Drummond & Lance, 1984; Griffen et al., 2003). In other cases, the attack originates in the cortex in response to stress or excessive afferent stimulation such as noise, flickering light (Cao et al., 2002), or the smell of strong perfumes.

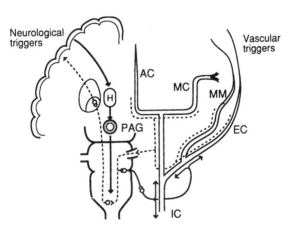

FIGURE 8.3 The mechanism of migraine headache. Migraine can be initiated by a central generator, probably in the vicinity of the hypothalamus (H) or triggered by afferent stimulation such as noise, flickering light, or strong smells. Descending fibers influence the processing of head pain and originate in the upper brainstem, periaqueductal gray matter (PAG), and dorsolateral pontine tegmentum. Migraine can also be triggered by stimulation of vascular afferents (vasodilator drugs, arteriography) that induce excessive neural activity in central pathways released from modulation by the pain control system as well as increasing vasodilation by the trigeminovascular reflex illustrated in Figure 8.4. Arteries: internal carotid (IC), anterior cerebral (AC), middle cerebral (MC) middle meningeal (MM), external carotid (EC).

Some trigger factors—for example, injecting a contrast medium into the carotid or vertebrobasilar circulations or ingesting vasodilator agents—appear to act primarily on the cranial blood vessels (see Figure 8.3). Nitrates cause vasodilation by conversion to nitric oxide (NO). Craniovascular afferents may then excite central pathways (see Figures 8.3 and 8.4). Interestingly sildenafil, which activates cGMP downstrean of NO, triggers migraine in the absence of vascular changes (Kruuse et al., 2003).

THE MIGRAINOUS AURA

Attention has been lavished on the migrainous aura because of the spectacular and often frightening nature of the symptoms, although most patients with migraine never have an aura. Only 10% of patients experience the classic "slow march" of symptoms such as fortification spectra, whereas in about 25% less specific disturbances of "spots in front of the eyes" or "shimmering vision" cover the whole visual field simultaneously (Lance & Anthony, 1966).

Lashley (1941) plotted the expansion of his own visual scotoma in migraine and calculated that the visual cortex was being compromised by some process

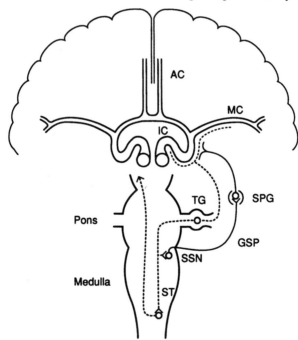

FIGURE 8.4 Interaction between brainstem and cerebral vessels. Parasympathetic fibers arising from the superior salivatory nucleus (SSN) pass in the greater superficial petrosal (GSP) nerve, synapse in the sphenopalatine ganglion (SPG), and supply the cerebral arteries with vasodilator fibers. Afferent fibers from the vessels traverse the trigeminal ganglion (TG), descend in the spinal tract (ST), and send collaterals to the SSN, completing the trigeminovascular reflex. Arteries: internal carotid (IC), anterior cerebral (AC), middle cerebral (MC).

advancing at about 3 mm each minute. A similar conclusion was reached by Lauritzen et al. (1983), who demonstrated by blood flow studies that oligemia spread from the occipital lobe forward over the cortex with much the same speed, between 2 and 6 mm each minute (Figure 8.5).

In some patients with migrainous aura (Olesen, Larsen, & Lauritzen, 1981), patchy areas of increased blood flow have been seen before cerebral blood flow diminished. Diminution of the flow starts in the occipital region or watershed area at the occipitoparietal junction and extends forward as a "spreading oligemia" (Olesen et al., 1981). The wave of oligemia progresses over the cortex at about 2 to 3 mm per minute, irrespective of arterial territories, stopping short at the central and lateral sulci, although the frontal lobes also become oligemic independently in some patients (Lauritzen et al., 1983). Spreading oligemia typically begins before the patient notices focal neurologic symptoms and reaches the sensorimotor area only after the appropriate symptoms have started and outlasts these symptoms. Oligemia lasts for several hours and is followed by delayed hyperemia (Andersen et al., 1988). The headache usually starts while cerebral blood flow is still diminished (Olesen et al., 1990) (Figure 8.6).

From these studies, the authors concluded that the migrainous aura was a manifestation of cortical spreading depression (CSD), described in the animal brain by the Brazilian neurophysiologist Leão (1944). This phenomenon is a progressive cortical shutdown, suppressing normal activity at a speed of 2 to 3 mm each minute and lasting 5 to 60 minutes. Leão speculated that this might be the mechanism of fortification spectra. Fifty years later his idea gained acceptance (Lauritzen, 1994).

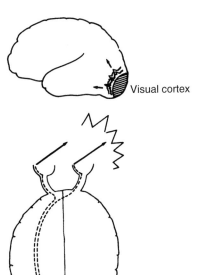

Visual cortex

FIGURE 8.5 Mechanism of fortification spectra. A wave of excitation followed by inhibition moves slowly over the visual cortex, causing scintillations and scotomas in the contralateral half of the visual field. (From Lance, 1986, by permission of the publishers, Charles Scribner's Sons, New York.)

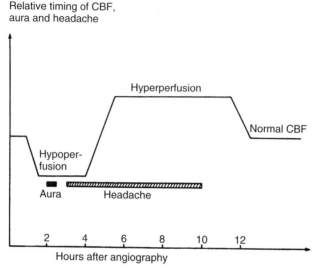

FIGURE 8.6 Relationship of aura and headache to changes in regional cerebral blood flow (CBF). (From Olesen et al., 1990, by permission of the editor of *Annals of Neurology*.)

The possibility that CSD might be a feature in some patients with migraines without an overt aura arose when Woods, Iacoboni, and Mazziotta (1994) by chance recorded the changes taking place in the brain of a patient undergoing a positron emission tomography (PET) scan for another purpose. This patient experienced transient blurring of vision but no traditional aura symptoms, yet occipital oligemia spread forward in the same way it does during a classical aura. This observation may explain the impairment of concentration and memory as well as the confusional state that may accompany migraine without aura.

Sramka et al. (1977) described spreading depression in human hippocampus and caudate nucleus during stereotaxic surgery, but the finding could not be confirmed by Piper et al. (1991) from our department, who sought evidence of CSD in nine anesthetized patients undergoing neurosurgery and found suggestive but not diagnostic changes in only two. McLachlan and Girvin (1994) tried but failed to elicit CSD in the cortex of 23 unanesthetized patients having localized cortical ablation for epilepsy. Gloor (1986) in his vast experience had never observed EEG changes suggestive of CSD during neurosurgical procedures.

Nevertheless, Barkley et al. (1990), using magnetoencephalography, demonstrated long-duration decrements in EEG amplitude and other changes during migraine headache similar to those seen in animals during CSD.

CSD does not necessarily imply cortical ischemia. Functional magnetic resonance imaging (MRI) demonstrates blood flow changes in CSD without blood oxygenation level–dependent (BOLD) MRI finding significant ischemia (Cutrer et al., 1998). Hadjikhani et al. (2001) found BOLD MRI changes suggestive of CSD in three patients studied during the evolution of a visual aura. An initial increase in signal, possibly reflecting vasodilation, was detected progressing slowly at 3.5 ± 1.1 mm/min over the occipital cortex in parallel with the visual symptoms, followed by a diminution in the BOLD signal. This is the most convincing evidence thus far for an event such as CSD generating the visual aura. Perhaps for the development of CSD the human brain requires priming by a migrainous susceptibility lowering the threshold. In patients studied by Cao et al. (2002), hyperoxia and blood volume increase in the red nucleus and substantia nigra preceded visually triggered migrainous aura or headache.

The photopsia experienced during a migraine aura resembles those produced by electrical stimulation of the visual cortex (Penfield & Perot, 1963; Brindley & Lewin, 1968). Zigzag fortification spectra can be explained by a wave of excitation passing over the columns of cells in the striate cortex, which Hubel and Weisel (1968) described as responding selectively to the presentation of bars at various angles to the field of vision, followed by inhibition causing a scotoma.

An interesting pharmacotherapeutic correlate between experimental work and aura is that in some species blockading nitric oxide synthase (NOS) can attenuate or eliminate the cerebral blood-flow changes associated with spreading depression (Goadsby, Kaube, & Hoskin, 1992), and Olesen's group has demonstrated that NOS blockade can abort acute migraine attacks, including headache and other symptoms (Lassen et al., 1997). When these various observations are taken together, spreading depression or the human equivalent, made somewhat different by the cytoarchitecture of the human brain, is the most likely explanation for the migrainous aura.

The Relationship of the Aura to Migraine Headache

Although auras may occur without an ensuing headache, and migraine headache usually occurs without any aura, it is tempting to seek some connection between the two phenomena. Could the cortical events responsible for the aura also set in train the neurovascular disturbance that causes headache?

Moskowitz thought that spreading depression of the cortex during the aura phase of migraine may depolarize trigeminal nerve fibers surrounding the pial arteries and thus initiate the headache phase of migraine (Moskowitz, Nozaki, & Kraig, 1993). CSD was reported to enhance blood flow in the middle meningeal artery with plasma protein leakage within the dura mater (Bolay et al., 2002). These authors predicted that headache should develop especially on the side of the affected hemisphere. If this were the case, headache would always develop on the side of the head responsible for the cerebral symptoms; that is, a left visual field aura would be followed by a right-sided headache. Most authors agree that the headache may appear on the apparently inappropriate side (Peatfield & Clifford Rose, 1991).

Olesen et al. (1990) have also sought to link the phenomena underlying the aura phase with the development of headache. Most patients they studied did have headache on the side relevant to aura production, but even so, 3 of their 38 patients experienced their unilateral headache on the "wrong" side. Of 19 patients with bilateral headache, aura symptoms were bilateral in 6 and unilateral in 13. Of 10 patients with bilateral aura, 6 developed bilateral and 4 unilateral headache. An earlier prospective study of the Copenhagen group had found aura symptoms ipsi-lateral to the headache in 19 patients and contralateral in 18 (Jensen et al., 1986).

Ebersberger et al. (2001) studied the possible relationship between CSD and neurogenic inflammation in rats, with findings contrary to those of Bolay et al. CSD did not alter plasma extravasation in the dura mater or neuronal activity in trigeminal pathways.

Thus no consistent laboratory or clinical evidence supports the notion that CSD alone could initiate headache. We must account for the many patients who experience migraine headache without aura and the few who experience aura without headache. The common linkage between aura and headache can be explained in one of two ways.

1. That CSD is an intrinsic property of the migrainous cerebral cortex, triggered by excessive afferent bombardment such as flickering light or by intrinsic mechanisms in response to emotion or stress. In this event downstream projections from the cortex could be responsible for releasing the endogenous pain-control pathway to initiate migraine headache on one side of the head or the other.
2. That projections from the brainstem to cortex may trigger CSD in a susceptible subject and also be responsible for the changes in pain perception and vascular control underlying migraine headache. This model would account for the dissociation between aura and headache and for the switching of headache from one side to another during a migraine attack.

THE SOURCE OF PAIN IN MIGRAINE

Migraine headache often starts as a dull pain in the frontotemporal region, upper neck, or occipital area and becomes pulsatile in character only as the severity of the attack increases. Because of the throbbing quality of the pain, the conspicuous dilation of extracranial arteries in some instances, and the known pain sensitivity of cranial blood vessels, migraine has long been considered as a "vascular headache."

Pain-Producing Structures

Our knowledge of pain-producing structures in the human head owes much to the work of Harold G. Wolff and his colleagues, who studied the reaction of conscious subjects to the probing, stimulation, or distension of the brain, meninges, and blood vessels (Wolff, 1963). Direct stimulation of the cerebral cortex, the ependymal lining of the ventricles, choroid plexuses, and much of the dura and pia arachnoid does not cause pain, although selective stimulation of certain areas in the brain may augment or diminish the perception of pain. The floor of the anterior and posterior fossa gives rise to pain, but the middle cranial fossa is sensitive only in the vicinity of the middle cerebral artery. The most important structures that register pain are the blood vessels, particularly the proximal part of the cerebral and dural arteries, and the large veins and venous sinuses (Ray & Wolff, 1940).

Cranial bone is insensitive, but pain is experienced when the periosteum is stretched (Wolff, 1963). Distension of the middle meningeal artery causes referred pain to the back of the eye as well as the overlying area (Figure 8.7).

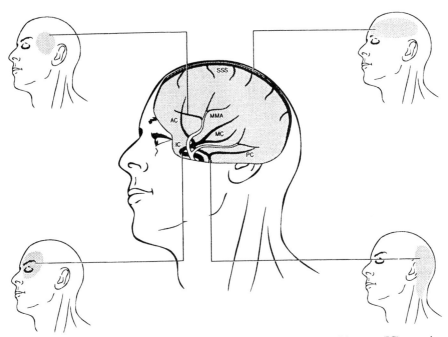

FIGURE 8.7 Referral of pain from intracranial vessels. Internal carotid artery (IC), anterior cerebral artery (AC), middle cerebral artery (MC), posterior cerebral artery (PC), middle meningeal artery (MMA), and superior sagittal sinus (SSS). (Fields of referral are based on the observations of Wolff, 1963.)

Stimulation of the intracranial segment of the internal carotid artery and the proximal 2 cm of the middle cerebral and anterior cerebral arteries causes referred pain to the area in and around the eye, including forehead and temple. The vertebral artery causes referred pain to the occiput. Pain elicited from the superior sagittal sinus is less intense than that evoked from cerebral arteries and is felt in the frontoparietal area on the side stimulated (Wolff, 1963) (see Figure 8.7). Inflation of a balloon in the internal carotid and middle cerebral arteries (Nichols et al., 1993) during embolization of arteriovenous malformations has given additional localizing information. The distal internal carotid artery and proximal part of the middle cerebral artery causes discomfort or pain in an area lateral to the eye, whereas the middle third causes retro-orbital pain, and the distal third of the middle cerebral artery causes referred pain above the ipsilateral eye. In general terms, pain arising from the anterior and middle fossae is felt anterior to a line drawn vertically above the ear, whereas pain from the posterior fossa or neck is felt behind that line, although referral of pain from one to the other region is common (Figure 8.8).

Nociceptive Pathways from Dural and Intracranial Vessels

The trigeminal nerve transmits pain from the upper surface of the tentorium and the anterior and middle cranial fossae. In 1851, Arnold described the tentorial

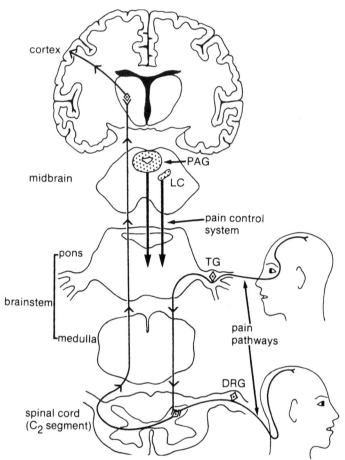

FIGURE 8.8 Pathways serving head pain. The main afferent pathway for the anterior two thirds of the head is the ophthalmic division of the trigeminal nerve. The central axon of the cell body in the trigeminal ganglion (TG) descends in the spinal tract of the trigeminal nerve to the second cervical cord segment, where fibers from the occipital region traverse the dorsal root ganglion (DRG) to converge on second-order neurons. Transmission at this synapse is modulated by the endogenous pain-control system descending from the periaqueductal gray matter (PAG) and the region of the locus coeruleus (LC). (From Lance, 1986, by permission of the publishers, Charles Scribner's Sons, New York.)

nerve, which supplies the superior surface of the tentorium, falx, and venous sinuses. Most of its fibers originate from the ophthalmic division (McNaughton, 1938), so that pain from these structures is referred to the eye and frontoparietal area (see Figure 8.8). In monkeys, trigeminal and sympathetic fibers from the superior cervical ganglion mingle in the wall of the cavernous sinus, forming the cavernous plexus from which the tentorial nerve arises (Ruskell, 1988).

Some parasympathetic fibers from the pterygopalatine (sphenopalatine) ganglion, as well as some fibers from the second trigeminal division, join the plexus anteriorly. Horseradish peroxidase (HRP) tracer studies in cats have shown that recurrent parasympathetic fibers are distributed to the middle cerebral artery (Walters, Gillespie, & Moskowitz, 1986) (Figure 8.9). Applying HRP to the proximal segment of the middle cerebral artery in cats labeled cell bodies in that part of the trigeminal ganglion receiving afferents from the ophthalmic division (Mayberg et al., 1981) (see Figure 8.9). The internal carotid artery and the anterior part of the circle of Willis in monkeys is innervated by branches of the cavernous plexus containing trigeminal and autonomic fibers (Ruskell & Simons, 1987). Other branches of the cavernous plexus pass back with the sixth cranial (abducens) nerve to its origin from the pons, where they join the basilar artery to be distributed to the posterior half of the circle of Willis and vertebral arteries. It is probable that branches of the vagal and glossopharyngeal nerves contribute to the innervation of the posterior circulation.

Afferent fibers from the middle meningeal artery are of trigeminal origin, mainly from the second and third divisions (McNaughton, 1938). The tentorium is the

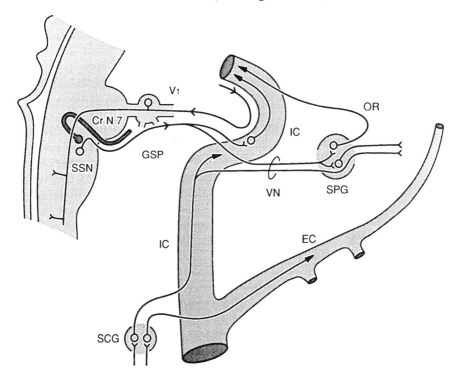

FIGURE 8.9 Autonomic control of the cranial circulation. Parasympathetic fibers arise in the superior salivatory nucleus (SSN) and accompany the facial nerve (CrN7) before branching off as the greater superficial petrosal (GSP) nerve to synapse on cells in the wall of the internal carotid (IC) artery while other fibers pass on with sympathetic fibers in the Vidian nerve (VN) to the sphenopalatine ganglion (SPG). Postganglionic neurons innervate branches of the external carotid (EC) artery, as well as loop back to the internal carotid artery, via orbital rami (OR). Sympathetic fibers from the superior cervical ganglion (SCG) form a plexus in the walls of both internal and external carotid arteries. Afferent fibers from the internal carotid circulation traverse the first division of the trigeminal nerve (V1).

watershed for dural innervation, because its superior surface is supplied by the trigeminal nerve and refers pain to the eye and forehead, whereas its inferior surface and the posterior fossa are supplied primarily by the upper three cervical roots and so refer pain to the occiput and upper neck (see Figure 8.8). The glossopharyngeal and vagal nerves make a small contribution to the dura of the posterior fossa, so that pain may sometimes be referred to the back of the throat or ear.

Transmission of painful impulse at the synapses in the trigemenal nucleus caudalis or dorsal horn is regulated by inhibitory neurones under the control of the endogenous pain-control system (see Figures 8.8 and 8.10).

Neurogenic Plasma Protein Extravasation

Neurogenic plasma extravasation (PPE) can be seen during electrical stimulation of the trigeminal ganglion in the rat (Markowitz, Saito, & Moskowitz,

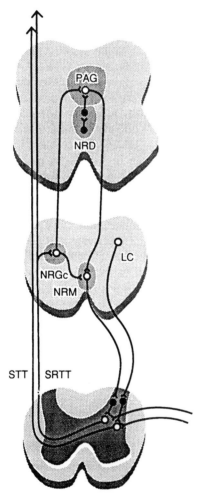

FIGURE 8.10 Simplified version of the endogenous pain-control system. The descending pathway from the periaqueductal gray matter (PAG) excites the nucleus raphe magnus (NRM), which projects together with descending fibers from the region of the locus coeruleus (LC), to inhibitory interneurons in the spinal trigeminal nucleus and dorsal horn of the upper cervical spinal cord. The pain suppression system is activated by ascending fibers in the spinoreticulothalamic tract (SRTT), which accompanies the spinothalamic tract (STT) and synapses in the nucleus reticularis gigantocellularis (NRGc), and is inhibited by neurons from the nucleus raphe dorsalis (NRD) and adjacent reticular formation. O = exciting neurons; ● = inhibitory neurons.

1987). Plasma extravasation can be blocked by ergot alkaloids (Markowitz, Saito, & Moskowitz, 1988), indomethacin, acetylsalicylic acid (Buzzi, Sakas, & Moskowitz, 1989), the serotonin 5-HT$_{1B/1D}$, receptor agonist sumatriptan (Buzzi & Moskowitz, 1990), γ-aminobutyric acid (GABA) agonists such as valproate and benzodiazepines (Lee et al., 1995), neurosteroids (Limmroth et al., 1995), and substance P (SP) antagonists (Cutrer et al., 1995; Lee, Moussaoui, & Moskowitz, 1994). PPE is a plausible explanation for the aggravation of migraine pain by movement and arterial pulsation. It is unlikely to be the fundamental element of dysfunction, nor does it explain all aspects of the syndrome. The phenomenon has not been observed in humans and has been sought with sensitive MRI techniques (Nissila et al., 1996). Furthermore, although bosentan, a potent endothelin antagonist (Clozel et al., 1994), blocks PPE (Brandli et al., 1995), it was ineffective in double-blind placebo-controlled studies in patients with migraine (May et al., 1996). Similarly, substance P, neurokinin-1, receptor antagonists are potent inhibitors of PPE (Lee et al., 1994) but do not work as either acute (Goldstein et al., 1997, Connor et al., 1998; Norman et al., 1998; Diener and The RPR 100893 Study Group, 2003) or preventive (Goldstein et al., 2001) treatments in migraine.

Perhaps most difficult to reconcile in terms of an important role for PPE in migraine is the fact that the highly potent blocker of PPE (Lee & Moskowitz, 1993), the conformationally restricted analog of sumatriptan, CP122,288 (Gupta et al., 1995), is also ineffective in treating acute migraine attacks (Roon et al., 2000). It may be of relevance that both SP antagonists (Hoskin & Goadsby, 1997) and CP122,288 (Knight, Edvinsson, & Goadsby, 1997) are ineffective inhibitors of trigeminocervical complex activation in experimental conditions designed to activate intracranial pain-producing nerves.

Pain and the Intracranial Vessels

Headache does not depend on increased cortical perfusion, because migraine without aura (common migraine) is not usually associated with alteration of regional cerebral blood flow (Olesen et al., 1981), and the headache of migraine with aura (classical migraine) usually starts while blood flow is still reduced (Lauritzen et al., 1983; Olesen et al., 1990) (see Figure 8.6). Kobari et al. (1989) found that cerebral blood flow was increased during migraine headache, but this increase was not related to the side on which headache was experienced. Geraud et al. (1989) described areas of hypoperfusion (clinically silent oligemic areas), as well as regions of hyperperfusion coexisting in patients with migraine without aura. Migrainous headache may be relieved by ergotamine (Norris, Hachinski, & Cooper, 1975) or codeine (Sakai & Meyer, 1978), although cerebral perfusion remains increased.

Transcranial Doppler sonography has been used to assess velocity of flow in proximal branches of the internal carotid artery. Friberg et al. (1991) found that flow in the middle cerebral artery was reduced on the side affected by headache. Because regional cerebral blood flow in the territory supplied by that artery was unaltered, they deduced that dilation of the middle cerebral artery reduced the velocity. The intravenous infusion of 2 mg of the 5-HT agonist sumatriptan relieved the headache within 30 minutes, and the velocity of flow in the middle cerebral artery returned to normal. These observations are reminiscent of comments by Graham and Wolff (1938) concerning the effect of ergotamine on extracranial arteries. They indicate that vascular dilation accompanies some migraine attacks, but it does not necessarily follow that the distension of vessels is entirely responsible for headache. After injecting sumatriptan 4 mg subcutaneously, Diener et al. (1991) could not demonstrate any change of blood flow velocity in the extracranial portions of the internal or external carotid arteries, nor in the middle cerebral or basilar arteries.

Moskowitz (1992) has pointed out that sumatriptan and the ergot alkaloids attenuate the release of neuropeptides from trigeminovascular fibers and may thus play a wider role than vasoconstriction by reducing the "sterile inflammatory response" of migraine headache. The level of the vasodilator substance CGRP in the jugular venous blood, which is elevated during migraine headache, returns to baseline after the headache is relieved by sumatriptan (Goadsby & Edvinsson, 1993). The IV infusion of alpha CGRP in 10 patients prone to migraine precipitated headache, resembling migraine without aura, in three cases after a latent period, suggesting that vasodilation may play a role mediated by CGRP (Lassen et al., 2002) although Kruuse et al.'s observation of migraine triggered by sildenafil without any vascular change suggests dilation is not necessary for an attack to be triggered. The observations of Goltman (1935–1936) on a patient with migraine with a cranial bone defect are interesting in this context. The skull defect was depressed before the headache started and bulged during the headache phase. Lance (1995) has also reported the latter effect.

Pain from Extracranial Arteries

Pain from the supraorbital, frontal, and superficial temporal arteries is mediated by the trigeminal nerve. Afferent fibers from extracranial arteries pursue their course to the trigeminal ganglion separate from the intracranial innervation and are not collaterals of intracranial fibers (Borges & Moskowitz, 1983), so that referred pain must depend on their convergence centrally on second-order neurons. Pain may be referred to the temple in the distribution of the zygomaticotemporal nerve, a branch of the second division of the trigeminal nerve, and the auriculotemporal nerve, which derives from the third division. The upper cervical roots mediate pain from the postauricular and occipital arteries.

Graham and Wolff (1938) recorded the pulsation of branches of the superficial temporal artery during migraine headache and observed that after injection of ergotamine tartrate the amplitude of the pulse wave declined as the intensity of headache diminished. The concept of migraine being an "extracranial vascular headache" appeared to be strengthened by the studies of Tunis and Wolff (1953), who reported that the mean amplitude of temporal artery pulsations was greater during headache than in periods of freedom. This conclusion may have been biased by the fact that after examining 5000 recordings from 75 patients, they selected 10 patients for analysis. In any event, vascular dilation by itself would not cause headache. In periarterial fluid sampled during migraine headache, Chapman et al. (1960) found a substance similar to the polypeptide found in blister fluid, which they named "neurokinin." This bradykinin-like substance was postulated to set up a sterile inflammatory response in the vessel, which thus became pain-producing.

Sakai and Meyer (1978) found that extracranial blood flow increased by about 20% on the side affected by headache. Elkind, Friedman, and Grossman (1964) observed increased clearance of sodium-24 from the skin of the frontotemporal region during migraine attacks. Jensen and Olesen (1985) reported that temporal muscle blood flow increased by about one third during headache, but this did not reach statistical significance, and there was no difference between headache and nonheadache sides. Nevertheless, arteries and veins do become prominent in the temple during migraine, and pressure over them eases the pain.

Blau and Dexter (1981) assessed the contribution of extracranial arteries to migraine headache by inflating a sphygmomanometer cuff around the patient's head. Of 47 patients, only 21 experienced relief from headache after inflation of the pericranial cuff, whereas the majority complained that their headaches were aggravated by coughing, jolting, or holding their breath, indicating an intracranial component to head pain. Drummond and Lance (1983) compared the pulse amplitude of the superficial temporal artery and its main frontotemporal branch with the intensity of pain felt in the temple while the ipsilateral common carotid and temporal arteries were compressed alternately. Of 62 patients, selected only by the presence of a unilateral migrainous headache, the pain appeared to be of extracranial vascular origin in about one third, was of mainly intracranial vascular origin in one third, and had no detectable vascular component in the remaining third. In the subgroup with increased arterial pulsation in the frontotemporal region, thermography demonstrated increased heat loss from this area, and temporal artery compression eased the headache briefly. Although the frontal branches of the temporal artery were found to dilate in one third of patients, Drummond and Lance (1983) could not detect any change in the pulsation of the superficial temporal artery itself. Iversen et al. (1990) have since demonstrated by Doppler studies that the lumen of the temporal artery is increased during ipsilateral migraine headache relative to that of the opposite side and the lumen of peripheral arteries. They interpreted this as a generalized vasoconstriction, sparing the temporal artery on the headache side. These studies make clear that the extracranial circulation contributes to the pain of migraine headache in only a minority of patients.

Neuropeptides and Headache: Linking Experimental and Human Observations

Studies of cranial venous neuropeptide levels have proved valuable in elucidating some of the mechanisms involved in primary headaches (Figures 8.11 and 8.12). Stimulation of the trigeminal ganglion in the cat leads to a rise in cranial venous levels of both SP and CGRP. Similarly, stimulation of the trigeminal ganglion in humans undergoing thermocoagulation for trigeminal neuralgia leads to increases in the cranial venous outflow of both peptides (Goadsby, Edvinsson, & Ekman, 1988). More specific stimulation of pain-producing intracranial structures, such as the superior sagittal sinus, also results in cranial venous release of CGRP but not of SP (Zagami, Goadsby, & Edvinsson, 1990). During migraine, CGRP is elevated in the external jugular vein blood, whereas SP is not, both in

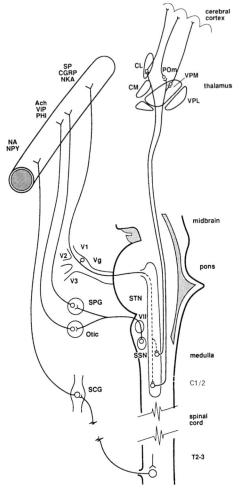

FIGURE 8.11   Peptide neurotransmitters associated with afferent and efferent pathways in the trigeminovascular system. Vascular afferent fibers have their cell bodies in the Gasserian ganglion (V_g) and descend in the spinal tract of the trigeminal nerve before synapsing in the nucleus caudalis and the upper cervical (C1–2) segments of the spinal cord, the trigeminocervical complex. The second-order neurons project to the ventroposterome-dial (VPM) nucleus, the intralaminar or centrolateral (CL) nuclei of the thalamus, and the medial nucleus of the posterior complexes (POm). The centromedian (CM) and the ventro-posterolateral (VPL) nuclei are also marked on the diagram. Other structures that take part in migraine are the trigeminovascular system, marked by the neuropeptides substance P (SP), calcitonin gene–related peptide (CGRP), and neurokinin A (NKA); sympathetic fibers origi-nating in the superior cervical ganglion (SCG) marked by noradrenaline (NA), and neuropep-tide Y (NPY); and parasympathetic fibers arising in the superior salivatory nucleus (SSN) that emerge in the seventh cranial nerve (VII) and traverse the ptyergopalatine, (sphenopalatine ganglion) (SPG) and otic ganglion, marked by vasoactive intestinal polypeptide (VIP), pep-tide histidine methionine (PHM), and acetylcholine (ACh). (From Goadsby, Zagami, & Lambert, 1991, by permission of the editor of *Headache*.)

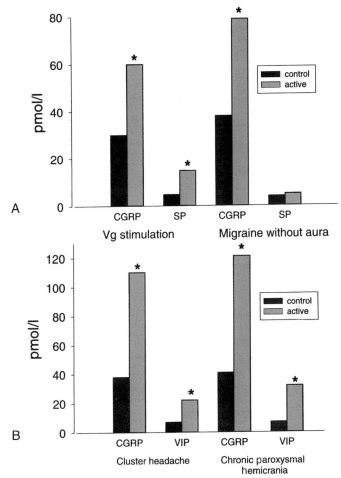

FIGURE 8.12 Neuropeptide release during primary headaches. Trigeminovascular activation with direct stimulation of the trigeminal ganglion and in migraine *(A)* and cluster headache and chronic paroxysmal hemicrania *(B)*, as reflected by elevations in calcitonin gene–related peptide (CGRP) but not substance P (SP) compared with elevation of both peptides during trigeminal ganglion (Vg) stimulation in humans.

adults (Goadsby, Edvinsson, & Ekman, 1990) and in adolescents (Gallai et al., 1995).

These data clearly demonstrate activation of trigeminovascular neurons during migraine with or without aura. Similarly, CGRP but not SP is elevated during acute attacks of cluster headache, both spontaneous (Goadsby & Edvinsson, 1994) and provoked (Fanciullacci et al., 1995), and during the pain of chronic paroxysmal hemicrania (Goadsby & Edvinsson, 1996). To understand the pathophysiology of cluster headache, note that vasoactive intestinal polypeptide (VIP), a marker for cranial parasympathetic nerve activation, is also elevated in cluster headache and paroxysmal hemicrania (Goadsby & Edvinsson, 1994; Goadsby & Edvinsson,

1996). Moreover, treatment with sumatriptan reduces CGRP levels in humans as their migraine subsides and in experimental animals during trigeminal ganglion stimulation (Goadsby & Edvinsson, 1993). Similarly, treatment with avitriptan, a potent clinically effective 5-HT agonist (Couch, Saper, & Meloche, 1996; Ryan, Elkind, & Goldstein, 1997), blocks CGRP release in experimental animals, whereas administration of the potent blocker of neurogenic PPE CP122,288 is not effective at doses specific for PPE (Knight, Edvinsson, & Goadsby, 1997). The release of these peptides offers the prospect of a marker for migraine that can be measured in a venous blood sample. Immunoreactivity to 5-HT$_{1D}$, CGRP, and SP is co-localized on fibers in the spinal trigeminal tract of human brainstem, suggesting that 5-HT mechanism are involved in the release of these vasoactive peptides (Smith et al., 2002).

Pain from Other Extracranial Structures

Disorders of the upper cervical spine refer pain to the occiput related to the distribution of the second and third cervical roots. Pain may also be felt behind the eye of the same side (Kerr, 1961), because pain fibers from the upper cervical roots converge with those in the spinal tract of the trigeminal nerve on neurons in the dorsolateral quadrant of the upper cervical cord (Goadsby & Hoskin, 1997; Goadsby, Hoskin, & Knight, 1997) (see Figure 8.8). The interaction of these inputs is presented on page 100 (Bartsch & Goadsby, 2002, 2003).

Trigeminal and cervical distribution overlap much more than previously realized. Denny-Brown and Yanagisawa (1973) sectioned the sensory root of one trigeminal nerve in a monkey and found the expected sensory loss over the anterior two thirds of the face and scalp. When the animal was given a subconvulsive dose of strychnine, the area of anesthesia receded until the only unresponsive region was around the eye, cheek, and upper lip, apparently the only area innervated exclusively by the fifth cranial nerve. Conversely, sections of the second, third, and fourth cervical dorsal roots produced a sensory loss over the occipital region and upper neck, which after administration of strychnine shrank to a thin band around the neck. When trigeminal and cervical inflow were both destroyed, there was still an area of innervation by the vagus and facial nerves around the ear, which under the influence of strychnine spread in a wedge shape to supply the posterior half of the scalp. It has not been appreciated that the vagus nerve, through its communication with auriculotemporal and posterior temporal branches, supplies the ear and a large part of the scalp. Whether this can be applied to help the patient with headache remains to be seen.

Muscle Contraction

Pain from muscle contraction may add a nonvascular component to migraine headache. Excessive contraction of the temporal, masseter, and neck muscles is common in patients with migraine (Lous & Olsen, 1982), more so than in patients with "tension headache," and becomes evident just before the headache reaches its maximum (Bakke et al., 1982). Tfelt-Hansen, Lous, and Olesen (1981) found that infiltration of tender muscle areas with local anesthetic or normal saline relieved migraine headaches within 70 minutes in 28 of 48 patients.

Serotonin (5-HT) and bradykinin potentiated the pain-producing effects of one another when injected into the temporal muscle of normal volunteers but did not evoke headache (Jensen et al., 1990). The sites of muscle contraction in migraine correlate with the spatial distribution of pain and tenderness, suggesting that muscle contraction is a secondary phenomenon but one that nonetheless contributes to headache.

Central Trigeminal Pain Pathways

The sites within the brainstem that are responsible for craniovascular pain have now begun to be mapped. Using c-Fos-immunocytochemistry, a method for looking at activated cells, after meningeal irritation with blood, expression is reported in the trigeminal nucleus caudalis (Nozaki, Boccalini, & Moskowitz, 1992). After stimulation of the superior sagittal sinus, Fos-like immunoreactivity is seen in monkey (Goadsby & Hoskin, 1997), cat (Kaube et al., 1993), and rat (Strassman, Mineta, & Vos, 1994) subjects in the trigeminal nucleus caudalis and in the dorsal horn at the C1 and C2 levels. These latter findings are in accord with similar data using 2-deoxyglucose measurements with superior sagittal sinus stimulation (Goadsby & Zagami, 1991) and more recent studies demonstrating a similar organization in the monkey (Goadsby & Hoskin, 1997).

These data contribute to our view of the trigeminal nucleus as extending beyond the traditional nucleus caudalis to the dorsal horn of the high cervical region in a functional continuum that includes a cervical extension that could be regarded as a trigeminal nucleus cervicalis. The entire group of cells may be usefully regarded as the trigeminocervical complex, to place emphasis on the integrative role that these neurons have in head pain. The data clearly demonstrate that a substantial portion of trigeminovascular nociceptive information comes by way of the most caudal cells.

The rather diffuse activation of neurons in the trigeminal nucleus in visceral pain, such as that arising from intracranial vessels, is to be contrasted with what is seen when pain stimuli are applied to discrete facial structures. Neuronal activation is more restricted (Strassman & Vos, 1993; Strassman et al., 1993) in line with the relatively good spatial localization of more superficial pain. This concept provides an anatomic explanation for the referral of pain to the back of the head in migraine.

Further direct evidence for the trigeminocervical complex as the site of referred pain comes from an animal study in which the greater occipital nerve, a branch of C2, was directly stimulated and 2-deoxyglucose activation was observed in the entire complex, including the trigeminal nucleus caudalis (Goadsby, Hoskin, & Knight, 1997).

Bartsch and Goadsby (2002) examined cells in the C2 spinal dorsal horns of rats that responded both to stimulation of the supratentorial dura and the greater occipital nerve (GON), to study the interaction between the two inputs. The neuronal responses to dural stimulation were enhanced by stimulating the GON or by applying the C-fiber activator mustard oil to the cutaneous or muscular territories innervated by the GON. In contrast, neurons with combined input that were identified as projecting to the contralateral thalamus by antidromic stimulation responded more readily to GON stimulation when the background activation from the dura was augmented by applying mustard oil to it (Bartsch &

Goadsby, 2003). This mutual sensitization of input from neck and dura under-scores the reciprocal relationship underlying the referral of pain from trigeminal territory to the neck and vice-versa. It is relevant that suboccipital stimulators have been successful in relieving chronic migraine (Matharu et al., 2004).

Autoradiographic studies have demonstrated that $5\text{-HT}_{1B/1D/1F}$ receptors are all present in the trigeminocervical complex (Castro et al., 1997; Goadsby & Knight, 1997). Various antimigraine drugs such as ergots, acetylsalicylic acid, naratriptan, eletripton zolmitriptan, rizatriptan, and sumatriptan (after disruption of the blood–brain barrier) reduce activity of these second-order neurons, which have the potential of being sites for their central action.

Researchers had assumed that triptans blocked trigeminal transmission by a presynaptic mechanism, but Goadsby, Akerman, and Storer (2001) showed that second-order neurons excited by the iontophoresis of a glutamine agonist were significantly less responsive when sumatriptan was co-injected.

Following transmission in the caudal brainstem and high cervical spinal cord, information is relayed in a group of fibers (the quintothalamic tract) to the thalamus (see Figure 8.11). Processing of vascular pain in the thalamus occurs in the ventroposteromedial thalamus, medial nucleus of the posterior complex, and intralaminar thalamus (Zagami & Goadsby, 1991; Zagami & Lambert, 1990). Zagami and Lambert (1991) have shown, by applying cap-saicin to the superior sagittal sinus, that trigeminal projections with a high degree of nociceptive input are processed in neurons particularly in the ventro-posteromedial thalamus and in its ventral periphery. The properties and further higher-center connections of these neurons are the subject of ongoing studies that will help build a more complete picture of the trigeminovascular pain pathways.

The Role of Central Nervous System Modulation in Migraine Pain

Even in periods of freedom from migraine, people with migraine carry with them susceptibility to head pain. Raskin and Knittle (1976) found that cold drinks or ice cream evoked headache in 93% of patients with migraine, com-pared with only 31% of control subjects. One third of patients with ice cream headache state that this pain involves precisely the same part of the head as their habitual migraine headaches (Drummond & Lance, 1984). Moreover, 42% of patients with migraine are prone to sudden jabs of pain in the head ("ice-pick pains" or primary stabbing headache), compared with 3% of controls without headache (Raskin & Schwartz, 1980). Drummond and Lance (1984) found that ice-pick pains coincided with the site of the customary headache in 40% of patients. The trigeminal pathways may thus become activated spontaneously in paroxysms lasting a fraction of a second (ice-pick pains) or may be activated reflexively for seconds or minutes by sudden cooling of the pharynx (ice cream headache). This indicates a persisting disinhibition of a segment of the trigemi-nal pathways in patients with migraine, suggesting that the trigeminal system could also discharge excessively for hours or days to provide a neural origin for migraine headache. During headache, sensitivity to pressure is increased over the areas where pain is felt but can be normal or increased in the fingers

(Drummond, 1987), so that any defect in pain control mechanisms appears localized to the affected areas.

Stimulation of the periaqueductal gray matter (PAG) by indwelling electrodes is used in the control of otherwise intractable bodily pain (Baskin et al., 1986). Raskin, Hosobuchi, and Lamb (1987) reported that 15 of 175 patients developed migraine-like headaches after the electrode insertion. This observation was confirmed by Veloso and Kumer (1996), who found that 15 of 64 patients implanted had developed unilateral headaches for the first time. Thus the endogenous pain-control system can apparently be switched on or off from the periaqueductal gray matter (see Figure 8.10), and switching off can permit the development of headache with the characteristics of migraine.

Weiller et al. (1995) demonstrated by PET scan an area of activation in the midbrain and upper pons encompassing the nucleus raphe dorsalis, locus ceruleus, and PAG contralateral to the side of migraine headache in nine patients. Bahra et al. (2001) found activation in the dorsolateral pens glyceryl trinitrate precipitated migraine without aura. Activation persists after pain subsides under the influence of sumatriptan, suggesting that it was not simply a response to pain but may have some "generator function" for migraine. This view is supported by the fact that the same changes do not arise in pain from other sources such as cluster headache or the injection of capsaicin into the forehead of experimental subjects (May et al., 1998).

Suboccipital stimulation, which relieves chronic migraine (Matharu et al., 2004), increases regional cerebral blood flow demonstrated by PET scanning in the dorsal rostral pons and anterior cingulate cortex, areas activated in episodic migraine. The upper pontine/midbrain area (PAG) is implicated in the endogenous pain-control system but does not differ in MRI morphometry between migrainous and control subjects (Matharu et al., 2003). Microinjecting a P/Q-type calcium channel-blocking agent into the rat ventrolateral PAG increases the response of trigeminal second-order neurons in nucleus caudalis to dural stimulation (Knight et al., 2002), suggesting that dysfunctional P/Q-type calcium channels may play a part in the increased pain perception of migraine headache.

Neural Control of the Cranial Circulation and Endogenous Pain-Control Systems

The brainstem nuclei innervating the cerebral circulation are in a unique position to influence brain blood flow while also being involved in nociceptive processing from pain-producing craniovascular structures. This dual role provides a focus for special attention to neurovascular anatomy and physiology in the context of *neurovascular headache.*

Brainstem Influences

Cerebral vascular resistance increases (that is, blood flow falls) by about 20% with low-frequency stimulation of the locus ceruleus (LC) in the monkey (Goadsby, Lambert, & Lance, 1982). Regional cerebral blood flow diminishes in the cat, particularly in the occipital cortex (Goadsby & Duckworth, 1987).

However, external carotid resistance diminishes (i.e., blood flow increases) as the frequency of LC stimulation increases. The extracranial vasodilator effect was later shown to be mediated by the greater superficial petrosal (GSP) branch of the facial nerve (Goadsby, Lambert, & Lance, 1983) (see Figure 8.9). These changes, which were predominantly ipsilateral, bear a striking resemblance to the vascular changes accompanying migraine with aura. This effect of LC stimulation is presumably exerted on the microcirculation, because it does not produce any consistent change in the discharge frequency of cells in the cat occipital cortex (Adams, Lambert, & Lance, 1989). In contrast, stimulating the nucleus raphe dorsalis increases cerebral blood flow in the monkey; in the cat and monkey, it dilates both internal and external carotid circulation through connections with the facial (GSP) nerve (Goadsby et al., 1985a, 1985b). The degree of extracranial vasodilation is comparable with the reflex effects of LC stimulation.

Extrinsic (Autonomic) Influences

Thermocoagulation of the Gasserian ganglion for tic douloureux, a procedure that would be very painful if the patient was not anesthetized, produces a facial flush in the distribution of the division or divisions coagulated (Drummond, Gonski, & Lance, 1983) (see Figure 18.1). Lambert et al. (1984) showed that electrical stimulation of the Gasserian ganglion in cats diminished carotid resistance and increased blood flow and facial temperature by a reflex pathway traversing the trigeminal root, as its afferent limb, and the GSP branch of the facial nerve, as its efferent limb, a phenomenon known as the "trigeminovascular reflex" (see Figures 8.3 and 8.4). A minor component of the response, particularly that elicited from the third division, persisted after section of the trigeminal root, almost certainly caused by the liberation of vasoactive peptides from antidromic activation of trigeminal nerve terminals. The main reflex vasodilator response to stimulation of the LC, raphe nuclei, or the trigeminal nerve is mediated by the sphenopalatine and otic ganglia (Goadsby, Lambert, & Lance, 1984) and employs vasoactive intestinal polypeptide (VIP) as its neurovascular transmitter (Goadsby & Macdonald, 1985).

A pathway has therefore been established that can account for extracranial vascular dilation accompanying a primary pain-producing excitation of trigeminal pathways, a mechanism that is relevant to the vascular changes of migraine.

Interrelationship Between Intrinsic and Extrinsic Craniovascular Innervation

Activation of the trigeminal nerve or nucleus raphe dorsalis or high-frequency stimulation of the LC increases cerebral and extracranial blood flow through their connections with the GSP nerve (Lance et al., 1983; Goadsby & Lance, 1988) (see Figures 8.1 and 8.2). Trigeminal nerve terminals can also release vasodilator peptides antidromically to increase cerebral blood flow in cats (Lambert et al., 1984) and promote the leakage of plasma protein from blood vessels in the rat dura mater (Markowitz, Saito, & Moskowitz, 1987).

There are thus two ways in which pain-mediating trigeminal pathways can cause cerebral, dural, and extracranial blood flow to increase: reflexively via the parasympathetic outflow in the GSP nerve and directly by the antidromic release of vasodilator peptides (Goadsby, Edvinsson, & Ekman, 1988, 1990; Goadsby & Edvinsson, 1993, 1994).

The vascular effects evoked from the LC and nucleus raphe dorsalis, which are predominantly unilateral, simulate flow changes reported in patients with migraine headache, which could therefore be secondary to neural changes in the brainstem. The LC appears to exert an inhibitory influence on the contralateral locus (Buda et al., 1975), which could be the basis for unilateral cerebral changes alternating from hemisphere to hemisphere in migraine. The identification, using PET, of areas of activation in humans during migraine in regions of the periaqueductal gray matter and dorsolateral pontine tegmentum (Weiller et al., 1995), which contain the nucleus raphe dorsalis and LC, respectively, is consistent with an aminergic dysmodulation in the brainstem, accounting for many features of the migraine syndrome.

The Implication of 5-Hydroxytryptamine (5-HT, Serotonin) in the Migraine Syndrome

5-Hydroxytryptamine has long been considered as a possible mediator of the migraine syndrome because of its action on blood vessels, renal function, and the gastrointestinal tract. It became a serious contender when Sicuteri (1959) reported that methysergide, a known 5-HT antagonist, was of value in preventing migraine. Kimball, Friedman, and Vallejo (1960), in a brief but influential paper, noted that the intramuscular injection of 2.5 mg of reserpine, which releases 5-HT from body stores, induced a typical headache in 10 of 15 patients with migraine. They also found that the intravenous injection of 5-HT 5 mg relieved migraine headache in five patients with spontaneous attacks but caused transient dyspnea, faintness, flushing, and paraesthesias.

Sicuteri et al. (1961) showed that the urinary output of the principal catabolite of 5-HT, 5-hydroxyindoleacetic acid (5-HIAA), increased during migraine headache, with the mean daily excretion rising from 4 mg to 10.6 mg. Curran, Hinterberger, and Lance (1965) confirmed this, finding that 5-HIAA excretion increased in 15 of 22 headaches and also reported that the content of 5-HT in platelets fell at the onset of migraine headache. Anthony et al. (1967) followed this up in 15 patients, finding that the 5-HT level dropped in 20 of 21 headaches studied, by an average of 45% (Figure 8.13). No change was found in patients with headache following pneumoencephalography or in those undergoing stressful procedures such as angiography. The content of 5-HT in platelets fell, as would be expected, in 9 out of 10 patients after the intravenous injection of reserpine 2.5 mg, which caused a typical headache in patients with migraine but only a dull ache in subjects not prone to migraine. The intravenous injection of 5-HT 2 to 7.5 mg eased both spontaneous and reserpine-induced migraine. Anthony, Hinterberger, and Lance (1969) went on to show that the incubation of platelets with platelet-free plasma taken during headache caused 5-HT to be released, but this did not occur when platelets were incubated with postheadache plasma. This observation, that a 5-HT–releasing factor was present in the plasma during migraine headache, was supported by findings from other laboratories (Dvilansky et al., 1976; Muck-Zeler, Deanovic, & Dupelj, 1979; Launay & Pradalier, 1985) but could not be replicated by Ferrari et al. (1987). The latter

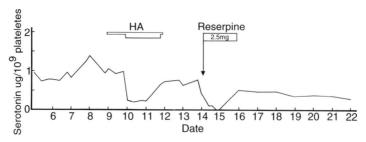

FIGURE 8.13 Blood platelets discharge serotonin at the onset of spontaneous or induced migraine headache. The bar labeled *HA* indicates a sensation of heaviness in the head followed by typical migraine headache. (From Anthony, Hinterberger, & Lance, 1967, by permission of the editor of *Archives of Neurology*.)

group reported that platelet 5-HT content fell only in migraine without aura but that the level of free 5-HT in plasma increased by more than 100% during migraine headache regardless of whether it was preceded by an aura (Ferrari et al., 1989). Platelet dense bodies, the storage organelles for 5-HT, are increased in migraine with aura (D'Andrea et al., 1989b). The 5-HT–releasing factor in migraine has not been identified but is of molecular weight less than 50,000. Free fatty acids are possible contenders (Anthony, 1978).

AN ATTEMPTED SYNTHESIS

The cardinal features of migraine are recurrent headache and its association with transient neurologic symptoms. The headache, usually felt in the region of distribution of the trigeminal nerve and upper cervical roots, implies unrestrained firing of cells in the spinal trigeminal nucleus and its extension into the upper cervical cord. On occasions, migrainous pain may spread to the shoulder, arm, and even to the lower limb, suggesting that cells in the basal nuclei of the thalamus may also be involved. The frequency of "ice-pick pains" and "ice cream headache" in patients with migraine indicates that this part of their pain control system is defective, permitting a high-frequency neuronal discharge spontaneously or in response to a cold stimulus. Such an unstable system may then respond by a continuous discharge when subjected to stimulation from higher centers (cortex, hypothalamus) as the result of stress or by excessive afferent input from the special senses or from cerebral or extracranial vessels.

The aura phase of migraine may take the form of a slow advance of neurologic symptoms, explicable by a phenomenon similar to the spreading cortical depression of Leão, or may affect cortical function more diffusely without any stepwise progression of symptoms being apparent. If spreading depression is responsible for fortification spectra in migraine, the way in which it is produced remains uncertain. Does it arise in the cortex, or is it induced by subcortical structures?

An animal model is available for the reported vascular changes of migraine (Goadsby & Lance, 1988). As outlined earlier, the LC can induce cerebral vasoconstriction and extracranial vasodilation in monkeys, and the nucleus raphe dorsalis can dilate both circulations. A similar mechanism in human patients could account for the vascular changes of migraine being secondary to brainstem activity. Once activated centrally or peripherally, the trigeminal system may promote the leakage of plasma protein from dural vessels and increase blood flow intracranially and extracranially by antidromic discharge and by a reflex connection with the parasympathetic outflow through the GSP nerve (see Figure 8.9).

Following a phase of monoaminergic excitation, a phase of depletion could follow, thus reducing the activity of the endogenous pain-control system, removing the remaining restraint on the discharge of neurons in the spinal tract of the trigeminal nerve. The resulting headache could be aggravated by afferent impulses from dilated cerebral and extracranial arteries.

This explanation of the interaction between the brain and its vascular supply in the causation of migraine is speculative but even in light of newer human functional imaging studies remains plausible and consistent with clinical observations and the information gained from animal experimentation.

SUMMARY

Migraine is a neurovascular reaction in response to sudden changes in the internal or external environment. Each individual has a hereditary migrainous threshold, with the degree of susceptibility depending on the balance between excitation and inhibition at various levels of the nervous system. Such a balance may be influenced by magnesium deficiency, excitatory amino acids, monoamines, opioids, and other factors outlined earlier. Neural and vascular elements both contribute to headache.

The mechanism of migraine has been presented as an unstable trigeminovascular reflex with a segmental defect in the pain control pathway, thus permitting excessive discharge of part of the spinal nucleus of the trigeminal nerve and its thalamic connections in response to excessive afferent input or corticobulbar drive. The end result is interaction between brainstem and cranial blood vessels, with the afferent impulses from the latter intensifying pain perception through the trigeminovascular reflex. Diffuse projections from the LC to the cerebral cortex could initiate cortical oligemia and possibly spread depression. Activity in this system could account for the migrainous aura, which may occur quite independently of the headache, although one commonly follows the other. The headache phase may be interrupted by therapy aimed at either the central or peripheral end of the trigeminovascular reflex.

There is strong evidence that 5-HT plays an important part in the genesis of migraine. It remains uncertain whether the place of 5-HT lies in central pain-control pathways, in the serotonergic projection to the cerebral cortex, in a direct action on the cranial blood vessels, or in its action at all three sites. Probably the primary action of specific antimigraine treatments, such as sumatriptan or ergotamine, in terminating migraine headache is exerted on the cerebral and extracranial vascular and dural structures and their trigeminal innervation, whereas preventive medications may act centrally.

References

Adams, R. W., Lambert, G. A., & Lance, J. W. (1989). Stimulation of brain stem nuclei in the cat: Effect on neuronal activity in the primary visual cortex of relevance to cerebral blood flow and migraine. *Cephalalgia, 9*, 107–118.

Ambrosini, A., de Noordhout, A. M., Sándor, P. S., & Schoenen, J. (2003). Electrophysiological studies in migraine: A comprehensive review of their interest and limitations. *Cephalalgia, 23*(Suppl. 1), 13–31.

Andersen, A. R., Friberg, L., Skyhöj-Olsen, T., & Olesen, J. (1988). SPECT demonstration of delayed hyperemia following hypoperfusion in classic migraine. *Arch Neurol, 45*, 154–159.

Anthony, M. (1978). Role of individual free fatty acids in migraine. In A. P. Friedman, Granger, M. E. Critchley, M. (Eds.), *Research and clinical studies in headache* (vol. 6, pp 110–116). Basel: Karger.

Anthony, M., Hinterberger, H., & Lance, J. W. (1967). Plasma serotonin in migraine and stress. *Arch Neurol, 16*, 544–552.

Anthony, M., Hinterberger, H., & Lance, J. W. (1969). The possible relationship of serotonin to the migraine syndrome. In A. P. Friedman (Ed.), *Research and clinical studies in headache* (Vol. 2, pp. 29–59). Basel: Karger.

Bach, F. W., Jensen, K., Blegvad, N., Fenger, M., Jordal, R., & Olesen, J. (1985). β-Endorphin and ACTH in plasma during attacks of common and classic migraine. *Cephalalgia, 5*, 177–182.

Bahra, A., Matharu, M. S., Buchel, C., Frackowiak, R. S., & Goadsby, P. J. (2001). Brainstem activation specific to migraine headache. *Lancet, 357*, 1016–1017.

Bakke, M., Tfelt-Hansen, P., Olesen, J., & Möller, E. (1982). Action of some pericranial muscles during provoked attacks of common migraine. *Pain, 14*, 121–135.

Barkley, G. L., Tepley, S., Nagel-Leiby, S., Moran, J. E., Simkins, R. T., & Welch, K. M. (1990). Magnetoenceph- ographic studies of migraine. *Headache, 30*, 428–434.

Bartsch, T., & Goadsby, P. J. (2002). Stimulation of the greater occipital nerve induces increased central excitability of dural afferent input. *Brain, 125*, 1496–1509.

Bartsch, T., & Goadsby, P. J. (2003). Increased responses in trigeminocervical nociceptive neurons to cervical input after stimulation of the dura mater. *Brain, 126*, 1801–1813.

Baskin, D. S., Mehler, W. R., Hosobuchi, Y., Richardson, D. E., Adams, J. E., & Flitter, M. A. (1986). Autopsy analysis of the safety, efficacy and cartography of electrical stimulation of the central gray in humans. *Brain Res, 371*, 231–236.

Blau, J. N. (1980). Migraine prodromes separated from the aura; complete migraine. *BMJ, 21*, 658–660.

Blau, J. N., & Dexter, S. L. (1981). The site of pain origin during migraine attacks. *Cephalalgia, 1*, 143–147.

Bolay, H., Reuter, U., Dunn, A. K., Huang, Z., Boas, D. A., & Moskowitz, M. A. (2002). Intrinsic brain activity triggers trigeminal meningeal afferents in a migraine model. *Nat Med, 8*, 136–142.

Borges, L. F., & Moskowitz, M. A. (1983). Do intracranial and extracranial trigeminal afferents represent divergent axon collaterals? *Neurosci Lett, 35*, 265–70.

Brandli, P., Loffler, B. M., Breu, V., Osterwalder, R., Maire, J. P., & Clozel, M. (1996). Role of endothelin in mediating neurogenic plasma extravasation in rat dura mater. *Pain, 64*, 315–322.

Brindley, G. S., & Lewin, W. S. (1968). The sensations produced by electrical stimulation of the visual cortex. *J Physiol, 196*, 479–493.

Buda, M., Roussel, B., Renard, B., & Pujol, J.-F. (1975). Increase in tyrosine hydroxylase activity in the locus coeruleus of the rat brain after contralateral lesioning. *Brain Res, 93*, 564–569.

Buzzi, M. G., & Moskowitz, M. A. (1990). The antimigraine drug, sumatriptan (GR43175), selectively blocks neurogenic plasma extravasation from blood vessels in dura mater. *Br J Pharmacol, 99*, 202–206.

Buzzi, M. G., Sakas, D. E., & Moskowitz, M. A. (1989). Indomethacin and acetylsalicylic acid block neurogenic plasma protein extravasation in rat dura mater. *Eur J Pharmacol, 165*, 251–258.

Cao, Y., Aurora, S. K., Nagesh, V., Patel, S. C., & Welch, K. M. (2002). Functional MRI-BOLD of brainstem structures during visually triggered migraine. *Neurology, 59*, 72–78.

Castro, M. E., Pascual., J., Romon, T., del Arco, C., del Olmo, E., & Pazos, A. (1997). Differential distribution of sumatriptan binding sites (5-HT1B, 5-HT1D and 5-HT1F receptors) in human brain: Focus on brainstem and spinal cord. *Neuropharmacology, 36*, 535–542.

Chapman, L. F., Ramos, A. O., Goodell, H., Silverman, G., & Wolff, H. G. (1960). A humoral agent implicated in vascular headache of the migrainous type. *Arch Neurol, 3*, 223–229.

Clozel, M., Breu, V., & Gray, A. G. (1994). Pharmacological characterisation of bosentan, a new potent orally active nonpeptide endothelin receptor antagonist. *J Pharmacol Exp Ther, 270*, 228–235.

Conner, H. E., Bertin, L., Gillies, S., Beattie, D. T., & Ward, P. (1998). The GR205171 Clinical Study Group. Clinical evaluation of a novel, potent, CNS penetrating NK_1 receptor antagonist in the acute treatment of migraine. *Cephalalgia, 18,* 392.

Couch, J. R., Saper, J., & Meloche, J. P. (1986). Treatment of migraine with BMS180048: Response at 2 hours. *Headache, 36,* 523–530.

Curran, D. A., Hinterberger, H., & Lance, J. W. (1965). Total plasma serotonin, 5-hydroxyindoleacetic acid and *p*-hydroxy-m-methoxymandelic acid excretion in normal and migrainous subjects. *Brain, 88,* 997–1010.

Cutrer, F. M., Garret, C., Moussaoui, S. M., & Moskowitz, M. A. (1995). The non-peptide neurokinin-1 antagonist, RPR 100893, decreases c-Fos expression in trigeminal nucleus caudalis following noxious chemical meningeal stimulation. *Neuroscience, 64,* 741–750.

Cutrer, F. M., Sorensen, A. G., Weisskoff, R. M., Ostergaurd, L., Sanchez del Rio, M., Lee, E. J., et al. (1998). Perfusion-weighted imaging defects during spontaneous migrainous aura. *Ann Neurol, 43,* 25–31.

D'Andrea, G., Cananzi, A. R., & Joseph, R. (1989a). Platelet excitatory amino acids in migraine. *Cephalalgia, 9*(Suppl. 10), 105–106.

D'Andrea, G. K., Welch, K. M. A., Riddle, J. M., Grunfeld, S., & Joseph, R. (1989b). Platelet serotonin metabolism and ultrastructure in migraine. *Arch Neurol, 46,* 1187–1189.

De Fusco, M., Marconi, R., Silvestri, L., Atorino, L., Rampoldi, L., Morgante, L., et al. (2003). Haploinsufficiency of ATP1A2 encoding the Na^+/K^+ pump $\alpha2$ subunit associated with familial hemiplegic migraine type 2. *Nature Genetics, 33,* 192–196.

Denny-Brown, D., & Yanagisawa, N. (1973). The function of the descending root of the fifth nerve. *Brain, 96,* 783–814.

Diener, H. C. (1996). Substance-P antagonist RPR100893-201 is not effective in human migraine attacks. In J. Olesen & P. Tfelt-Hansen (Eds.), *Proceedings of the VIth International Headache Seminar, Copenhagen.* New York: Lippincott-Raven.

Diener, H. C. (2003). The RPR100893 Study Group. RPR100893, a substance-P antagonist is not effective in the treatment of migraine attacks. *Cephalalgia, 23,* 183–185.

Diener, H. C., Haab, J., Peters, C., Reid, S., Dichgars, J., & Pilgrim, A. (1991). Subcutaneous sumatriptan in the treatment of headache during withdrawal from drug-induced headache. *Headache, 31,* 205–209.

Drummond, P. D. (1982). Extracranial and cardiovascular reactivity in migrainous subjects. *J Psychosom Res, 26,* 317–331.

Drummond, P. D. (1987). Scalp tenderness and sensitivity to pain in migraine and tension headache. *Headache, 27,* 45–50.

Drummond, P. D., Gonski, A., & Lance, J. W. (1983). Facial flushing after thermocoagulation of the Gasserian ganglion. *J Neurol Neurosurg Psychiatry, 46,* 611–616.

Drummond, P. D., & Lance, J. W. (1981). Extracranial vascular reactivity in migraine and tension headache. *Cephalalgia, 1,* 149–155.

Drummond, P. D., & Lance, J. W. (1983). Extracranial vascular changes and the source of pain in migraine headache. *Ann Neurol, 13,* 32–37.

Drummond, P. D., & Lance, J. W. (1984). Neurovascular disturbances in headache patients. *Clin Exp Neurol, 20,* 93–99.

Ducros, A., Joutel, A., Vahedi, K., Cecillon, M., Lopez de Munain, A., Bernard, E., et al. (1997). Familial hemiplegic migraine: Mapping of the second gene and evidence for a third locus. *Cephalalgia, 17,* 232.

Dvilansky. A., Rishpon, S., Nathan, I., Zolotow, Z., & Korczyn, A. D. (1976). Release of platelet 5-hydroxytryptamine by plasma taken from patients during and between migraine attacks. *Pain, 2,* 315–318.

Ebersberger, A., Schaible, H.-G., Averbeck, B., & Richter, F. (2001). Is there a correlation between spreading depression, neurogenic inflammation and nociception that might cause migraine headache? *Ann Neurol, 49,* 7–13.

Elkind, A. H., Friedman, A. P., & Grossman, J. (1964). Cutaneous blood flow in vascular headache of the migrainous type. *Neurology, Minneap, 14,* 24–30.

Evers, S., Quibeldey, F., Grotemeyer, K. H., Suhr, B., & Husstedt, I. W. (1999). Dynamic changes of cognitive habituation and serotonin metabolism during the migraine interval. *Cephalalgia, 19,* 485–491.

Fanciullacci, M., Alessandri, M., Figini, M., Geppetti, P., & Michelacci, S. (1995). Increases in plasma calcitonin gene–related peptide from extracerebral circulation during nitroglycerin-induced cluster headache attack. *Pain, 60,* 119–123.

Fanciullacci, M., Franchi, G., & Sicuteri, F. (1974). Hypersensitivity to lysergic acid diethylamide (LSD-25) and psilocybin in essential headache. *Experentia, 30,* 1441–1442.

Fanciullacci, M., Michelacci, S., Curradi, C., & Sicuteri, F. (1980). Hyper-responsiveness of migraine patients to the hypotensive action of bromocriptine. *Headache, 20,* 99–102.

Ferrari, M. D., Frolich, M., & Odink, J., (1987). Methionine-enkephalin and serotonin in migraine and tension headache. In F. Clifford Rose (Ed.), *Current Problems in Neurology. Vol. 4. Advances in headache research* (pp. 227–234). London: John Libbey.

Ferrari, M. D., Odink, J., Box, K. D., Malessy, M. J., & Bruyn, G. W. (1990). Neuroexcitatory plasma amino acids are elevated in migraine. *Neurology, 40,* 1582–1586.

Ferrari, M. D., Odink, J., Tapparelli, C., Van Kampen, G. M., Pennings, E. J., & Bruyn, G. W. (1989). Serotonin metabolism in migraine. *Neurology, 39,* 1239–1242.

Friberg, L., Olesen, J., Iversen, H. K., & Sperling, B. (1991). Migraine pain associated with middle cerebral artery dilatation-reversal by sumatriptan. *Lancet, 338,* 13–17.

Gallai, V., Sarchielli, P., Floridi, A., Franceschini, M., Codini, M., Glioti, G., et al. (1995). Vasoactive peptide levels in the plasma of young migraine patients with and without aura assessed both interictally and ictally. *Cephalalgia, 15,* 384–390.

Géraud, G., Besson, M., Fabre, M., Danet, B., & Bes, A. (1989). Heterogenous cerebral blood flow during spontaneous attacks of migraine with and without aura: a Tc-99m HMPAO SPECT study. *Cephalalgia, 9*(Suppl. 10), 31–32.

Gloor, P. (1986). Migraine and regional cerebral blood flow. *Trends Neurosci, 2,* 21.

Goadsby, P. J. (1992). The oligemic phase of cortical spreading depression is not blocked by tirilazad mesylate (U-74006F). *Brain Res, 588,* 140–143.

Goadsby, P. J. (1997). Bench to bedside: What have we learnt recently about headache? *Curr Opin Neurol, 10,* 215–220.

Goadsby, P. J., & Duckworth, J. W. (1987). Locus coeruleus stimulation leads to reductions in regional cerebral blood flow in the cat. *J Cereb Blood Flow Metabol, 7,* S221.

Goadsby, P. J., & Edvinsson, L. (1993). The trigeminovascular system and migraine: studies characterising cerebrovascular and neuropeptide changes seen in man and cat. *Ann Neurol, 33,* 48–56.

Goadsby, P. J., & Edvinsson, L. (1994). Human in vivo evidence for trigeminovascular activation in cluster headache. *Brain, 117,* 427–434.

Goadsby, P. J., & Edvinsson, L. (1996). Neuropeptide changes in a case of chronic paroxysmal hemicrania—evidence for trigemino-parasympathetic activation. *Cephalalgia, 16,* 448–450.

Goadsby, P. J., Edvinsson, L., & Ekman, R. (1988). Release of vasoactive peptides in the extracerebral circulation of man and the cat during activation of the trigeminovascular system. *Ann Neurol, 23,* 193–196.

Goadsby, P. J., Edvinsson, L., & Ekman, R. (1990). Vasoactive peptide release in the extracerebral circulation of humans during migraine headache. *Ann Neurol, 28,* 183–187.

Goadsby, P. J., & Gundlach, A. L. (1991). Localization of dihydroergotamine binding sites in the cat central nervous system: Relevance to migraine. *Ann Neurol, 29,* 91–94.

Goadsby, P. J., & Hoskin, K. L. (1997). The distribution of trigeminovascular afferents in the non-human primate brain Macaca nemestrina: A c-Fos immunocytochemical study. *J Anat, 190,* 367–375.

Goadsby, P. J., & Knight, Y. E., & Hoskin, K. L. (1997). Stimulation of the greater occipital nerve increases metabolic activity in the trigeminal nucleus caudalis and cervical dorsal horn of the cat. *Pain, 73,* 23–28.

Goadsby, P. J., Kaube, H., & Hoskin, K. L. (1992). Nitric oxide synthesis couples cerebral blood flow and metabolism. *Brain Res, 595,* 167–170.

Goadsby, P. J., & Knight, Y. E. (1997). Direct evidence for central sites of action of zolmitriptan (311C90): An autoradiographic study in cat. *Cephalalgia, 17,* 153–158.

Goadsby, P. J., Lambert, G. A., & Lance, J. W. (1982). Differential effects on the internal and external carotid circulation of the monkey evoked by locus coeruleus stimulation. *Brain Res, 249,* 247–254.

Goadsby, P. J., Lambert, G. A., & Lance, J. W. (1983). Effects of locus coeruleus stimulation on carotid vascular resistance in the cat. *Brain Res, 278,* 175–183.

Goadsby, P. J., Lambert, G. A., & Lance, J. W. (1984). The peripheral pathway for extracranial vasodilatation in the cat. *J Auto Nerv Syst, 10,* 145–155.

Goadsby, P. J., & Lance, J. W. (1988). Brainstem effects on intra- and extracerebral circulations. Relation to migraine and cluster headache. In J. Olesen & L. Edvinsson (Eds.), *Basic mechanisms of headache* (pp. 413–427). Amsterdam: Elsevier Science.

Goadsby, P. J., & Macdonald, G. J. (1988). Extracranial vasodilatation mediated by VIP (vasoactive intestinal polypeptide). *Brain Res, 329,* 285–288.

Goadsby, P. J., Piper, R. D., Lambert, G. A., & Lance, J. W. (1985a). The effect of activation of the nucleus raphe dorsalis (DRN) on carotid blood flow. I. The Monkey. *Am J Physiol, 248,* R257–R262.

Goadsby, P. J., Piper, R. D., Lambert, G. A., & Lance, J. W. (1985b). The effect of activation of the nucleus raphe dorsalis (DRN) on carotid blood flow. II. The Cat. *Am J Physiol, 248,* R263–R269.

Goadsby, P. J., & Zagami, A. S. (1991). Stimulation of the superior sagittal sinus increases metabolic activity and blood flow in certain regions of the brainstem and upper cervical spinal cord of the cat. *Brain, 114,* 1001–1011.

Goadsby, P. J., Zagami, A. S., & Lambert, G. A. (1991). Neural processing of craniovascular pain: A synthesis of the central structures involved in migraine. *Headache, 31,* 365–371.

Goldstein, D. J., Offen, W. W., Klein, E. G., Phebus, L. A., Hipskind, P., Johnson, K. W., et al. (2001). Lanepitant, an NK-1 antagonist, in migraine prevention. *Cephalalgia, 21,* 102–106.

Goldstein, D. J., Wang, O., Saper, J. R., Stoltz, R., Silberstein, S. D., & Mather, N. T. (1997). Ineffectiveness of neurokini-1 antagonist in acute migraine: a crossover study. *Cephalalgia, 17,* 785–790.

Goltman, A. M. (1935–1936). The mechanism of migraine. *J Allergy, 7,* 351–355.

Graham, J. R., & Wolff, H. G. (1938). Mechanism of migraine headache and action of ergotamine tartrate. *Arch Neurol Psychiatry, 39,* 737–763.

Griggs, R. C., & Nutt, J. G. (1995). Episodic ataxias as channelopathies. *Ann Neurol, 37,* 285–287.

Gupta, P., Brown, D., Butler, P., Ellis, P., Grayson, K. L., Land, G. C., et al. (1995). The in vivo pharmacological profile of a 5-HT1 receptor agonist, CP122,288, a selective inhibitor of neurogenic inflammation. *Br J Pharmacol, 116,* 2385–2390.

Hadjikhani, N., Sanchez del Rio, M., Wu, O., Schwartz, D., Bakker, D., Fischl, B., et al. (2001). Mechanisms of migraine aura revealed by functional MRI in human visual cortex. *PNAS, 98,* 4687–4692.

Hoskin, K. L., & Goadsby, P. J. (1997). The substance P antagonist, GR205171, does not inhibit trigeminal neurons activated by stimulation of the sagittal sinus: Does NK1 blockade have a role in migraine? *Cephalalgia, 17,* 347.

Hubel, D. H., & Weisel, T. N. (1968). Receptive fields and functional architecture of monkey striate cortex. *J Physiol, 195,* 215–243.

Iversen, H. K., Nielsen, T. H., Olesen, J., & Tfelt-Hansen, P. (1990). Arterial responses during migraine headache. *Lancet, 336,* 837–839.

Jensen, K., & Olesen, J. (1985). Temporal muscle blood flow in common migraine. *Acta Neurol Scand, 71,* 561–570.

Jensen, K., Tuxen, C., Pederson-Bjergaard, U., Jansen, I., Edvinsson, L., & Olesen, J. (1990). Pain and tenderness in human temporal muscle induced by bradykinin and 5-hydroxytryptamine. *Peptides, 11,* 1127–1132.

Jensen, K., Tfelt-Hansen, P., Lauritzen, M., & Olesen, J. (1986). Classic migraine. A prospective reporting of symptoms. *Acta Neurol Scand, 73,* 359–362.

Katsarava, Z., Giffin, N., Diener, H-C., & Kaube, H. (2003). Abnormal habituation of "nociceptive" blink reflex in migraine-evidence for increased excitability of trigeminal nociception. *Cephalalgia, 23,* 814–819.

Kaube, H., Katsarava, Z., Kaufer, T., Diener, H. C., & Ellrich, J. (2000). A new method to increase the nociception specificity of the human blink reflex. *Clinicl Neurophysiology, 111,* 413–416.

Kaube, H., Katsarava, Z., Pizywara, S., Drepper, J., Ellrich, J., Diemer, H. C. (2002). Acute migraine headache: possible sensitization of neurons in the spinal trigeminal nucleus? *Neurology, 58,* 1234–1238.

Kaube, H., Keay, K., Hoskin, K. L., Bandler, R., & Goadsby, P. J. (1993). Expression of c-Fos-like immunoreactivity in the caudal medulla and upper cervical cord following stimulation of the sagittal sinus in the cat. *Brain Res, 629,* 95–102.

Kerr, F. W. L. (1961). A mechanism to account for frontal headache in cases of posterior fossa tumours. *J Neurosurg, 18,* 605–609.

Kimball, R. W., Friedman, A. P., & Vallejo, E. (1960). Effect of serotonin in migraine patients. *Neurology, Minneap, 10,* 107–111.

Knight, Y. E., Bartsch, T., Kaube, H., & Goadsby, P. J. (2002). P/Q-type calcium-channel blockade in the periaqueductal gray facilitates trigeminal nociception: A functional genetic link for migraine? *J Neurosci, 22: RC213,* 1–6.

Knight, Y. E., Edvinsson, L., & Goadsby, P. J. (1997). Blockade of release of CGRP after superior sagittal sinus stimulation in cat: A comparison of avitriptan and CP122,288. *Cephalalgia, 17,* 248.

Kobari, M., Meyer, J. S., Ichjo, M., Imai, A., & Oravez, W. T. (1989). Hyperperfusion of cerebral cortex, thalamus and basal ganglia during spontaneously occurring migraine headaches. *Headache, 29,* 282–289.

Kruuse, C., Thomsen, L. L., Birk, S., & Olesen, J. (2003). Migraine can be induced by sildenafil without changes in middle cerebral artery diameter. *Brain, 126,* 241–247.

Kupfermann, I. (1985). Hypothalamus and limbic system. II: Motivation. In E. R. Kandel & J. H. Schwartz (Eds.), *Principles of neural science* (pp. 626–635). Amsterdam: Elsevier Science.

Lambert, G. A., Bogduk, N., Goadsby, P. J., Duckworth, J. W., & Lance, J. W. (1984). Decreased carotid arterial resistance in cats in response to trigeminal stimulation. *J Neurosurg, 61,* 307–315.

Lance, J. W. (1986). *Migraine and other headaches.* New York: Scribner's.

Lance, J. W. (1995). Swelling at the site of a skull defect during migraine headache. *J Neurol Neurosurg Psychiatry, 59,* 641.

Lance, J. W., & Anthony, M. (1966). Some clinical aspects of migraine: A prospective survey of 500 patients. *Arch Neurol, 15,* 356–361.

Lance, J. W., Lambert, G. A., Goadsby, P. J., & Duckworth, J. W. (1983). Brainstem influences on cephalic circulation: Experimental data from cat and monkey of relevance to the mechanism of migraine. *Headache, 23,* 258–265.

Lance, J. W., Lambert, G. A., Goadsby, P. J., & Zagami, A. S. (1989). Contribution of experimental studies to understanding the pathophysiology of migraine. In M. Sandler & G. M. Collins (Eds.), *Migraine: A spectrum of ideas* (pp. 21–39). Oxford, Oxford University Press.

Lashley, K. S. (1941). Patterns of cerebral integration indicated by the scotomas of migraine. *Arch Neurol Psychiat, 46,* 331–339.

Lassen, L. H., Ashina, M., Christiansen, I., Ulrich, V., & Olesen, J. (1997). Nitric oxide synthesis inhibition in migraine. *Lancet, 349,* 401–402.

Lassen, L. H., Haderslev, P. A., Jacobsen, V. B., Iversen, H. K., Sperling, B., & Olesen, J. (2002). CGRP may play a causative role in migraine. *Cephalalgia, 22,* 54–61.

Launay, J. M., & Pradalier, A. (1985). Common migraine attack: Platelet modifications are mainly due to plasma factor(s). *Headache, 25,* 262–268.

Lauritzen, M. (1994). Pathophysiology of the migraine aura. The spreading depression theory. *Brain, 117,* 199–210.

Lauritzen, M., Skyhöj-Olsen, T., Lassen, N. A., & Paulson, O. B. (1983). The changes of regional cerebral blood flow during the course of classical migraine attacks. *Ann Neurol, 13,* 633–641.

Leão, A. A. P. (1944). Spreading depression of activity in cerebral cortex. *J Neurophysiol, 7,* 359–390.

Lee, W. K., Limmroth, V., Ayata, C., Cutrer, F. M., Waeber, C., Yn, X., et al. (1995). Peripheral GABA-A receptor mediated effects of sodium valproate on dural plasma protein extravasation to substance P and trigeminal stimulation. *Br J Pharmacol, 116,* 1661–1667.

Lee, W. S., & Moskowitz, M. A. (1993). Conformationally restricted sumatriptan analogues, CP-122,288 and CP-122,638, exhibit enhanced potency against neurogenic inflammation in dura mater. *Brain Res, 626,* 303–305.

Lee, W. S., Moussaoui, S. M., & Moskowitz, M. A. (1994). Blockade by oral or parenteral RPR100893 (a non-peptide NK1 receptor antagonist) of neurogenic plasma protein extravasation in guinea-pig dura mater and conjunctiva. *Br J Pharmacol, 112,* 920–924.

Limmroth, V., Lee, W. S., Cutrer, F. M., Waeber, C., & Moskowitz, A. (1995). Progesterone and its ring-A-reduced metabolites suppress dural plasma protein extravasation by activation of peripheral GABAA receptors. *Cephalalgia, 15*(Suppl. 14), 98.

Lous, I., & Olsen, J. (1982). Evaluation of pericranial tenderness and oral function in patients with common migraine, muscle contraction headache and "combination headache." *Pain, 12,* 385–393.

Markowitz, S., Saito, K., & Moskowitz, M. A. (1987). Neurogenically mediated leakage of plasma proteins occurs from blood vessels in dura mater but not brain. *J Neurosci, 7,* 4129–4136.

Markowitz, S., Saito, K., & Moskowitz, M. A. (1988). Neurogenically mediated plasma extravasation in dura mater: Effect of ergot alkaloids. A possible mechanism of action in vascular headache. *Cephalalgia, 8,* 83–91.

Matharu, M. S., Bartsch, T., Ward, N., et al. (2003). Central neuromodulation in chronic migraine patients with suboccipital stimulators: A PET study. *Brain, 127,* 220–230.

Matharu, M. S., Good, C. D., May, A., Bahra, A., & Goadsby, P. J. (2003). No change in the structure of the brain in migraine: A voxel-based morphometric study. *Eur J Neurol, 10,* 53–57.

May, A., Gijsman, H. J., Wallnofer, A., Jones, R., Diener, H. C., & Ferrari, M. D. (1996). Endothelin antagonist bosentan blocks neurogenic inflammation, but is not effective in aborting migraine attacks. *Pain, 67,* 375–378.

May, A., Kaube, H., Buchel, C., Eichten, C., Rijntjes, M., Juptner, M., et al. (1998). Experimental cranial pain elicited by capsaicin: A PET study. *Pain, 74,* 61–66.

May, A., Ophoff, R. A., Terwindt, G. M., Urban, C., Van Eijk, R., Haan, J., et al. (1995). Familial hemiplegic migraine locus on chromosome 19p13 is involved in common forms of migraine with and without aura. *Human Genet, 96,* 604–608.

Mayberg, M., Langer, R. S., Zervas, N. T., & Moskowitz, M. A. (1981). Perivascular meningeal projections from cat trigeminal ganglia: Possible pathway for vascular headaches in man. *Science, 213,* 228–230.

McLachlan, R. S., & Girvin, J. P. (1994). Spreading depression of Leao in rodent and human cortex. *Brain Res, 666,* 133–136.

McNaughton, F. L. (1938). The innervation of the intracranial blood vessels and dural sinuses. *Proc Assoc Res Nervous Mental Dis, 18,* 178–200.

Moskowitz, M. A. (1992). Neurogenic versus vascular mechanisms of sumatriptan and ergot alkaloids in migraine. *Trends Pharmacol Sci, 13,* 307–311.

Moskowitz, M. A., & Buzzi, M. G. (1991). Neuroeffector functions of sensory fibres: implications for headache mechanisms and drug actions. *J Neurol, 238,* S18–S22.

Moskowitz, M. A., & Cutrer, F. M. (1993). Sumatriptan: A receptor-targeted treatment for migraine. *Ann Rev Med, 44,* 145–154.

Mosnaim, A. D., Wolf, M. E., Chevesich, J., Callaghan, O. H., & Diamond, S. (1985). Plasma methionine enkephalin levels. A biological marker for migraine? *Headache, 25,* 259–261.

Mraovitch, S., Calando, Y., Goadsby, P. J., & Seylaz, J. (1992). Subcortical cerebral blood flow and metabolic changes elicited by cortical spreading depression in rat. *Cephalalgia, 12,* 137–141.

Muck-Seler, D., Deanovic, Z., & Dupelj, M. (1979). Platelet serotonin (5-HT) and 5-HT releasing factor in plasma of migrainous patients. *Headache, 19,* 14–17.

Nichols, F. T., Mawad, M., Mohr, J. P., Hilal, S., & Adams, R. J. (1993). Focal headache during balloon inflation in the vertebral and basilar arteries. *Headache, 33,* 87–89.

Nissila, M., Parkkola, R., Sonninen, P., & Salonen, R. (1996). Intracerebral arteries and gadolinium enhancement in migraine without aura. *Cephalalgia, 16,* 363.

Norman, B., Panebianco, D., & Block, G. A. (1998). A placebo-controlled, in-clinic study to explore the preliminary safety and efficacy of intravenous L-758,298 (a prodrug of the NK1 receptor anagonist L-754,030) in the acute treatment of migraine. *Cephalalgia, 18,* 407.

Norris, J. W., Hachinski, V. C., & Cooper, P. W. (1975). Changes in cerebral blood flow during a migraine attack. *BMJ, 3,* 676–677.

Nozaki, K., Boccalini, P., & Moskowitz, M. A. (1992). Expression of c-Fos-like immunoreactivity in brainstem after meningeal irritation by blood in the subarachnoid space. *Neuroscience, 49,* 669–680.

Olesen, J., Friberg, L., Skyhöj-Olsen, T., Iversen, H. K., Lassen, N. A., & Andersen, A. R. (1990). Timing and topography of cerebral blood flow, aura and headache during migraine attacks. *Ann Neurol, 28,* 791–798.

Olesen, J., Larsen, B., & Lauritzen, M. (1981). Focal hyperemia followed by spreading oligemia and impaired activation of rCBF in classic migraine. *Ann Neurol, 9,* 344–352.

Olesen, J., Tfelt-Hansen, P., Henriksen, L., & Larsen, B. (1981). The common migraine attack may not be initiated by cerebral ischemia. *Lancet, ii,* 438–440.

Ophoff, R. A., Terwindt, G. M., Vergouwe, M. N., van Eijk, R., Oefner, P. J., Hoffman, S. M., et al. (1996). Familial hemiplegic migraine and episodic ataxia type-2 are caused by mutations in the Ca2+ channel gene CACNL1A4. *Cell, 87,* 543–552.

Peatfield, R. C., & Clifford Rose, F. (1991). Prospective study of unilateral classical migraine. In F. Clifford Rose (Ed.), *New advances in headache research* (Vol. 2). London: Smith-Gordon.

Penfield, W., & Perot, P. (1963). The brain's record of auditory and visual experience. *Brain, 86,* 595–696.

Peroutka, S. J. (1997). Dopamine and migraine. *Neurology, 49,* 650–656.

Piper, R. D., Matheson, J. M., Hellier, M., Vanau, M., Lambert, G. A., Olausson, B., et al. (1991). Cortical spreading depression is not seen intraoperatively during temporal lobectomy in humans. *Cephalalgia, 11*(Suppl. 11), 1.

Ramadan, N. M., Halvorson, H., Vande-Linde, A., Levine, S. R., Helpem, J. A., & Welch, K. M. (1989). Low brain magnesium in migraine. *Headache, 29,* 416–419.

Raskin, N. H., Hosobuchi, Y., & Lamb, S. (1987). Headache may arise from perturbation of brain. *Headache, 27,* 416–420.

Raskin, N. H., & Knittle, S. C. (1976) Ice cream headache and orthostatic symptoms in patients with migraine headache. *Headache, 16,* 222–225.

Raskin, N. H., & Schwartz, R. K. (1980). Icepick-like pain. *Neurology, 30,* 203–205.

Ray, B. S., & Wolff, H. G. (1940). Experimental studies on headache. Pain sensitive structures of the head and their significance in headache. *Arch Surg, 41,* 813–856.

Roon, K. I., Olesen, J., Diener, H. C., Ellis, P., Hettiarachchi, J., Poole, P. H., et al. (2000). No acute antimigraine efficacy of CP-122 288, a highly potent inhibitor of neurogenic inflammation: Results of two randomized, double-blind, placebo-controlled clinical trials. *Ann Neurol, 47,* 238–241.

Ruskell, G. L. (1988) The tentorial nerve in monkeys is a branch of the cavernous plexus. *J Anat, 157,* 67–77.

Ruskell, G. L., & Simons, T. (1987). Trigeminal nerve pathways to the cerebral arteries in monkeys. *J Anat, 155,* 23–37.

Russell, M. B., Rassmussen, B. K., Fenger, K., & Olesen, J. (1996). Migraine without aura and migraine with aura are distinct clinical entities: A study of four hundred and eight-four male and female migraineurs from the general population. *Cephalalgia, 16,* 239–245.

Ryan, R. E., Elkind, A., & Goldstein, J. (1997). Twenty-four hour effectiveness of BMS 180048 in the acute treatment of migraine headaches. *Headache, 37,* 245–248.

Sakai, F., & Meyer, J. S. (1978). Regional cerebral hemodynamics during migraine and cluster headaches measured by the 133. Xe inhalation method. *Headache, 18,* 122–132.

Sakai, F., & Meyer, J. S. (1979). Abnormal cerebrovascular reactivity in patients with migraine and cluster headache. *Headache, 19,* 257–266.

Sicuteri, F. (1959). Prophylactic and therapeutic properties of UML-491 in migraine. *Int Arch Allergy, 15,* 300–307.

Sicuteri, F. (1977). Dopamine, the second putative protagonist in headache. *Headache, 17,* 129–131.

Sicuteri, F., Boccuni, M., Fanciullacci, M., & Gatto, G. (1983). Naloxone effectiveness on spontaneous and induced perceptive disorders in migraine. *Headache, 23,* 179–183.

Sicuteri, F., Testi, A., & Anselmi, B. (1961). Biochemical investigations in headache: Increase in hydrox-yindoleacetic acid excretion during migraine attacks. *Int Arch Allergy, 19,* 55–58.

Smith, D., Hill, R. G., Edvinsson, L., & Longmore, J. (2002). An immunocytochemical investigation of human trigeminal nucleus caudalis: CGRP, substance P., & 5HT1D-receptor immunoreactivities are expressed by trigeminal sensory fibres. *Cephalalgia, 22,* 424–431.

Sramka, M., Brozek, G., Bures, J., & Nadvornik, P. (1977). Functional ablation by spreading depression: Possible use in human stereotactic neurosurgery. *App Neurophysiol, 40,* 48–61.

Strassman, A. M., Mineta, Y., & Vos, B. P. (1994). Distribution of Fos-like immunoreactivity in the medullary and upper cervical dorsal horn produced by stimulation of dural blood vessels in the rat. *J Neurosci, 14,* 3725–3735.

Strassman, A. M., & Vos, B. P. (1993). Somatotopic and laminar organization of Fos-like immunoreactivity in the medullary and upper cervical dorsal horn induced by noxious facial stimulation in the rat. *J Comp Neurol, 331,* 495–516.

Strassman, A. M., Vos, B. P., Mineta, Y., Naden, S., Borsook, D., & Burstein, R. (1993). Fos-like immunoreactivity in the superficial medullary dorsal horn induced by noxious and innocuous thermal stimulation of the facial skin in the rat. *J Neurophysiol, 70,* 1811–1821.

Swaab, D. F., Hofman, M. A., Lucassen, P. J., Purba, J. S., Raadsheer, F. C., & Van de Nes, J. A. (1993). Functional neuroanatomy and neuropathology of the hypothalamus. *Anat Embryol, 187,* 317–330.

Tfelt-Hansen, P., Lous, I., & Olesen, J. (1981). Prevalence and significance of muscle tenderness during common migraine attacks. *Headache, 21,* 49–54.

Tunis, M. M., & Wolff, H. G. (1953). Long term observations of the reactivity of the cranial arteries in subjects with vascular headache of the migraine type. *Arch Neurol Psychiat, 70,* 551–557.

Veloso, F., & Kumar, K. (1996). Deep brain implant migraine. *J Neurol Neurosurg Psychiatry, 46*(Suppl. 7), A168–A169.

Walters, D. W., Gillespie, S. A., & Moskowitz, M. (1986). Cerebrovascular projections from the sphenopalatine and otic ganglia to the middle cerebral artery of the cat. *Stroke, 17,* 488–494.

Weiller, C., May, A., Limmroth, V., Juptner, M., Kaube, H., Schayck, R. V., et al. (1995). Brain stem activation in spontaneous human migraine attacks. *Nat Med, 1,* 658–660.

Welch, K. M., & Ramadan, N. M. (1995). Mitochondria, magnesium and migraine. *J Neurol Sci, 134,* 9–14.

Wolff, H. G. (1963). *Headache and other head pain.* New York: Oxford University Press.

Woods, R. P., Iacoboni, M., & Mazziotta, J. C. (1994). Bilateral spreading cerebral hypoperfusion during spontaneous migraine headache. *N Engl J Med, 331,* 1689–1692.

Zagami, A. S., & Goadsby, P. J. (1991). Stimulation of the superior sagittal sinus increases metabolic activity in cat thalamus. In F. Clifford Rose (Ed.), *New advances in headache research* (Vol. 2, pp. 169–171). London: Smith-Gordon.

Zagami, A. S., Goadsby, P. J., & Edvinsson, L. (1990). Stimulation of the superior sagittal sinus in the cat causes release of vasoactive peptides. *Neuropeptides, 16,* 69–75.

Zagami, A. S., & Lambert, G. A. (1990). Stimulation of cranial vessels excites nociceptive neurones in several thalamic nuclei of the cat. *Exp Brain Res, 81,* 552–566.

Zagami, A. S., & Lambert, G. A. (1991). Craniovascular application of capsaicin activates nociceptive thalamic neurons in the cat. *Neurosci Lett, 121,* 187–190.

Chapter 9
Migraine: Treatment

Migraine is a horrid disability and deserves to be taken seriously (Menken et al., 2000). It very rarely kills (Kors et al., 2001) but can destroy many of the pleasures of life. It can ruin marriages, families, and careers. It is a disorder that warrants full attention from the physician or general practitioner and can be very rewarding to treat.

At present there is no cure for migraine, and perhaps there never will be. It is important to explain to patients at the outset that they have been born with a *tendency to have headaches* that overreacts to internal changes or external stimuli and that there is a very good chance the condition can be brought under control by advice and judicious medication. It is useful to point out that *migraine* as a term can refer to the typical attack that many have read about with a mixture of visual disturbance, nausea, or sensitivity to light and sound, or *migraine* can refer to the disease. Migraine the disease is marked by a general dysfunction in sensory processing. Thus attacks may include dizziness and impaired concentration, a general intolerance for repetitive stimuli, and allodynia (the development of scalp or facial sensitivity) (Selby & Lance, 1960; Burstein et al., 2000).

Many people seek "natural" methods of treatment and resent the need to take pills. They want to know the cause of their headaches and what lifestyle changes will prevent them. Some patients find the genetic explanation unsatisfactory, because it implies they cannot just take a pill or avoid some magical trigger substance. Perhaps meditation, manipulation, or removal of some superfluous viscus would do the trick. We all wish it were that simple. Doctors should feel empathy toward their patients with headache and take some time to make sure they understand the principles of management. A patient with *difficult* migraine has a complex biologic problem that requires a doctor's full attention.

If the history is typical of migraine headache, the patient should be assured that there is no suggestion a cerebral tumor or other progressive disease is causing the symptoms and therefore there is no need for extensive and expensive investigations (Quality Standards Subcommittee of the American Academy of Neurology, 1994). The history and physical examination may have disclosed precipitating or aggravating factors that require attention.

The following common factors may increase the frequency and severity of migraine attacks:

- Anxiety or depressive state
- Onset of systemic hypertension
- Use of oral contraceptive pills or vasodilator drugs
- Excessive consumption of analgesics, caffeine, or ergotamine

General advice includes some guidance on lifestyle that can be given to the patient:
- Try to spread your workload evenly to avoid peaks and troughs of stress at work or at home.
- Do not sleep in (later than your normal hour of waking) during weekends, because this often causes a "let-down" headache.
- Avoid excessive fatigue.
- Eat at regular times, and do not miss meals. Eliminate any item in your diet that you believe may precipitate an attack. This applies to the intake of alcohol, particularly red wines, in susceptible people.
- Limit your consumption of tea, coffee, and analgesics, because these may lead to rebound headaches.
- Watch your posture. Avoid craning your neck forward. Think tall.
- Keep your muscles as relaxed as possible when not physically active. Do not frown or clench your jaw.
- Exercise daily, but restrict physical exertion on a hot day.
- Avoid glare or exposure to flickering light, noise, or strong smells if these are triggers.
- Bear in mind the classic Greek admonition "Moderation in all things."

GENERAL (NONPHARMACEUTICAL) METHODS OF TREATMENT

Psychological Management

Psychological counseling is an important part of migraine management. Often, the doctor of first contact is the family physician or general practitioner. In such cases the doctor likely knows the patient in his or her family setting and is in the best position to give advice. Sometimes, however, patients may be reluctant to discuss embarrassing personal problems with a doctor who knows them and their family socially. Thus the doctor and patient must invest time and patience in the initial discussion, understanding that solutions may not be found for all of the problems that emerge. The goals of this initial discussion are to provide patients with a chance to unburden themselves, the opportunity to gain objective advice, and the knowledge that their problem is not unique and has been overcome by many others. Changing the patient's personality or life pattern is not always possible, but the open discussion itself helps patients and reinforces that doctors understand that they are dealing with individuals. Patients may also learn that they can rearrange their daily routine to minimize stress and then more easily adjust to those fluctuations that inevitably occur. The external environment can be stabilized to some extent as well, which will allow patients to concentrate on themselves and their reactions to change.

Although physicians generally agree that psychological factors are important in triggering headache, few carefully controlled trials demonstrate the effectiveness of psychological management in general and the comparative merits of the various forms of treatment used.

Physiological Management (Relaxation and Biofeedback)

Simple relaxation training, as described in Appendix B, can help patients with migraine reduce the frequency and severity of headache.

Relaxation training is often augmented by feedback from an electromyogram (EMG) of the frontal and temporal muscles, from skin temperatures of scalp and hand, or from recordings of the temporal artery pulsations. Spontaneous recovery from migraine headache is associated with increased blood flow and skin temperature in the hands. A study of treatments such as relaxation and thermal biofeedback demonstrated significant improvement over headache-monitoring control subjects, but the addition of cognitive therapy conferred no further advantage (Blanchard et al., 1990). Keep in mind that migraine tends to improve when a patient is under supervision in a clinical trial. In our own clinics, placebo results in controlled trials of drug therapy have varied from 20% to 60% improvement, the latter figure being achieved when psychological counseling and relaxation training were part of general management. Also, clear evidence from meta-analysis in headache (Ferrari et al., 2001; Diener, 2003) and in pain more widely (Hrobjartsson & Gotzsche, 2001) shows that the placebo response must be considered. We considered it a bonus from a clinical viewpoint. The results of nonpharmacologic treatments of migraine have been summarized by Holroyd and Penzien (1990), who concluded that biofeedback/relaxation therapy was as effective as propranolol in managing migraine, each reducing headache by 43%, whereas placebo produced only a 14% reduction. It is probable that biofeedback achieves no more than relaxation therapy alone, and indeed may be less satisfactory, but both fulfill the requirements of patients who demand relief without drugs and are satisfied with only a modest improvement in their headache pattern.

Transcendental Meditation and Hypnotherapy

Any means of achieving emotional equilibrium and physical relaxation might be expected to help a migraine, but transcendental meditation benefited only 6 of 17 patients studied by Benson, Klemchuk, and Graham (1974). The results of hypnotherapy are more encouraging. Anderson, Basker, and Dalton (1975) compared 23 patients undergoing hypnotherapy with a control group of 24 treated with prochlorperazine. The hypnosis group (in six sessions at intervals of 10 to 14 days) were given "ego-strengthening" suggestions that they would have less tension, anxiety, and apprehension; they were also given specific suggestions about constricting the arteries in their heads. Patients were asked to practice hypnosis daily and to use it to abort a threatened attack of migraine. The trial extended for 12 months, and in the last 3 months of the trial, 44% of patients in the hypnotherapy group were free of headache, compared with 13% of patients in the control group. The median number of attacks per month dropped from 4.5 to 0.5 in the patients treated with hypnosis, compared with 3.3 to 2.9 of patients in the prochlorperazine group.

Acupuncture

Acupuncture has been practiced in China for more than 2000 years and is currently a vogue in the Western world. Loh and colleagues (1984) studied the effect of acupuncture in 55 patients with migraine and tension headache who had not responded to "every kind of drug that had been fashionable at that time." Of the 41 patients who completed a 3-month course, 9 improved greatly, 7 moderately, 8 slightly, and 17 not at all. Baischer (1995) described the effect of acupuncture, courses averaging 10 treatments, in 26 patients. An improvement of more than 33% was achieved by 18 patients. A meta-analysis of the use of acupuncture that included 15 trials in migraine concluded the evidence for an effect was weak (Melchart et al., 1999). Our own impression is that the response to acupuncture is inconsistent and not usually sustained after treatment ceases.

Exercise

Strenuous exertion may precipitate migraine in some patients, but a gradual increase in exercise, particularly if it is disguised by some agreeable sport or occupation, is usually beneficial.

Prevention of Salt and Water Retention

Fluid retention is common for several days before the menstrual period and is also common immediately before migraine headache. That menstruation and migraine often coincide (Stewart et al., 2000) led to the use of salt restriction and diuretics in the treatment of migraine, regardless of whether it tended to occur with the menses. Fluid retention may indeed be prevented by such measures, but migraine usually continues unabated.

Elimination Diets

In Chapter 7 we discussed dietary factors as possible precipitants of migraine headache. McQueen and associates (1989) reviewed this subject in presenting the results of a controlled trial of dietary modification in 95 patients, of whom 26 considered that their headaches could be precipitated by specific foods, 14 by alcohol, and 10 by both. The protocol consisted of an elimination diet for 4 to 6 weeks (during which time 37 patients improved, 22 did not, and 36 dropped out), followed by blinded food challenges and the prescription of diets containing, and diets avoiding, provoking factors in a randomized fashion. Of the 19 patients who completed this rigorous program, 9 had fewer and less severe headaches while on the therapeutic diet than while on the control diet, whereas 6 were no different and 4 were worse. It is therefore unlikely that food allergy plays any part in adult migraine, but it is quite possible that simplifying the diet, like other aspects of lifestyle, may exert a benign but nonspecific influence on the course of migraine.

Spinal Manipulation

Success has been claimed for manipulation of the neck in treating migraine headache, as in many other fields, but objective evidence is lacking. Cyriax (1962) stated that "an attack of migraine can sometimes be instantly aborted by strong traction on the neck. Half a minute's traction in some cases is regularly successful, in others not. The mechanism is obscure (it may be connected with stretching of the carotid and vertebral arteries) and the phenomenon would clearly repay further study." Cyriax goes on to say, "a minority of patients have reported to me, some years after the reduction by manipulation of a cervical disc, that since that time attacks of obvious migraine have ceased."

A controlled trial (Parker, Tupling, & Pryor, 1978) has evaluated manipulation of the cervical spine. Patients with migraine were allocated randomly to three groups: one group treated by chiropractic manipulation, a second group in which patients underwent manipulation by a doctor or physiotherapist, and a control group in which participants had a course of cervical mobilization by a doctor or physiotherapist. Treatment of the last group involved a number of the nonspecific therapeutic ingredients common to other groups. Migraine symptoms were reduced by about 28% in all groups, but no one group improved significantly more than the other over the 6-month trial, although the severity of headache was less in the chiropractic group. Twenty months after the course of treatment, migraine attacks had diminished by an additional 19%, which the authors attributed to the natural history of the disorder (Parker, Pryor, & Tupling, 1980).

Surgical Procedures

Operations on sympathetic or parasympathetic nerve pathways and ligation of branches of the external carotid or middle meningeal arteries, or both, have not provided any lasting benefit (Rowbotham, 1949). The painful component of the migraine attack can be reduced or abolished by lesions of the trigeminal ganglion or root or section of the spinal tract and nucleus of the trigeminal nerve (White & Sweet, 1955). However, such destructive surgery is rarely, if ever, warranted, and follow-up of such cases is limited. Therefore we do not recommend such an approach.

Injection of local anesthetic and corticosteroids into the region of the greater occipital nerve was pioneered by Anthony (1987, 1992), who has suggested its use in unilateral primary headache as well as secondary headaches, typically cervicogenic headache. Some believe a positive response proves a diagnosis of *occipital neuralgia*. It seems more likely, based on previous work (Wirth & van Buren, 1971; Goadsby, Hoskin, & Knight, 1997) and recent experimental work (Bartsch & Goadsby, 2002, 2003), that modulation of occipital input can alter brain processing of primary headache. Functional imaging studies of patients with chronic migraine, by the IHS definition (Headache Classification Committee of the International Headache Society, 2004), implanted with suboccipital nerve stimulators show both remarkable control of the headache and alteration in the pattern of brain activation when the stimulator is on (Matharu et al., 2004). A locus of action in the thalamus is postulated (Matharu et al., 2004). These stimulators are subcutaneous and have a low morbidity. They

require detailed evaluation but are reversible and may replace destructive procedures as options in the treatment of medically intractable migraine.

PHARMACOTHERAPY

The pharmacotherapy of migraine falls into two distinct classes: (1) preventive
or prophylactic measures that seek primarily to reduce headache frequency and
(2) abortive or acute attack treatments, whose purpose is to stop attacks when
they occur. Some patients who have frequent headache require preventive therapy, and the decision to start such therapy must be made after careful consulta-
tion and discussion between the patient and physician. In general, patients who
have two or fewer headaches a month do reasonably well with acute attack medications alone, whereas patients who have more than four attacks a month often
benefit from preventive therapy. Decisions for patients in the middle—and for
patients with more or less frequent attacks—are driven by patient response to
acute attack medications, including tolerability, efficacy, and safety of the acute
attack medications. Ultimately, the decision amalgamates the perceptions and
views of both the patient and managing physician, although a golden rule is that
it is the patient who suffers and who must be involved completely in the decision
to begin preventive therapy.

Agents Used in the Treatment of Acute Attacks

The development of acute attack treatments over the past fifteen years has been a
major advance in the management of migraine. Treatments for acute attacks may
be divided into two broad categories: nonspecific (i.e., analgesics with antipain
actions that are not specific to migraine) and specific compounds (i.e., drugs
with antimigraine actions but no general antipain actions) (Goadsby & Olesen,
1996).

Specific Treatments of Acute Migraine Attacks

Current specific antimigraine drugs derive in a broad pharmacologic sense
from the ergot alkaloids. The triptans, serotonin 5-HT$_{1B/1D}$ receptor agonists,
first studied as AH25086B (Doenicke et al., 1987) and subsequently developed and marketed in the form of sumatriptan (Humphrey et al., 1990), represent a sharpened pharmacologic focus on certain subclasses of serotonin
(5-hydroxytryptamine, 5-HT) receptors (Goadsby, 2000). There are currently
seven classes of 5-HT receptors (Table 9.1), with the 5-HT$_1$ subclass being
the major focus of recent drug development (Table 9.2). Comparison of the
pharmacology of dihydroergotamine and sumatriptan (Table 9.3) shows that
the synthesis of newer compounds has basically been aimed at removing
unwanted effects at receptor sites associated with the side effects of serotonin
administration.

ERGOTAMINE TARTRATE.   Ergotamine has been used for more than 75 years in the
management of migraine headache (Maier, 1926) and should be given in optimal
dosage orally, rectally, or by inhalation or injection at the first sign of an attack

TABLE 9.1   Classification of serotonin (5-HT) receptors

5-HT receptor class	Second messenger	Antagonist	Comments
1	↓ Adenylate cyclase		See Table 9.2 for details
2	↑ Phosphoinositide turnover	Methysergide Pizotifen	Contraction of smooth muscle Central nervous system excitation
			Subtypes: 2_A, 2_B, 2_C
3	K^+	Granisetron	Membrane depolarization
	Ca^{2+}	Ondansetron	
	Na^+	Tropisetron	
4	↑ Adenylate cyclase	GR113808	Stimulates GI contraction Atria Brain Four splice variants: a, b, c, d (Blondel et al., 1998)
5		-	Subclasses A, B
6	↑ Adenylate cyclase	Ro 04-6790 (Bentley et al., 1999)	Single receptor
7	↑ Adenylate cyclase	SB-258719 (Thomas et al., 1998)	Splice variants (Jasper et al., 1997) Role in circadian rhythms

GI, gastrointestinal.
From Hoyer et al., 1994.

(Tfelt-Hansen et al., 2000c). A double-blind crossover study (Hakkarainen et al., 1979) has confirmed the effectiveness of ergotamine. Ergotamine tartrate is an agonist of 5-HT$_1$ receptors and a competitive antagonist with partial agonism at α-adrenergic receptors (Muller-Schweinitzer & Fanchamps, 1982). The intramuscular injection of 0.25 to 1.0 mg or the intravenous injection of 0.5 mg ergotamine or 1 mg dihydroergotamine does not alter regional cerebral blood flow in humans (Andersen et al., 1987). The pharmacokinetics of ergotamine when administered orally are unpredictable (Tfelt-Hansen, Ibraheem, & Paalzow, 1982; Ibraheem, Paalzow, & Tfelt-Hansen, 1983; Tfelt-Hansen & Johnson, 1993).

TABLE 9.2   Classification of serotonin (5-HT) subclass 1 receptors

Subtype of 5-HT$_1$ receptor	Agonist	Antagonist	Function
A	8-OH-DPAT*	WAY100165*	Hypotension
	Dihydroergotamine		Behavioral (satiety)
	Sumatriptan		
	Donitriptan		
	Eletriptan		
	Frovatriptan		
	Naratriptan		
Rat B Human B	CP-93,129* Dihydroergotamine All triptans	GR127935* SB-216641	Central autoreceptor (rat) Craniovascular receptor
D	Dihydroergotamine All triptans	GR127935* BRL 15572	Trigeminal Neuronal receptor
E	—	—	?
F	Sumatriptan	—	?
	Almotriptan		
	Eletriptan		
	Frovatriptan		
	Naratriptan		
	Zolmitriptan		
	LY334370[†]	—	?

*8-OH-DPAT (8-hydroxy-2-(di-n-propylamino)tetralin), WAY100165, CP-93,129, and GR127935 are all compounds used in the laboratory for pharmacologic purposes and have no current clinical indications.
[†]Clinically effective although specificity in clinical trials unclear (Goldstein et al., 2001).
From Hartig et al., 1996; John et al., 2000; Goadsby, 2000.

The clinical use of ergotamine is usually restricted to managing single acute episodes, because overdose causes nausea, vomiting, malaise, rebound headache, and peripheral vasoconstriction, which may, rarely, be severe enough to cause arterial obstruction (Magee, 1991). The excessive use of ergotamine-containing suppositories has been reported to cause anorectal ulceration (Jost, Raulf, & Muller-Loeck, 1991). Ergotamine should be avoided in patients with ischemic or thyrotoxic heart disease (Benedict & Robertson, 1979) and in patients with known arterial or venous insufficiency. Patients are generally advised not to exceed intake of 10 mg weekly, but patient tolerance varies widely

TABLE 9.3   Comparison of the pharmacology of dihydroergotamine (DHE) and sumatriptan

	DHE	*Sumatriptan*
Serotonergic (5-HT)		
1_A	+++	+
1_B	++	++
1_D	++	++
1_e	++	−
1_f	++	+
$2_{A/C}$	+	−
3	−	−
Adrenergic		
α_1	+	−
α_2	+	−
β	+/−	−
Dopaminergic		
D_1	−	−
D_2	+/−	−

From Berde & Schild, 1978; Humphrey et al., 1991.

and each patient must be assessed individually. Some may control their migraine without side effects while using larger amounts, whereas others may be unable to tolerate lower dosages because of side effects.

DIHYDROERGOTAMINE.   Dihydroergotamine (DHE) has a broad spectrum of pharmacologic effects (see Table 9.3), an elimination half-life of about 2.5 hours when administered intravenously, and poor bioavailability when administered orally because of inadequate absorption and high first-pass metabolism in the liver (Little et al., 1982). DHE has important effects in the central nervous system, binding 5-HT receptors in the endogenous pain-control system (Goadsby & Gundlach, 1991), and it inhibits trigeminocervical neurons when administered peripherally in experimental animals (Hoskin, Kaube, & Goadsby, 1996). DHE shares with sumatriptan an affinity for the 5-HT$_{1B/1D}$ receptors (Peroutka, 1990) and the ability to inhibit neuropeptide release in the trigeminovascular system (Goadsby & Edvinsson, 1993; Tognetto et al., 2001). It is used mainly to manage acute migraine attacks in doses of 0.5 to 0.75 mg intravenously or 1 mg intramusucularly, and it has become available for intranasal application in some countries (Gallagher, 1996; Massiou, 1996; Touchon et al., 1996).

Raskin (1986) has advocated the use of DHE 0.3 to 1 mg intravenously (the dose depending on patient tolerance, particularly the absence of nausea), in conjunction with metoclopramide 10 mg every 8 hours in patients with intractable migraine. Of 55 patients treated, 49 became headache free within 24 hours. In another study, 37 patients seen in an emergency department with acute migraine were all treated with prochlorperazine 5 mg intravenously initially and then randomized to receive intravenous DHE 0.75 mg or placebo (Callaham & Raskin, 1986). There was no difference between the result in each group at 30 minutes, but pain was significantly less in the first group 60 minutes after receiving DHE. Of patients treated with prochlorperazine and DHE, 13.5% required parenteral narcotics, compared with 45% of patients with migraine headache not enrolled in this study. DHE performs favorably compared with subcutaneous sumatriptan; it has a slower onset of action, but significantly fewer patients report recurrent headache. Thus the response rate when judged at 24 hours after dosing is equal to that of sumatriptan (Winner et al., 1996).

DHE can be administered by a nasal spray (Ziegler et al., 1994), which gives about 40% bioavailability compared with the intravenous route. In double-blind trials, complete relief of pain was achieved in 38% of patients treated with intranasal DHE, compared with 17% of those using placebo (Lataste, Taylor, & Notte, 1989). DHE nasal spray is inferior to subcutaneous sumatriptan (Touchon et al., 1996), although again it has a lower recurrence rate in patients who respond. Compared with the sumatriptan nasal spray, DHE nasal spray is probably slower in onset but again has a lower recurrence rate (Massiou, 1996). DHE, like ergotamine tartrate and methysergide, may, rarely, cause retroperitoneal or pleural fibrosis after repeated usage (Malaquin et al., 1989).

TRIPTANS.   Triptans are serotonin $5\text{-HT}_{1B/1D}$ receptor agonists (Table 9.2 and Figure 9.1). Sumatriptan was the first in the class of triptans that bind specifically to the $5\text{-HT}_{1B/1D}$ receptor (Feniuk, Friedman, & Vallejo, 1991) used in routine clinical practice. Triptans replicate the beneficial effect of 5-HT in the relief of migraine headache without the severe side effects that prevented the therapeutic use of the parent substance (Kimball et al., 1960; Anthony, Hinterberger, & Lance, 1967). The mechanisms of action of the triptans are covered in Chapter 8. They have some particular differences in pharmacokinetics and metabolic pathways that can be used in some clinical settings (Table 9.4). There are insufficient data from randomized controlled trials to determine whether newer medicinal approaches, such as rapidly dissolving oral (Ahrens et al., 1999; Pascual et al., 2001; Dowson et al., 2002) or upper gastrointestinal (GI) tract (Carpay et al., 2004) formulations, truly represent an important advance.

Selection of a migraine-specific therapy entails gaining an understanding of what the patient's current therapy is *not* delivering and then tailoring the triptan to the patient's needs (Table 9.5). The triptans have been compared extensively in meta-analyses (Tfelt-Hansen et al., 2000b; Ferrari et al., 2001, 2002; Oldman et al., 2002), and their place in migraine therapy has recently been assessed

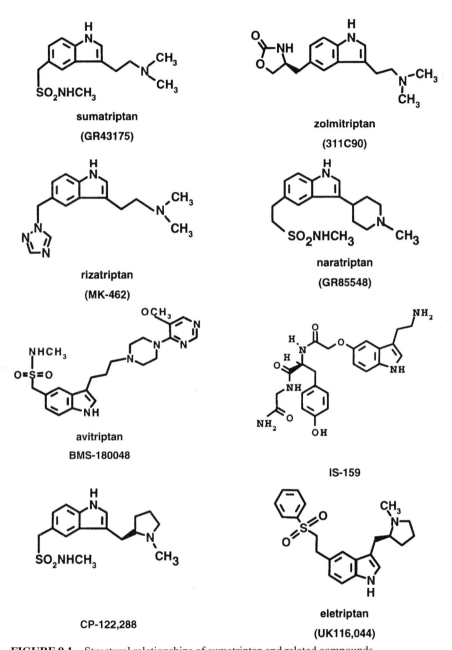

FIGURE 9.1   Structural relationships of sumatriptan and related compounds.

TABLE 9.4 Comparative pharmacokinetics of triptans

	Sumatriptan (Fowler et al., 1991)	Almotriptan (Cabarrocas & Salva, 1997)	Eletriptan	Frovatriptan*	Naratriptan	Rizatriptan	Zolmitriptan
$T_{1/2}$ (hours)	2	3.5	5 (Milton et al., 1997)	25	6 (Kempsford, Baille, & Fuseau, 1997)	2–3	3 (Seaber et al.,1996)
T_{max} (hours)							
Out	2	2–3	1 (Morgan et al., 1997)	2–4	2–3 (Kempsford, Baille, & Fuseau, 1997)	1(Goldberg et al., 2000)	1 (Thomsen et al., 1996)
In	1.5		(Morgan et al., 1997)			1	
Oral bioavailability (%)	14	70	50 (Morgan et al., 1997)	24–30	63–74 (Fuseau et al., 1997)	40–45	40 (Palmer & Spencer, 1997)
Metabolism/excretion (main route)	MAO	P450/MAO	P450	Renal 50%	Renal/P450 (Fuseau et al., 1997)	MAO	P450/MAO (Palmer & Spencer, 1997)
Log $D_{pH7.4}$ (Rance et al., 1997)	−1.3	+0.35	+0.5		−0.2	−0.7	−0.7

MAO, monoamine oxidase; P450, liver P450 metabolism.
*VML251 or SB209509.

TABLE 9.5   Clinical stratification of acute specific migraine therapies

Clinical situation	Treatment options
Failed analgesics/NSAIDs	*First tier*
	Sumatriptan 50 mg or 100 mg PO
	Almotriptan 12.5 mg PO
	Rizatriptan 10 mg PO
	Eletriptan 40 mg PO
	Zolmitriptan 2.5 mg PO
	Slower effect/better tolerability
	Naratriptan 2.5 mg PO
	Frovatriptan 2.5 mg PO
	Infrequent headache
	Ergotamine 1–2 mg PO
	Dihydroergotamine nasal spray 2 mg
Early nausea or difficulties taking tablets	Zolmitriptan 5 mg nasal spray
	Sumatriptan 20 mg nasal spray
	Rizatriptan 10 mg wafer
	Zolmitriptan 2.5 mg wafer
Headache recurrence	Ergotamine 2 mg (most effective pr ± caffeine)
	Naratriptan 2.5 mg PO
	Almotriptan 12.5 mg PO
	Eletriptan 80 mg
Tolerating acute treatments poorly	Almotriptan 12.5 mg
	Naratriptan 2.5 mg
	Frovatriptan 2.5 mg
Early vomiting	Zolmitriptan 5 mg nasal spray
	Sumatriptan 25 mg PR
	Sumatriptan 6 mg SC
Menstruation-related headache	Prevention
	Ergotamine PO nocte
	Oestrogen patches
	Tripacking oral contraceptive
	Treatment
	Triptans
	Dihydroergotamine nasal spray
Very rapidly developing symptoms	Zolmitriptan 5 mg nasal spray
	Sumatriptan 6 mg SC
	Dihydroergotamine 1 mg imi

PO, oral; PR, rectal; SC, subcutaneous.

(Goadsby, Lipton, & Ferrari, 2002). Using triptans correctly requires a combination of understanding their pharmacokinetics and formulation advantages and can be clinically very rewarding.

Nonspecific Treatments of Acute Migraine Attacks

Nonsteroidal Anti-inflammatory Drugs (NSAIDs)

ASPIRIN.   Aspirin reduces prostaglandin synthesis, but it is unknown whether this is related to its action in relieving headache. Aspirin can be an effective agent in migraine, providing it can be adequately absorbed. Volans (1974) showed that absorption of aspirin was impaired in 19 of 42 migraine patients during headache, which has led to the use of metoclopramide 10 mg orally or intramuscularly to facilitate absorption of ergotamine tartrate and aspirin in the management of the acute attack of migraine. An intravenous form of aspirin (D,L-lysine-acetylsalicylate), each vial containing about 500 mg, has been used in Japan and Europe (Fukuda & Izumikawa, 1988), and the oral form is particularly effective when combined with metoclopramide (Chabriat et al., 1994), as Wilkinson (1983) advocated.

FENEMATES.   Flufenamic acid at dosages of 250 mg every 2 hours, up to a maximum of 1000 mg, provided symptomatic relief in 195 of 200 migraine headaches (Vardi et al., 1976), although 8 of 26 patients experienced upper abdominal discomfort and 2 others had severe nausea and vomiting, 1 with melena.

Tolfenamic acid in doses of 200 mg was found to be as effective as ergotamine tartrate 1 mg in relieving migraine (Hakkarainen et al., 1979). Both drugs were more effective than aspirin, which in turn was superior to placebo. The efficacy of tolfenamic acid in its rapid-release version is comparable to that of oral sumatriptan (Myllyla et al., 1998).

INDOMETHACIN.   Indomethacin, given at high dosages (150 to 200 mg daily), is said to be beneficial in preventing migraine (Sicuteri, Michelacci, & Anselmi, 1964) but produces a high incidence of GI side effects. We did not find it helpful in more modest dosages of 25 mg three times daily (Anthony & Lance, 1968). Indomethacin finds a place in the management of paroxysmal hemicrania (see Chapter 12), hemicrania continua (see Chapter 11), in primary stabbing headache and exertional vascular headache (see Chapter 13).

OTHER NSAIDS.   Davis and colleagues (1995) found ketorolac 60 mg intramuscularly to be as effective as meperidine (pethidine) 75 mg and promezathine 25 mg intramuscularly in relieving migraine. Ibuprofen (Codispoti et al., 2001), naproxen (Welch, 1986; Treves, Streiffler, & Korczyn, 1992), and diclofenac (Karachalios et al., 1992; Diclofenac-K/Sumatriptan

Migraine Study Group, 1999) have also proved useful for treating migraine headache.

Other Agents

LIGNOCAINE (LIDOCAINE).   Lignocaine 100 mg intravenously has been reported to relieve migraine and cluster headache for approximately 20 minutes (Maciewicz et al., 1988). We typically continue a lignocaine infusion at 2 mg/min for as long as necessary to control pain (Kaube, Hoskin, & Goadsby, 1994). This can be combined with DHE 0.5 mg intravenously given every 8 hours. Reutens and associates (1991) failed to confirm the usefulness of lignocaine when given at a lower dosage of 1 mg/kg intravenously. During lignocaine infusion, patients should be under observation, with regular blood pressure recordings.

PHENOTHIAZINES.   Chlorpromazine 12.5 mg intravenously repeated at 20-minute intervals to a total of 37.5 mg was compared with DHE 1 mg intravenously (repeated in 30 minutes if necessary) and lignocaine 50 mg intravenously (repeated at 20-minute intervals to a maximum of 150 mg if needed) in managing acute migraine headache (Bell et al., 1990). Chlorpromazine-treated patients fared significantly better than those receiving the two other medications, with 15 of the 24 patients reporting persistent relief when contacted 12 to 24 hours later. Lane, McLellan, and Baggoley (1989) reported the use of chlorpromazine 0.1 mg/kg intravenously as adjuvant therapy in 24 patients, with 6 responding to one injection, 9 requiring two doses, and 9 needing three doses at 15-minute intervals. Prochlorperazine 10 mg intravenously is also an effective agent for treating acute migraine headache (Jones et al., 1989). Of 42 patients treated with prochlorperazine, 80% had complete or partial relief of headache, compared with 45% relief in those given placebo.

Metoclopramide 10 mg intramuscularly or a 20-mg suppository relieved nausea more effectively than placebo in a double-blind trial but did not by itself improve migraine headache (Tfelt-Hansen et al., 1980). Dystonic reactions may occur after many phenothiazines, and benztropine mesylate (1.0 to 2.0 mg intravenously) should be available to counter this problem if it arises.

5-HT$_3$ ANTAGONISTS.   Thus far, no 5-HT$_3$ antagonist has proved both safe and clearly effective in managing migraine, either as acute or prophylactic medications. Granisetron is a potent antiemetic in cancer chemotherapy and a selective 5-HT$_3$ receptor antagonist (Joss & Dott, 1993). We find both granisetron and ondansetron useful in the adjunctive management of migraine to control nausea and vomiting.

THE PLACE OF OPIOIDS IN THE MANAGEMENT OF ACUTE ATTACKS.   Using narcotics, particularly pethidine (meperidine), to relieve migraine is common in general practice in the United States, as in many countries (Ziegler, 1997), but it is very unusual in Europe. The case for injection of opioids rests on the presence of opioid receptors in the brain's endogenous pain-control pathways and on the fact that some patients claim their migraine headaches respond rapidly to injection of a narcotic agent but not to the other measures described earlier. When its use is confined to infrequent attacks of migraine accompanied by obvious signs of distress in a stable personality, pethidine appears to be a safe, cheap, and often effective remedy. The case against using narcotics rests on the short duration of their action and their tendency to induce tolerance, dependence, or addiction if used often.

A number of comparative trials have sought to show that other treatments, such as dihydroergotamine and metoclopramide, are as effective or more effective than pethidine (Klapper & Stanton, 1993; Scherl & Wilson, 1995), but the fact remains that some patients do respond to opioids and do not respond to other therapies without showing any indication of addiction. Pethidine may be the treatment of choice during pregnancy, when the use of ergotamine or similar preparations is to be avoided.

It is difficult to formulate a set of rules governing when and how often a narcotic should be administered to a particular patient. If patients are manipulative, seeking injections of narcotics more and more frequently, or visiting different doctors to obtain narcotics, they are best referred to a drug and alcohol advisory clinic. However, if a patient is known to be emotionally stable and to suffer genuine migraine that responds solely to narcotics, it is only humane to administer them appropriately. One cardinal rule is that the patient should have a single prescribing practitioner or medical practice. If the patient requires attention during nonbusiness hours and seeks treatment at a 24-hour medical clinic or emergency service, the primary prescriber should be notified if narcotics are used in treatment so that a check is maintained on frequency of administration.

Agents Used for Prophylactic (Interval) Therapy

If migrainous headaches occur twice a month or more and do not respond to ergotamine, sumatriptan, or other agents discussed earlier, consideration should be given to the daily administration of medication with the goal of reducing the frequency or severity of attacks (Table 9.6). The International Headache Society Committee on Clinical Trials in Migraine (Tfelt-Hansen et al., 2000a) has published guidelines for designing controlled trials to determine the effectiveness of a particular medication. Bear in mind, a drug that proves more effective than placebo in a double-blind trial may still be fairly useless clinically, leaving the patient with a slightly reduced frequency of devastating headaches. The results of clinical trials can also be confounded by the patient's unwillingness or inability to follow the regimen prescribed.

TABLE 9.6   Preventive therapy for migraine*

Drug	*Dose*	*Selected side effects*
Proven or very-well-accepted treatments (Silberstein & Goadsby, 2002)		
Beta-Adrenergic receptor antagonists		
Propranolol	40–120 mg bid	Reduced energy, tiredness, postural symptoms
Metoprolol	100–200 mg daily	Contraindicated in asthma
Tricyclic antidepressants		
Amitriptyline	25–75 mg nocte	Drowsiness
		Note: Some patients are very sensitive and may only need a total dose of 10 mg, although often 1 mg/kg body weight is required for a response.
Valproate (Divalproex) (Silberstein, 1996)	400–600 mg bid	Drowsiness, weight gain, tremor, hair loss, fetal abnormalities, and hematologic and liver abnormalities
Flunarizine (Leone et al., 1991)	5–15 mg daily	Tiredness, weight gain, depression, parkinsonism
Topiramate (Diener et al., 2003b; Brandes et al., 2004; Silberstein et al., 2004)	100–200 mg daily	Cognitive impairment, paresthesia, weight loss
Methysergide	1–6 mg daily	Drowsiness, leg cramps, hair loss, retroperitoneal fibrosis (a 1-month drug holiday is required every 6 months)
Widely used with poor evidence		
Verapamil	160–320 mg daily	Constipation, leg swelling, and A-V conduction disturbances
SSRIs: fluoxetine	20 mg daily	
Promising[†]		
Gabapentin (Mathew et al., 2001)	900–2400 mg daily	Tiredness, dizziness

*Commonly used preventive drugs are listed with reasonable doses and common side effects. Local prescribing information should be checked.

[†]Positive placebo-controlled study but more data are required.

Beta-Adrenergic Antagonists

Beta-blocking agents have been used to prevent migraine for more than 30 years and remain the first line of defense in nonasthmatic patients. Agents without intrinsic sympathomimetic (agonist) activity have proved effective, but whether they act by beta-blockade or a 5-HT agonist effect remains an open question. They consist of the nonselective beta-blockers propranolol, nadolol, and timolol as well as the selective beta-blockers atenolol and metoprolol (Tfelt-Hansen, 1989; Silberstein & Goadsby, 2002). Beta-blockers are best avoided in patients with a prolonged aura or severe focal neurologic symptoms, because some have reportedly suffered migrainous stroke (Bardwell & Trott, 1987).

Drugs Acting on 5-HT Mechanisms

PIZOTIFEN AND CYPROHEPTADINE.   Pizotifen (pizotyline) is a benzocycloheptathiophene derivative that is structurally similar to cyproheptadine and the tricyclic antidepressants. It has an elimination half-life of about 23 hours and can therefore be given as a single nocturnal dose. Pizotifen and cyproheptadine are 5-HT$_2$ and histamine-1 antagonists. They probably have a similar efficacy in preventing migraine and share the same side effects of drowsiness, increased appetite, and weight gain. Pizotifen has proved effective in controlled trials (Speight & Avery, 1972), although less potent than methysergide. A study comparing flunarizine 10 mg nocturnally and pizotifen 2 to 3 mg daily did not show any significant difference in the reduction of headache frequency, both compounds being effective (Louis & Spierings, 1982).

METHYSERGIDE.   Methysergide (L-methyl-D-lysergic acid butanolamide) is an ergot derivative with an elimination half-life of about 3 hours. It breaks down to methylergometrine (methylergonovine), which is probably responsible for its sustained beneficial effect in preventing migraine. Methysergide is a 5-HT antagonist but also has agonist properties on 5-HT$_2$ receptors. It has been proved effective in preventing migraine in double-blind trials (Lance, Fine, & Curran, 1963; Pedersen & Moller, 1966).

Graham (1967) reported that retroperitoneal fibrosis, pleural fibrosis, or cardiac valvular fibrosis had developed in about 100 patients of the half-million who were estimated to have been treated with methysergide at that time. In 35 years of extensively using methysergide, we have known eight patients with retroperitoneal fibrosis, three with pleural fibrosis, and one patient who under observation developed a cardiac murmur. Bear in mind that other agents may cause fibrotic syndromes and that in some cases no cause may be apparent. Lewis and colleagues (1975) reported a retrospective study of seven patients with retroperitoneal fibrosis from the London Hospital. None had ever taken methysergide, but four of the seven had taken excessive amounts of analgesics. Cases associated with methysergide usually resolve completely once treatment stops. The fibrotic complications of methysergide may result from its 5-HT–like action. Graham (1967) commented on the similarity of appearance at operation of valvular fibrosis in methysergide-treated patients to that seen in carcinoid syndrome. In this context the recent report of valvular fibrosis with fenfluramine treatment is of interest (Connolly et al., 1997). The administration of 5-HT to rats either decreases or increases granuloma formation, depending on adrenal gland function (Bianchine & Eade, 1967). Excessive fibrosis appears only if adrenal insufficiency is induced. This raises the question of whether there may be adrenal insufficiency in patients who develop fibrotic syndromes in response to 5-HT or methysergide. Perhaps any drug that relies on a 5-HT–simulating action to treat migraine has the potential for producing excessive fibrosis in susceptible people. To minimize the possibility of fibrotic complications, we recommend patients to cease medication with methysergide for 1 month every 6 months.

AMITRIPTYLINE.   Amitriptyline blocks reuptake of 5-HT and noradrenaline at central synapses. Apart from its use as an antidepressant, it has been used to manage tension-type headache (see Chapter 10) and other pain syndromes, such as postherpetic neuralgia (see Chapter 18). It is effective in preventing migraine (Gomersall & Stuart, 1973; Couch, Ziegler, & Hassanein, 1976; Ziegler et al., 1993) independent of its antidepressant effect. Individual responses to amitriptyline vary greatly. Some patients cannot tolerate as little as 10 mg given as a nocturnal dose, because of intolerable drowsiness the next day, whereas others experience no side effects while taking 150 mg in divided doses or a single nocturnal dose. Plasma levels on a given dosage vary widely (as much as 10-fold), but a steady state is reached 7 to 14 days after a fixed dosage is achieved (Ziegler, Clayton, & Biggs, 1977). Apart from drowsiness and a "drugged feeling," weight gain and dry mouth may be troublesome side effects. Adding amitriptyline to propranolol does not improve the results in migraine headache, but the combination is superior to either preparation alone in managing headaches that combine features of migraine and tension headache (Mathew, Stubits, & Nigam, 1982).

MONOAMINE OXIDASE INHIBITORS.   Because platelet 5-HT levels are lowered in migraine, using a drug that maintains or increases 5-HT levels is a logical form of treatment. Anthony and Lance (1969) treated 25 patients who had failed to respond to other forms of interval medication with phenelzine 45 mg daily for periods of up to 2 years. The frequency of headache fell to less than half in 20 of the 25 patients. Although mean platelet 5-HT increased by about 50%, there was no correlation between the 5-HT level and the response of each individual patient. We have continued to use this form of treatment in cases resistant to other therapy. Patients are given a notice specifying the foods and drugs to avoid while using monoamine oxidase (MAO) (A) inhibitors (Figure 9.2). Diamond (1995) has prescribed sumatriptan for acute attacks in patients maintained on phenelzine without encountering untoward reactions, but caution is advisable. Phenelzine has been used in conjunction with the beta-blocker atenolol, which has proved advantageous in that the side effect of postural hypotension is less frequent (Merikangas & Merikangas, 1995). The MAO (B) inhibitor selegiline, which prevents the breakdown of dopamine and phenylethylamine, is not helpful in managing migraine (Kuritzky, Zoldan, & Melamed, 1992).

Phenelzine prevents the breakdown of serotonin and noradrenaline in the body. You must avoid taking certain drugs and foods while you are on medication with phenelzine to avoid a serious increase in blood pressure.

Under no circumstances must you use nasal sprays or take tablets for sinusitis or blocked nostrils. No pethidine, morphine, reserpine, tranquillizers, sleeping tablets, blood pressure or weight reducing tablets or hypoglycaemic agents.

Avoid:
1. Cheese of any type
2. Meat or vegetable extracts such as Marmite
3. Red wines
4. Alcohol in excess
5. Broad beans
6. Pickled herrings
7. Chicken livers
8. Packet soups
9. Any other tablets or injections apart from those prescribed for migraine. Codeine, aspirin, paracetamol (acetaminophen), Migral, Ergodryl, Cafergot, and other ergotamine preparations are safe.

FIGURE 9.2   List of foods and drugs to avoid while taking monoamine oxidase inhibitors.

SPECIFIC SEROTONIN-REUPTAKE INHIBITORS.   The newer group of antidepressants called specific serotonin reuptake inhibitors (SSRIs) is not as effective in treating migraine as the tricyclics. The combination of the two is to be avoided, because cases of the "serotonin syndrome" have been reported, with agitation, myoclonus, and other movement disorders (Mathew, Tiejen, & Lucker, 1996). Fluoxetine is a high-profile antidepressant that specifically blocks 5-HT reuptake. A controlled trial involving 58 migraine patients given fluoxetine 20 mg daily (Saper et al., 1994) did not exhibit any improvement compared with placebo, although another group with chronic daily headache showed some response. Side effects of fluoxetine included sleep disturbance, tremor, and abdominal pain.

ANTICONVULSANTS.   The suggested link between migraine and epilepsy (Lipton et al., 1994) has led to paroxysmal outbursts of advocacy for anticonvulsant agents in managing migraine. Carbamazepine was mooted as being a useful prophylactic agent (Rompel & Bauermeister, 1970), but a comparative trial in our own clinic was unable to substantiate this (Anthony & Lance, 1972).

VALPROATE.   Sodium valproate was advocated as a means of suppressing migraine headache (Sorensen, 1988), and a controlled trial (Hering & Kuritzky, 1992) demonstrated that attack frequency fell to half the number and severity while patients were taking 400 mg twice daily over a 2-month period. The effectiveness of valproate (divalproex) has been confirmed in large controlled studies (Jensen, Brinck, & Olesen, 1994; Mathew et al., 1995; Klapper & Divalproex Sodium in Migraine Prophylaxis Study Group, 1997). Its efficacy is comparable to that of propranolol (Kaniecki, 1997). In practice, this effective compound is particularly useful in patients who experience frequent headache (Mathew & Ali, 1991). Silberstein (1996) has summarized clinical experience with valproate. Side effects include GI disturbances, weight gain, and either hyperexcitability or drowsiness. Tremor is a problem, especially in patients with a family history of tremor. About 3% of women complain of their hair falling out, but it grows back, very occasionally curly; we have never encountered baldness as a side effect. Hepatic toxicity has occurred in children on polypharmacy when there was an underlying liver problem but does not present a problem in adults on monotherapy (Silberstein & Wilmore, 1996).

Valproate has also been reported as overcoming the vexing problem of visual disturbance persisting for weeks or months after a migrainous aura (Rothrock, 1997). Unfortunately this is a complex issue, and Rothrock's report seems to contain two types of patients, who give clinically distinct histories. First, some patients describe a visual disturbance that is persistent and generally involves large areas, if not the entire visual field. Such patients report bright spots, sometimes colorful change or haziness, and often compare their vision to that of a poorly tuned television. The phrase *visual snow* is often used. Liu and colleagues (1995) seemed to be describing such patients in their initial report. Case 2 of Rothrock's (1997) also seems to fit this description. We have applied the term *primary persistent visual disturbance* to this clinical picture in two of our patients (Jager, Giffin, & Goadsby, 2004) to distinguish it from more typical cases with a visual disturbance of a migrainous type. The second group of patients have a more typical aura that persists, such as Haas's original description (Haas, 1982), case 1 of Rothrock (1997), and cases 3 and 4 of Jager and colleagues (2004). The latter cases seem best classified as migraine with persistent aura (Headache Classification Committee of the International Headache Society, 2004). We have had success with flunarizine in the former and have even seen a 10-year-old with visual snow phenomenon.

TOPIRAMATE.   Shuaib and colleagues (1999) reported a small open-label pilot study in which topiramate was effective in treating migraine. Subsequent small placebo-controlled studies corroborated this finding (Potter et al., 2000), particularly with regard to migraine with aura (Silberstein et al., 2002). Three large, well-powered, randomized, parallel-group, placebo-controlled studies have been done, two against placebo and a third against placebo and propranolol, and each has shown a significant effect for topiramate in preventing episodic migraine. In one study, 483 patients were randomized to receive topiramate 50, 100, and 200 mg daily, or placebo and compared using the change in mean monthly migraine frequency from baseline as the primary endpoint. There was significant effect against placebo for topiramate 100 and 200 mg daily, but no better 50% responder rate for the larger dose, 49% versus 47% (Brandes et al., 2004). In the second study the same doses were tested in 487 patients again randomized to the same dosing groups; again the results for the 100- and 200-mg topiramate doses were significant. Furthermore, again the topiramate 100-mg dose had a comparable 50% responder rate of 54% when compared with topiramate 200 mg at 52% (Silberstein et al., 2004). The third study has been reported in abstract form only at the time of this writing and showed a significant effect for topiramate 100 mg daily and propranolol 160 mg daily when compared with placebo and a comparable effect for the two active compounds (Diener et al., 2003b). Topiramate side effects include paresthesias in about 50% of treated patients because of its carbonic-anhydrase inhibition effect (Rosenfeld, 1997), cognitive impairment, and weight loss. The latter side effect is in marked contrast with many migraine preventive drugs. Caution in patients with a history of renal stones, glaucoma, or metabolic disorders is advised. It is unclear how topiramate works, but it does inhibit trigeminovascular neuronal traffic (Storer & Goadsby, 2004) and inhibits cortical spreading depression in cats and rats (Akerman & Goadsby, 2004). It is a useful addition in clinical practice.

GABAPENTIN.   An open trial of gabapentin (Mathew & Lucker, 1996) at dosages of 900 to 1800 mg/day gave promising results and was followed by a placebo-controlled study. In the controlled study, 98 patients took gabapentin at a maximum dosage of 2400 mg daily and 45 took placebo. Sixteen of the gabapentin and nine of the placebo-treated patients discontinued with adverse events, including dizziness. At the end of the 12-week treatment phase, there was a modified intention-to-treat analysis for the 2400-mg dose that demonstrated a significant 50% reduction in the 4-week migraine rate of 46% for the gabapentin-treated group and 16% for the placebo-treated group (Mathew et al., 2001). This was a methodologically weak analysis with a promising result that, taken with the data for chronic daily headache (see Chapter 11) (Beran & Spira, 2001), needs further exploration.

Calcium Channel Blocking Agents

Despite initial enthusiastic reports concerning the benefit of calcium channel blockers in treating migraine, the subject remains controversial. This probably relates to the remarkable differences in distribution and roles of the voltage-gated calcium channels (Ertel et al., 2000). It is best to consider these compounds separately.

Flunarizine is a calcium channel blocker with dopamine antagonist properties and a very long half-life. A number of double-blind studies summarized in a review by Leone and colleagues (1991) have demonstrated its efficacy at a dosage of 10 mg/day. Its efficacy is comparable to the efficacies of pizotifen (Louis & Spierings, 1982), propranolol (Wober et al., 1991; Diener et al., 2002), and valproate (Mitsikostas & Polychronidis, 1997). Flunarizine is particularly useful in some patients with migraine with prolonged aura, particularly sporadic hemiplegic (Thomsen et al., 2003) and familial hemiplegic migraine (Ducros et al., 2001), but its effects may take 4 to 6 months to commence. Patience in its use can be very rewarding for patient and clinician. Side effects include fatigue, depression, and the development of parkinsonian symptoms after prolonged use.

Solomon and colleagues (1983) reported 12 patients in a small crossover study of verapamil that had a nearly 50% dropout rate. Markley, Cleronis, and Piepko (1984) reported a placebo-controlled study with a 15% dropout rate. It was a small study ($n = 14$) and was positive against placebo. Solomon (1986) reported a study comparing propranolol and verapamil with a placebo arm. The study did not report a significant effect for verapamil against placebo and was not powered ($n = 15$) for equivalence to propranolol. Solomon and Diamond (1987) reported a study of two doses of verapamil, again in a small study ($n = 12$), with no placebo control. Neither of the latter two studies has been fully reported. Solomon (1989) summarized 5 years' experience and reported a study that is not in the English literature (Prusinski & Kozubski, 1987). This latter study had 23 patients, and 20 were said to have improved. Dropout rates and the primary endpoint are unclear. Thus there are three positive but small studies. One had a substantial dropout, and one is not fully reported in any accessible manner. The effect of verapamil in our hands has never been impressive. Constipation and swollen ankles are the main side effects in routine dosing.

The Migraine-Nimodipine European Study Group (1989) was unable to demonstrate any significant effect of nimodipine 40 mg three times daily over placebo in migraine with or without aura, although the group noted that a larger sample in the latter trial could have potentially yielded a positive result. A trial of cyclandelate did not show any advantage over placebo (Diener et al., 1996).

Nonsteroidal Anti-inflammatory Drugs in Prophylaxis

Aspirin has been used both to prevent and treat migraine attacks. Of a group of physicians taking low-dose aspirin (325 mg every 2 days), 6.0% reported suffering from migraine at some time after randomization, compared with 7.4% of those in the placebo group (Buring, Peto, & Hennekens, 1990). This reduction of 20% was modest but significant. Masel and associates (1980) conducted a controlled crossover trial of aspirin 325 mg twice daily, combined with dipyridamole 25 mg three times daily, finding that the frequency and severity of migraine attacks were significantly reduced compared with the placebo period.

A crossover double-blind trial established that naproxen 275 mg given in two tablets at morning and night gave significantly better results than placebo, with freedom from severe headaches being achieved in 59% of patients taking naproxen compared with 19% receiving placebo (Welch, 1986).

Other Medications

FEVERFEW.   The ancient herbal remedy feverfew, which inhibits the release of 5-HT from platelets, has been in vogue as a remedy for migraine. Six randomized controlled trials of feverfew leaf in the treatment of migraine have been published. Three were negative (Murphy, Heptinstall, & Mitchell, 1988; De Weerdt, Bootsma, & Hendriks, 1996; Pfaffenrath et al., 2002); two were positive, one published in full (Palevitch, Earon, & Carrasso, 1997) and one in abstract form

(Diener et al., 2003a); and another, which used an unorthodox design and uncertain patient population (Johnson et al., 1985), was positive. Even if the poor-quality studies are included, one might conclude there is a cloud over the subject (Goadsby, 2003). The most recent abstract is promising (Diener et al., 2003a), and further study is required.

MAGNESIUM.   There have been conflicting reports about the efficacy of oral magnesium. Peikert, Willimzig, and Kohne-Volland (1996) found that 600 mg of trimagnesium citrate daily reduced attack frequency by 42%, compared with 16% on placebo after 2 months. However, Pfaffenrath and colleagues (1996) could not demonstrate any benefit from a slightly smaller dose given over 3 months; as might be expected, diarrhea was the main side effect.

RIBOFLAVIN.   On the ground that mitochondrial phosphorylation is reduced in patients suffering from migraine (Welch & Ramadan, 1995), riboflavin 400 mg daily has been tested for efficacy. Schoenen, Jacquy, and Lenaerts (1998) showed that headache frequency and severity were reduced to half in the riboflavin group. The issue of energy failure as part of the explanation for migraine certainly deserves exploration, as does such a therapeutic approach.

COENZYME Q10.   After the study of riboflavin and based on a hypothesis of a deficit in mitochondrial energy reserve in migraine, coenzyme Q10 100 mg three times daily was studied in a double-blind, randomized, parallel-group study in patients with migraine (Sandor et al., 2003). After a 1-month baseline, participants were randomized to receive placebo ($n = 21$) or Q10 ($n = 21$) for 3 months. The reduction in attack frequency and headache days was significant in the Q10 group versus the placebo group. The 50% responder rate was 48% for Q10 and 14% for placebo. One patient from the Q10 group withdrew with cutaneous allergy. This is a promising approach with interesting implications for migraine biology.

HISTAMINE ANTAGONISTS.   In a carefully controlled double-blind trial, we were unable to demonstrate any worthwhile effects of the histamine-1 blocking agent chlorpheniramine or the histamine-2 blocking agent cimetidine in preventing migraine (Anthony, Lord, & Lance, 1978).

CLONIDINE.   Clonidine is an α_2-adrenoceptor agonist, which was proposed as a prophylactic agent for migraine. Initial optimistic reports were followed by a series of negative trials. Of 11 published reports, 1 gave positive results (Kallanranta et al., 1977), 4 gave negative results, 3 were equivocal, and 3 provided insufficient data to form an opinion. In practice, clonidine has no place in the management of migraine, although this may be because of its dose-limiting side effects rather than an incorrect mechanism of action.

THE PRACTICAL MANAGEMENT OF MIGRAINE

Pre-emptive Treatment

If premonitory symptoms give 6 to 12 hours' warning of a migraine attack, administering domperidone 30 to 40 mg at the onset of symptoms is said to prevent development of migraine headache in about 60% of cases (Waelkens, 1981, 1984). Patients who experience mood changes or a craving for sweet foods predictably on the evening before they awaken with migraine headache may prevent the development of headache by taking a nocturnal dose of ergotamine tartrate.

Treatment of the Acute Attack

Some patients respond rapidly to *aspirin* or a similar analgesic agent administered at the first sign of an attack, particularly if *metoclopramide* (10 mg) is given by mouth or by the intramuscular route at the same time to promote gastric absorption and reduce nausea. The intravenous use of aspirin is worth further exploration and is certainly useful in some patients. NSAIDs, such as naproxen 500 to 1000 mg or ibuprofen 600 to 800 mg, can be given orally, by suppository, or by syrup, as available formulations and age dictate, as an alternative to aspirin, and in preference to it in young patients. Ketorolac 60 mg intramuscularly can be effective in minimizing an attack (Davis et al., 1995). The patient should then rest and, preferably, sleep. Unfortunately, severe migraine headaches are usually resistant to these measures.

The *triptans* are now the most efficacious medications to terminate an acute attack of migraine. We have taught students for many years to use acute treatments early if the patient is confident the attack is a migraine, certainly before the headache is well established and perhaps related to the development of allodynia (Burstein, Collins, & Jakubowski, 2004). Evidence is now emerging for triptans (Cady et al., 2000; Klapper et al., 2002; Pascual & Cabarrocas, 2002; Winner et al., 2003), and indeed for other medicines against acute attack (Lipton & Goadsby, 2001), that when pain is mild early treatment is an effective approach. The major problem with studies done thus far is that patient groups have been selected for slowly developing attacks, and all the conclusions may not be generalizable to all migraine patients. One approach would involve sumatriptan 50 mg taken at the onset of symptoms. Some patients require 100 mg, whereas others may respond to 25 mg. A second or third tablet of any of the sumatriptan doses of equivalent strength can be taken within a 24-hour period if a headache recurs once the effect of sumatriptan wears off. Based on available evidence, rizatriptan 10 mg, eletriptan 40 or 80 mg, and almotriptan 12.5 mg offer the best chance of helping patients (Ferrari et al., 2002). Certain advantages to particular triptans are detailed in Table 9.5. Naratriptan 2.5 mg (Gunasekara & Wiseman, 1997) or frovatriptan 2.5 mg (McDavis & Hutchison, 1999) are useful in patients who, although responding to any of the other triptans, experience marked side effects. If oral medications fail or drug absorption is a particular problem, as in patients who vomit early on, sumatriptan 20 mg (Dahlof, 1999) or zolmitriptan 5 mg (Charlesworth et al., 2003) nasal spray can be very helpful, and where available the suppository formulation of sumatriptan (25 mg) (Dahlof, 2001) may also be useful. An autoinjector administering 6 mg subcutaneously (Ferrari & Subcutaneous Sumatriptan International Study Group, 1991) can be used if patients do not respond to oral medications or cannot tolerate or fail the intranasal route. The injection can be repeated within 24 hours if required. Some patients respond to sumatriptan on some occasions but not on others (Visser et al., 1996), so it is worth trying this medication for at least three attacks to ascertain its value for each individual.

The major indication for using triptans is for patients who are incapacitated by their migraine headache despite using nonspecific therapies or for those who do not tolerate those medicines. Certainly for many patients a triptan is cost effective, and many patients prefer these medications over ergotamine and analgesics. There remains an important place for regular prophylactic medication (tricyclic antidepressants, beta-blockers, pizotifen, methysergide, topiramate, and valproate) to treat patients who have very frequent attacks. It currently is advised not to use triptans in patients partly controlled by methysergide, although there is no evidence for imcompatibility (see Chapter 12), and there is no evidence of major interaction with propranolol, flunarizine, pizotifen, valproate, or dihydroergotamine (which acts mainly on venous-capacitance vessels). It is recommended that sumatriptan not be administered until 24 hours after the last dose of ergotamine tartrate, because the vasoconstrictive effects of each drug may be additive. However, ergotamine can be administered 6 hours after sumatriptan because of the latter's short half-life and similarly can be adjusted for the half-lives of the other triptans. In this setting it can be useful for preventing recurrence of headache once the effect of sumatriptan wears off.

The most remarkable effect of sumatriptan in our experience is the ability of the injectable form to abolish migraine headaches of a severity that previously required narcotic agents to provide relief. This has proved a boon to the harassed general practitioner or staff of an accident and emergency unit, who often are confronted with the dilemma of whether it is justifiable to administer narcotics to a particular patient. Sumatriptan has also proved useful in controlling migraine headaches during withdrawal from excessive use of ergotamine and analgesics (Diener et al., 1991).

Ergotamine tartrate is cheaper but less effective than sumatriptan and should be given at an optimal dosage at the first indication of an attack developing. If the patient is not nauseated, ergotamine 1 to 2 mg may be taken by mouth, alone or in combination with caffeine (Cafergot) or caffeine plus an antiemetic agent in a variety of preparations. Because gastric absorption is often impaired in migraine, the gastric route may be bypassed by a suppository. The most commonly available suppository is Cafergot, which contains 2 mg of ergotamine tartrate and may cause nausea and aching in the legs. This can be avoided by instructing the patient to put the suppositories in a refrigerator to harden, then slicing them in half. Half of the suppository can be inserted at the onset of an attack and the other half later on if the headache does not abate. It is said that no more than 10 mg of ergotamine should be taken in 1 week, but individual tolerance varies and vascular side effects are uncommon.

Patients who use ergotamine frequently may run into the problem of daily rebound headaches and feel generally unwell, in which case the drug is best stopped completely—at least for a period—to let the previous intermittent pattern of headache re-establish.

Dihydroergotamine (DHE) 1 mg intramuscularly can be given as the attack begins (Winner et al., 1996) or repeated every 8 hours if headache continues. Similarly, DHE can now be used intranasally and is particularly useful in patients who experience headache recurrence. DHE acts on venous-capacitance vessels rather than on arteries and is usually free of vasoconstrictive side effects. There is also evidence it has a central action on pain pathways (Goadsby & Gundlach, 1991; Hoskin et al., 1996).

Metoclopramide 10 mg intravenously or intramuscularly or prochlorperazine 12.5 mg intramuscularly may be given to relieve nausea and vomiting; prochlorperazine 10 mg intravenously has also been reported to abort headache. Chlorpromazine 12.5 mg intravenously has proved useful in treating headaches, as described earlier in this chapter.

We have found intravenous *lignocaine,* given slowly as a bolus of 100 mg, followed by an intravenous infusion of 2 mg/min, useful in terminating continuous migraine headache ("status migrainosus"). This can be combined with the intravenous injection of DHE 0.5 mg every 8 hours. There is less need for these measures with the advent of sumatriptan, because injecting sumatriptan 6 mg subcutaneously usually stops such headaches (Jauslin, Goadsby, & Lance, 1991).

Corticosteroids have been used in combination with other agents to treat intractable migraine headache (Gallagher, 1985).

The use of narcotic agents is to be avoided, because habituation can become a problem. One must beware of "smiling migraineurs" who assert they have an intolerable headache requiring injected narcotics while appearing to be in the best of health. For patients who do not respond to other measures and who exhibit objective signs of distress, narcotics should not be withheld. Morphine is usually less effective than meperidine (pethidine) in patients with migraine. Pentazocine may cause hallucinations.

PROPHYLACTIC THERAPY FOR FREQUENT MIGRAINE ATTACKS

If infrequent migraine headaches can be prevented from developing through the use of sumatriptan, ergotamine, or NSAIDs, there is no need for the patient to take prophylactic medication (interval therapy; see Table 9.4 and Figure 9.3). If these agents are not completely effective and the frequency of attacks warrants it (say two or more each month), it is worthwhile for the patient to take daily medication in an attempt to suppress headaches or reduce their frequency and severity. Many patients with frequent headache overuse analgesics, and overuse of compound analgesics, in particular, can make patients refractory to the effects of prophylactics medications. It is imperative that a careful drug history be obtained and that the patient's use of both prescription and nonprescription compounds be assessed so that he or she may be advised to reduce or eliminate

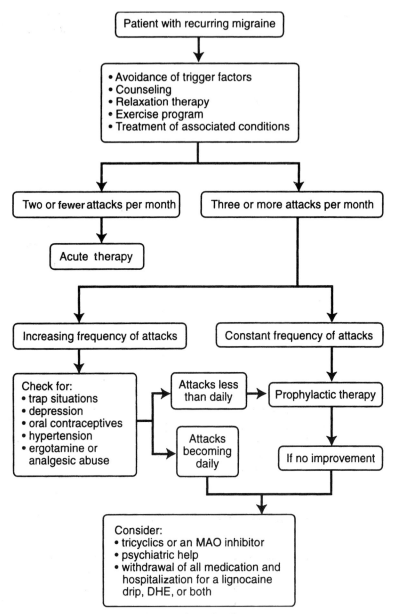

FIGURE 9.3   A possible approach to treating migraine.

the intake, thereby providing a window of opportunity for prophylactic medicines.

If the patient is not overweight, *pizotifen* or *cyproheptadine* is worth trying first. Tablets of pizotifen contain 0.5 mg, and the dosage can be increased slowly from 1 to 6 tablets at night if necessary, keeping at a level that does not cause morning drowsiness. Alternatively, cyproheptadine 4 mg divided in one or two tablets at night can be prescribed. Increase in appetite with resulting weight gain is a common side effect of both drugs. If the patient has not improved after 1 month on the optimum dosage, our own policy is to change to a *beta-blocker,* such as *propranolol,* after ensuring that the patient is not asthmatic. Some patients respond to as little as 10 mg twice daily of propranolol, but others require full beta-blocking dosages. Valproate is a useful preventive agent and often controls migraine in patients who have not responded to first-line agents, but the dosage must often be pushed to 1000 to 1500 mg and maintained for 6 to 8 weeks. Topiramate starting at 12.5 or 25 mg daily and increasing by 25 mg every 10 to 14 days to a dosage of 50 mg twice daily can be very useful, as can gabapentin slowly titrated to 2400 to 3600 mg daily taken in three divided doses. Flunarizine at 5 to 15 mg daily can also be helpful but is slow in its onset of action.

When migraine headache is frequent, tricyclic *antidepressants* are useful even for patients who are not depressed. *Amitriptyline* is probably the most effective; it should be given at night and the dosage increased slowly, because many patients complain of morning drowsiness. The patient can start with a tablet of 10 mg, or half a 25-mg tablet, at night and increase to 75 mg or even 150 mg each night if the medication is well tolerated. Its use may be limited by dry mouth and tremor as well as sedation. In this case dothiepin or imipramine can be used instead.

Methysergide is highly effective against migraine, but treatment must be started cautiously to minimize incidence of side effects. Patients are well advised to cut a pill in half as a small test dose, because about 40% of patients experience side effects, such as epigastric discomfort, muscle cramps, vasoconstrictive phenomena, or mood changes, if the full dosage schedule of 1 to 2 mg three times a day is taken immediately. Methysergide suppresses migraine completely in about 25% of patients and reduces headache frequency more than half in another 40%. If the patient's symptoms are substantially relieved, methysergide therapy is usually continued for 4 months and then reduced slowly and substituted by another prophylactic agent for 1 month before being recommenced. The reason for this precaution is the rare complication of retroperitoneal or pleural fibrosis.

Some patients choose to continue methysergide therapy, because attempts at withdrawal lead to a severe and debilitating recrudescence of migraine. In such cases the patient should be made aware of the possibility of fibrotic side effects and should report for a physical examination and a blood urea or creatinine estimation every 3 months; patients must be instructed to notify their medical adviser immediately if any symptoms appear. With these precautions, methysergide is a safe and useful form of migraine prophylaxis for many patients.

Some patients experience side effects, chiefly abdominal discomfort and muscle cramps, when treatment is first started, but these usually subside after days or weeks. Less common side effects include insomnia, depression, a sensation of swelling in the face or throat, increased venules over nose and cheeks, and weight gain (Curran, Hinterberger, & Lance, 1967). About 10% of patients cannot tolerate methysergide because of persistent unpleasant symptoms or the appearance of peripheral vasoconstriction with pallor of the extremities, intermittent claudication, or, very rarely, angina pectoris. Peripheral vascular disease, coronary artery disease, hypertension, a history of thrombophlebitis or peptic ulcer, and pregnancy are all contraindications to the use of methysergide. The reason for avoiding methysergide in the first four conditions is fairly clear—arterial vasoconstriction is a recognized side effect. Taking methysergide was found to double basal gastric secretion of hydrochloric acid in patients with peptic ulcer, so its use is best avoided in this condition. No evidence suggests methysergide is harmful to a pregnant mother or fetus, but we suspend its use if pregnancy is planned or occurs unexpectedly.

Some 80% of patients with migraine who have proved resistant to other forms of therapy respond to phenelzine 15 mg three times a day. A list of foods and drugs to avoid while taking MAO inhibitors should be given to each patient (see Figure 9.2). Particular mention should be made of oral or inhaled nasal decongestant or bronchodilator agents that commonly contain monoamines.

MIGRAINOUS AURAS (MIGRAINOUS EQUIVALENTS)

There are no clear evidence-based treatments of migraine aura in the acute phase. A capsule of nifedipine 10 mg can be bitten and several drops swallowed as soon as the visual disturbance or other neurologic symptoms begin. Inhalation of an isoprenaline spray or a tablet of glycerol trinitrate 0.6 mg may also hasten resolution of the aura. An open-label experience of ketamine, a glutamate NMDA (*N*-methyl-D-aspartate) blocker, has been reported, and this is a promising, avenue for study (Kaube et al., 2000).

MENSTRUAL MIGRAINE AND PREGNANCY

Hormonal methods of treating menstrual migraine are aimed at overcoming the sudden fall in plasma estradiol that precedes menstruation. Subcutaneous implantation of estradiol pellets, starting with 100 mg, inhibits ovulation and maintains estradiol levels, whereas regular monthly periods can be induced by cyclical oral progestogens. Using this method, Magos, Zilkha, and Studd (1983) rendered 20 of 24 patients virtually headache free over a follow-up period of 5 years. Applying a gel containing 1.5 mg estradiol to the skin 48 hours before the expected onset of menstruation prevented 18 of 26 menstrual headaches, compared with only 1 of 7 in the patients using a placebo gel (De Lignieres et al., 1986). The estrogen-containing oral contraceptive can be used to prevent menstrual migraine by so-called tripacking. The pill-free week is omitted twice so that the patient menstruates approximately every 3 months. This can be very effective, although certainly the trimonthly attack can require aggressive acute therapy when it happens.

Tamoxifen has complex effects on ovarian function, competing at estrogen and antiestrogen binding sites, as well as having calcium-channel–blocking properties. O'Dea and Davis (1990) reported a pilot open trial in which five of eight patients improved markedly and two improved moderately when treated with tamoxifen citrate 10 to 20 mg daily before and during menstruation. Continuous therapy with bromocriptine 2.5 mg three times daily reduced the frequency of premenstrual migraine in 18 of 24 women followed for a year (Herzog, 1997).

Our own practice is to use interval medication as described earlier for a few days before and during the menstrual period before attempting hormonal therapy.

Migraine headaches cease in the second and third trimesters of pregnancy in two thirds of women. There is no evidence that any of the agents used in treating migraine are harmful to the fetus, but we discontinue medication during pregnancy when possible. Ergotamine has only a weak oxytocic effect but is best avoided lest any natural complication of pregnancy be attributed to its use.

MIGRAINE IN CHILDHOOD

Episodic headaches in children and adolescents are often erroneously thought to be of the tension-type variety even though they are associated with nausea, photophobia, or other migrainous characteristics. Tensions at school and at home may certainly contribute to the frequency of migraine in childhood, and the excitement of a birthday party often triggers an attack. Good, Taylor, and Mortimer (1991) found that migrainous children wearing rose-tinted glasses reduced their monthly headache frequency from 6.2 to 1.6 per month over a period of 4 months, whereas wearing density-matched blue glasses had no effect. Improvement was attributed to the red tint reducing exposure to shortwave-length flicker from fluorescent lights. Attention must be paid to any psychological factors and to physical relaxation (Duckro & Cantwell-Simmons, 1989). The child's posture should be checked. If the height of chair and desk are mismatched, children may have to crane their heads awkwardly to write or see the board at school. Diet and regular mealtimes may play a more important part in childhood than in adult life, but the child should not be denied pharmacotherapy.

Although some children find their headaches are eased by an analgesic and disappear with sleep, many do not. In these children, triptans are effective. Controlled data show sumatriptan by nasal spray to be more effective than placebo (Hershey et al., 2001; Ahonen et al., 2004). Zolmitriptan 2.5 mg in the rapidly dissolving wafer formulation, with its agreeable taste, is also very easy to use in children. We have used ergotamine tartrate and dihydroergotamine in children, but they have little advantage over the triptans. When migraine recurs frequently in children, interval therapy can be used as in adults, usually starting with pizotifen or cyproheptadine (for children who are not overweight) or propranolol (if there is no tendency to asthma). Flunarizine is popular in many parts of Europe for childhood migraine and is safe and easy to use in this population, with a once-a-day dosage usually starting at 5 mg at bedtime. Once migraine is brought under control in children, it goes into remission in about 60% of cases, although it may recur in later years in about 20%.

CONCLUSION

The variety of medications used in treating migraine is an indication that none is entirely effective. Nevertheless, most patients can achieve relief with combined behavioral management and drug therapy. The advent of the selective 5-HT$_{1B/1D}$ agonists, the triptans, started a new era promising more specific and efficacious management of acute attacks. For patients who do not respond satisfactorily to a triptan, the newer ergotamine derivatives or analgesics and whose frequency of attacks exceeds two a month, a thorough trial of prophylactic therapy is indicated, with the aim of reducing the intensity and frequency of attacks or eliminating them completely.

References

Ahonen, K., Hamalainen, M. L., Rantala, H., & Hoppu, K. (2004). Nasal sumatriptan is effective in treatment of migraine attacks in children: A randomized trial. *Neurology, 62,* 883–887.

Ahrens, S. P., Farmer, M. V., Williams, D., Willoughby, E., Jiang, K., Block, G. A., & Visser, W. H. (1999). Efficacy and safety of rizatriptan wafer for the acute treatment of migraine. *Cephalalgia, 19,* 525–530.

Akerman, S., & Goadsby, P. J. (2004). Topiramate inhibits cortical spreading depression in rat and cat: A possible contribution to its preventive effect in migraine. *Cephalalgia, 24,* in press.

Andersen, A. R., Tfelt-Hansen, P., & Lassen, N. A. (1987). The effect of ergotamine and dihydroergotamine on cerebral blood flow in man. *Stroke, 18,* 120–123.

Anderson, J. A. D., Basker, M. A., & Dalton, R. (1975). Migraine and hypnotherapy. *Int J Exp Hypn, 23,* 48–58.

Anthony, M. (1987). The role of the occipital nerve in unilateral headache. In F. C. Rose (Ed.), *Current problems in neurology.* Vol. 4: *Advances in headache research* (pp. 257–262). London: John Libbey.

Anthony, M. (1992). Headache and the greater occipital nerve. *Clin Neur Neurosurg, 94,* 297–301.

Anthony, M., Hinterberger, H., & Lance, J. W. (1967). Plasma serotonin in migraine and stress. *Arch Neurol, 16,* 544–552.

Anthony, M., & Lance, J. W. (1968). Indomethacin in migraine. *Med J Aust, 1,* 56–57.

Anthony, M., & Lance, J. W. (1969). Monoamine oxidase inhibition in the treatment of migraine. *Arch Neurol, 21,* 263–268.

Anthony, M., & Lance, J. W. (1972). A comparative trial of pindolol, clonidine and carbamazepine in the interval therapy of migraine. *Med J Aust, 1,* 1343–1346.

Anthony, M., Lord, G. D. A., & Lance, J. W. (1978). Controlled trials of cimetidine in migraine and cluster headache. *Headache, 18,* 261–264.

Baischer, W. (1995). Acupuncture in migraine. Long term outcome and predicting factors. *Headache, 35,* 472–474.

Bardwell, A., & Trott, J. A. (1987). Stroke in migraine as a consequence of propranolol. *Headache, 27,* 381–383.

Bartsch, T., & Goadsby, P. J. (2002). Stimulation of the greater occipital nerve induces increased central excitability of dural afferent input. *Brain, 125,* 1496–1509.

Bartsch, T., & Goadsby, P. J. (2003). Increased responses in trigeminocervical nociceptive neurones to cervical input after stimulation of the dura mater. *Brain, 126,* 1801–1813.

Bell, R., Montoya, D., Shuaib, A., & Lee, M. A. (1990). A comparative trial of three agents in the treatment of acute migraine headache. *Ann Emerg Med, 19,* 1079–1082.

Benedict, C. R., & Robertson, D. (1979). Angina pectoris and sudden death in the absence of atherosclerosis following ergotamine therapy for migraine. *Am J Med, 67,* 177–178.

Benson, H., Klemchuk, H. P., & Graham, J. R. (1974). The usefulness of the relaxation response in the therapy of headache. *Headache, 14,* 49–52.

Bentley, J. C., Bourson, A., Boess, F. G., Fone, K. C., Marsden, C. A., Petit, N., & Sleight, A. J. (1999). Investigation of stretching behaviour induced by the selective 5-HT6 receptor antagonist, Ro 04-6790, in rats. *Br J Pharmacol, 126,* 1537–1542.

Beran, R. G., & Spira, P. J. (2001). Gabapentin in chronic daily headache. *Neurology, 56,* A220–A221.

Berde, B., & Schild, H. O. (1978). *Ergot alkaloids and related compounds* (Vol. 49). Berlin: Springer.

Bianchine, J. R., & Eade, N. R. (1967). The effect of 5-hyroxytryptamine on the cotton pellet local inflammatory response in the rat. *J Exp Med, 125,* 501–510.

Blanchard, E. B., Appelbaum, K. A., Radnitz, C. L., Morrill, B., Michulika, D., Kirsch, D., et al. (1990). A controlled evaluation of thermal biofeedback and thermal biofeedback combined with cognitive therapy in the treatment of vascular headache. *J Consult Clin Psychol, 58,* 216–224.

Blondel, O., Gastineau, M., Dahmoune, Y., Langlois, M., & Fischmeister, R. (1998). Cloning, expression and pharmacology of four human 5-HT4 receptor isoforms produced by alternative splicing in the carboxyl terminus. *J Neurochem, 70,* 2252–2261.

Brandes, J. L., Saper, J. R., Diamond, M., Couch, J. R., Lewis, D. W., Schmitt, J., Neto, W., Schwabe, S., Jacobs, D., & MIGR-002 Study Group (2004). Topiramate for migraine prevention: A randomized controlled trial. *JAMA, 291,* 965–973.

Buring, J. E., Peto, R., & Hennekens, & C. H. (1990). Low-dose aspirin for migraine prophylaxis. *JAMA, 264,* 1711–1713.

Burstein, R., Collins, B., & Jakubowski, M. (2004). Defeating migraine pain with triptans: A race against the development of cutaneous allodynia. *Ann Neurol, 55,* 19–26.

Burstein, R., Cutrer, M. F., & Yarnitsky, D. (2000). The development of cutaneous allodynia during a migraine attack. *Brain, 123,* 1703–1709.

Cabarrocas, X., & Salva, M. (1997). Pharmacokinetic and metabolic data on almotriptan, a new antimigraine drug. *Cephalagia, 17,* 421.

Cady, R. K., Sheftell, F., Lipton, R. B., O'Quinn, S., Jones, M., Putnam, D. G., Crisp, A., Metz, A., & McNeal, S. (2000). Effect of early intervention with sumatriptan on migraine pain: Retrospective analyses of data from three clinical trials. *Clin Ther, 22,* 1035–1048.

Callaham, M., & Raskin, N. (1986). A controlled study of dihydroergotamine in the treatment of acute migraine headache. *Headache, 26,* 168–171.

Carpay, J., Schoenen, J., Ahmad, F., Kinrade, F., & Boswell, D. (2004). Efficacy and tolerability of sumatriptan tablets in a fast-disintegrating, rapid-release formulation for the acute treatment of migraine: Results of a multicenter, randomized, placebo-controlled study. *Clin Ther, 26,* 214–223.

Chabriat, H., Joire, J. E., Danchot, J., Grippon, P., & Bousser, M. G. (1994). Combined oral lysine acetyl-salicylate and metoclopramide in the acute treatment of migraine: A multicentre double-blind placebo-controlled study. *Cephalalgia, 14,* 297–300.

Charlesworth, B. R., Dowson, A. J., Purdy, A., Becker, W. J., Boes-Hansen, S., & Farkkila, M. (2003). Speed of onset and efficacy of zolmitriptan nasal spray in the acute treatment of migraine: A double-blind, placebo-controlled, dose-ranging study versus zolmitriptan tablet. *CNS Drugs, 17,* 653–667.

Codispoti, J, R., Prior, M. J., Fu, M., Harte, C. M., & Nelson, E. B. (2001). Efficacy of nonprescription doses of ibuprofen for treating migraine headache. A randomized controlled trial. *Headache, 41,* 665–679.

Connolly, H. M., Crary, J. L., McGoon, M. D., Hensrud, D. D., Edwards, B. S., Edwards, W. D., & Schaff, H. V. (1997). Valvular heart disease associated with fenfluramine-phentermine. *N Engl J Med, 337,* 581–588.

Couch, J. R., Ziegler, D. K., & Hassanein, R. (1976). Amitriptyline in the prophylaxis of migraine. Effectiveness and relationship of antimigraine and antidepressant drugs. *Neurology, 26,* 121–127.

Curran, D. A., Hinterberger, H., & Lance, J. W. (1967). Methysergide. *Res Clin Stud Headache, 1,* 74–122.

Cyriax, J. (1962). *Textbook of orthopaedic medicine* (Vol. 1). London: Cassell.

Dahlof, C. (1999). Sumatriptan nasal spray in the acute treatment of migraine: A review of clinical studies. *Cephalalgia, 19,* 769–778.

Dahlof, C. (2001). Clinical efficacy and tolerability of sumatriptan tablet and suppository in the acute treatment of migraine: A review of data from clinical trials. *Cephalalgia, 21*(Suppl 1), 9–12.

Davis, C. P., Torre, P. T., Williams, C., Gray, C., Barrett, K., Krucke, G., Peake, D., & Bass, B., Jr. (1995). Ketorolac versus meperidine plus promethazine treatment of migraine headaches: Evaluation by patients. *Am J Emerg Med, 13,* 146–150.

De Lignieres, B., Mauvais-Javis, P., Mas, J. M., Toubout, P. J., & Bousser, M. G. (1986). Prevention of menstrual migraine by percutaneous oestradiol. *BMJ, 293,* 1540.

De Weerdt, C. J., Bootsma, H. P., & Hendriks, H. (1996). Herbal medicines in migraine prevention: Randomized double-blind placebo-controlled crossover trial of a feverfew preparation. *Phytomedicine, 3,* 225–230.

Diamond, S. (1995). The use of sumatriptan in patients on monoamine oxidase inhibitors. *Neurology, 45,* 1039–1040.

Diclofenac-K, Sumatriptan Migraine Study Group. (1999). Acute treatment of migraine attacks: Efficacy and safety of nonsteroidal anti-inflammatory drug, diclofenac-potassium, in comparison to oral sumatriptan and placebo. *Cephalalgia, 19,* 232–240.

Diener, H. C. (2003). Placebo in headache trials. *Cephalalgia, 23,* 485–486.

Diener, H. C., Foh, M., Iaccarino, C., Wessely, P., Isler, H. R., Strenge, H., Fischer, M., Wedekind, W., & Taneri, Z. (1996). Cyclandelate in the prophylaxis of migraine: A randomised parallel, double-blind study in comparison with placebo and propranolol. *Cephalalgia, 16,* 441–447.

Diener, H. C., Haab, J., Peters, C., Ried, S., Dichgans, J., & Pilgrim, A. (1991). Subcutaneous sumatriptan in the treatment of headache during withdrawal from drug-induced headache. *Headache, 31,* 205–209.

Diener, H. C., Matias-Guiu, J., Hartung, E., Pfaffenrath, V., Ludin, H. P., Nappi, G., & De Beukelaar, F. (2002). Efficacy and tolerability in migraine prophylaxis of flunarizine in reduced doses: A comparison with propranolol 160 mg daily. *Cephalalgia, 22,* 209–221.

Diener, H.-C., Pfaffenrath, V., Schnitker, J., Friede, M., Henneicke-von Zepelin, H.-H., & The Study Group. (2003a). Efficacy and safety of the feverfew co2-extract mig-99 in migraine prevention—A randomised, double-blind, multicentre, placebo-controlled study. *Cephalalgia, 23,* 691.

Diener, H. C., Tfelt-Hansen, P., Dahlof, C., Lainez, J. M., Sandrini, G., Wang, S. J., et al. (2003b). Topiramate in migraine prophylaxis: Results from a placebo-controlled trial including an active comparator—propranolol. *Cephalalgia, 23,* 691.

Doenicke, A., Siegel, E., Hadoke, M., & Perrin, V. L. (1987). Initial clinical study of AH25086B (5-HT$_1$-like agonist) in the acute treatment of migraine. *Cephalalgia, 7,* 437–438.

Dowson, A. J., Macgregor, E. A., Purdy, R, A., Becker, W. J., Green, J., & Levy, S. L. (2002). Zolmitriptan orally disintegrating tablet is effective in the acute treatment of migraine. *Cephalalgia, 22,* 101–106.

Duckro, P. N., & Cantwell-Simmons, E. (1989). A review of studies evaluating biofeedback and relaxation training in the management of paediatric headache. *Headache, 29,* 428–433.

Ducros, A., Denier, C., Joutel, A., Cecillon, M., Lescoat, C., Vahedi, K., Darcel, F., Vicaut, E., Bousser, M. G., & Tournier-Lasserve, E. (2001). The clinical spectrum of familial hemiplegic migraine associated with mutations in a neuronal calcium channel. *N Engl J Med, 345,* 17–24.

Ertel, E. A., Campbell, K. P., Harpold, M. M., Hofmann, F., Mori, Y., Perez-Reyes, E., Schwartz, A., Snutch, T. P., Tanabe, T., Birnbaumer, L., Tsien, R. W., & Catterall, W. A. (2000). Nomenclature of voltage-gated calcium channels. *Neuron, 25,* 533–535.

Feniuk, W., Humphrey, P. P., Perren, M. J., Connor, H. E., & Whalley, E. T. (1991). Rationale for the use of 5-HT1-like agonists in the treatment of migraine. *J Neurol, 238,* S57–S61.

Ferrari, M. D., Goadsby, P. J., Roon, K. I., & Lipton, R. B. (2002). Triptans (serotonin, 5-HT$_{1B/1D}$ agonists) in migraine: Detailed results and methods of a meta-analysis of 53 trials. *Cephalalgia, 22,* 633–658.

Ferrari, M. D., Roon, K. I., Lipton, R. B., & Goadsby, P. J. (2001). Oral triptans (serotonin, 5-HT$_{1B/1D}$ agonists) in acute migraine treatment: A meta-analysis of 53 trials. *Lancet, 358,* 1668–1675.

Ferrari, M. D., & Subcutaneous Sumatriptan International Study Group. (1991). Treatment of migraine attacks with sumatriptan. *N Engl J Med, 325,* 316–321.

Fowler, P. A., Lacey, L. F., Thomas, M., Keene, O. N., Tanner, R. J. N., & Baber, N. S. (1991). The clinical pharmacology, pharmacokinetics and metabolism of sumatriptan. *Eur Neurol, 31,* 291–294.

Fukuda, Y., & Izumikawa, K. (1988). Intravenous aspirin for intractable headache and facial pain. *Headache, 28,* 47–50.

Fuseau, E., Baille, P., & Kempsford, R. D. (1997). A study to determine the absolute oral bioavailability of naratriptan. *Cephalalgia, 17,* 417.

Gallagher, M. (1996). Acute treatment of migraine with dihydroergotamine nasal spray. Dihydroergotamine Working Group. *Arch Neurol, 53,* 1285–1291.

Gallagher, R. M. (1985). Emergency treatment of intractable migraine. *Headache, 25,* 164.

Goadsby, P. J. (2000). The pharmacology of headache. *Prog Neurobiol, 62,* 509–525.

Goadsby, P. J. (2003). Herbal remedies—feverfew is not effective in migraine. *N Engl J Med, 348,* 1499.

Goadsby, P. J., & Edvinsson, L. (1993). The trigeminovascular system and migraine: Studies characterizing cerebrovascular and neuropeptide changes seen in humans and cats. *Ann Neurol, 33,* 48–56.

Goadsby, P. J., & Gundlach, A. L. (1991). Localization of [^{3}H]-dihydroergotamine binding sites in the cat central nervous system: Relevance to migraine. *Ann Neurol, 29,* 91–94.

Goadsby, P. J., Hoskin, K. L., & Knight, Y. E. (1997). Stimulation of the greater occipital nerve increases metabolic activity in the trigeminal nucleus caudalis and cervical dorsal horn of the cat. *Pain, 73,* 23–28.

Goadsby, P. J., Lipton, R, B., & Ferrari, M. D. (2002). Migraine—current understanding and treatment. *N Engl J Med, 346,* 257–270.

Goadsby, P. J., & Olesen, J. (1996). Diagnosis and management of migraine. *BMJ, 312,* 1279–1282.

Goldberg, M. R., Lee, Y., Vyas, K. P., Slaughter, D. E., Panebianco, D., Ermlich, S. J., et al. Rizatriptan, a novel 5-HT1B/1D agonist for migraine: single- and multiple-dose tolerability and pharmacokinetics in healthy subjects. *Journal of Clinical Pharmacology* 2000; 40:74–83.

Goldstein, D. J., Roon, K. I., Offen, W. W., Ramadan, N. M., Phebus, L. A., Johnson, K. W., et al. (2001). Selective serotonin 1F (5-HT(1F)) receptor agonist LY334370 for acute migraine: A randomised controlled trial. *Lancet, 358,* 1230–1234.

Gomersall, J. D., & Stuart, A. (1973). Amitriptyline in migraine prophylaxis. Changes in pattern of attacks during a controlled clinical trial. *J Neurol Neurosurg Psychiatry, 36,* 684–690.

Good, P. A., Taylor, R. H., & Mortimer, M. J. (1991). The use of tinted glasses in childhood migraine. *Headache, 31,* 533–536.

Graham, J. R. (1967). Cardiac and pulmonary fibrosis during methysergide therapy for headache. *Am J Med Sci, 254,* 23–24.

Gunasekara, N. S., & Wiseman, L. R. (1997). Naratriptan. *CNS Drugs, 8,* 402–408.

Haas, D. C. (1982). Prolonged migraine aura status. *Ann Neurol, 11,* 197–199.

Hakkarainen, H., Vapaatolo, H., Gothoni, G., & Parantainen, J. (1979). Tolfenamic acid is as effective as ergotamine during migraine attacks. *Lancet, 2,* 326–328.

Hartig, P. R., Hoyer, D., Humphrey, P. P. A., & Martin, G. R. (1996). Alignment of receptor nomenclature with the human genome: Classification of 5HT-1B and 5-HT1D receptor subtypes. *Trends Pharmacol Sci, 17,* 103–105.

Headache Classification Committee of the International Headache Society. (2004). The International Classification of Headache Disorders (second edition). *Cephalalgia, 24,* 1–160.

Hering, R., & Kuritzky, A. (1992). Sodium valproate in the prophylactic treatment of migraine: A double blind study versus placebo. *Cephalalgia, 12,* 81–84.

Hershey, A. D., Powers, S. W., LeCates, S., & Bentti, A. L. (2001). Effectiveness of nasal sumatriptan in 5- to 12-year-old children. *Headache, 41,* 693–697.

Herzog, A. G. (1997). Continuous bromocriptine therapy in menstrual migraine. *Neurology, 48,* 101–102.

Holroyd, K. A., & Penzien, D. B. (1990). Pharmacological versus non-pharmacological prophylaxis of recurrent migraine headache: A meta-analytic review of clinical trials. *Pain, 42,* 1–13.

Hoskin, K. L., Kaube, H., & Goadsby, P. J. (1996). Central activation of the trigeminovascular pathway in the cat is inhibited by dihydroergotamine. A c-Fos and electrophysiology study. *Brain, 119,* 249–256.

Hoyer, D., Clarke, D. E., Fozard, J. R., Hartig, P. R., Martin, G. R., Mylecharane, E. J., Saxena, P. R., & Humphrey, P. P. (1994). International Union of Pharmacology classification of receptors for 5-hydroxytryptamine (serotonin). *Pharmacol Rev, 46,* 157–203.

Hrobjartsson, A., & Gotzsche, P. C. (2001). Is the placebo powerless? An analysis of clinical trials comparing placebo with no treatment. *N Engl J Med, 344,* 1594–1602.

Humphrey, P. P. A., Feniuk, W., Marriott, A. S., Tanner, R. J. N., Jackson, M. R., & Tucker, M. L. (1991). Preclinical studies on the anti-migraine drug, sumatriptan. *Eur Neurol, 31,* 282–290.

Humphrey, P. P. A., Feniuk, W., Perren, M. J., Beresford, I. J. M., Skingle, M., & Whalley, E. T. (1990). Serotonin and migraine. *Ann N Y Acad Sci, 600,* 587–598.

Ibraheem, J. J., Paalzow, L., & Tfelt-Hansen, P. (1983). Low bioavailability of ergotamine tartrate after oral and rectal administration in migraine sufferers. *Br J Clin Pharmacol, 16,* 695–699.

Jager, H. R., Giffin, N. J., & Goadsby, P. J. (2004). Diffusion- and perfusion-weighted MR imaging in persistent migrainous visual disturbances. *Cephalalgia, 24,* in press.

Jasper, J. R., Kosaka, A., To, Z. P., Chang, D. J., & Eglen, R. M. (1997). Cloning, expression and pharmacology of a truncated splice variant of the human 5-HT$_7$ receptor (h5-HT$_{7(b)}$). *Br J Pharmacol, 122,* 126–132.

Jauslin, P., Goadsby, P. J., & Lance, J. W. (1991). The hospital management of severe migrainous headache. *Headache, 31,* 658–660.

Jensen, R., Brinck, T., & Olesen, J. (1994). Sodium valproate has a prophylactic effect in migraine without aura: A triple blind, placebo-controlled crossover study. *Neurology, 44,* 647–651.

John, G. W., Perez, M., Pawels, P. J., Le Grand, B., Verscheure, Y., & Colpaert, F. C. (2000). Donitriptan, a unique high efficacy 5-HT$_{1B/1D}$ agonist: Key features and acute antimigraine potential. *CNS Drug Reviews, 6,* 278–289.

Johnson, E. S., Kadam, N. P., Hylands, D. M., & Hylands, P. J. (1985). Efficacy of feverfew as a prophylactic treatment of migraine. *BMJ, 291,* 569–573.

Jones, J., Sklar, D., Dougherty, J., & White, W. (1989). Randomized double-blind trial of intravenous prochlorperazine for the treatment of acute headache. *JAMA, 261,* 1174–1176.

Joss, R. A., & Dott, C. S. (1993). Clinical studies with granisetron, a new 5-HT3 receptor antagonist for the treatment of cancer chemotherapy-induced emesis. The Granisetron Study Group. *Eur J Cancer, 29A*(Suppl 1), S22–S29.

Jost, W. H., Raulf, F., & Muller-Loeck, H. (1991). Anorectal ergotism. Induced by migraine therapy. *Acta Neurol Scand, 84,* 73–74.

Kallanranta, T., Hakkarainen, H., Hokkanen, E., & Tuovinen, T. (1977). Clonidine in migraine prophylaxis. *Headache, 17,* 169–172.

Kaniecki, R. G. (1997). A comparison of divalproex with propranolol and placebo for the prophylaxis of migraine without aura. *Arch Neurol, 54,* 1141–1145.

Karachalios, G. N., Fotiadou, A., Chrisikos, N., Karabetsos, A., & Kehagioglou, K. (1992). Treatment of acute migraine attack with diclofenac sodium: A double-blind study. *Headache, 32,* 98–100.

Kaube, H., Herzog, J., Kaufer, T., Dichgans, M., & Diener, H. C. (2000). Aura in some patients with familial hemiplegic migraine can be stopped by intranasal ketamine. *Neurology, 55,* 139–141.

Kaube, H., Hoskin, K. L., & Goadsby, P. J. (1994). Lignocaine and headache: An electrophysiological study in the cat with supporting clinical observations in man. *J Neurol, 241,* 415–420.

Kempsford, R. D., Baille, P., & Fuseau, E. (1997). Oral naratriptan tablets (2.5 mg–10 mg) exhibit dose-proportional pharmacokinetics. *Cephalalgia, 17,* 408.

Kimball, R. W., Friedman, A. P., & Vallejo, E. (1960). Effect of serotonin in migraine patients. *Neurology, Minneap, 10,* 107–111.

Klapper, J., & Divalproex Sodium in Migraine Prophylaxis Study Group. (1997). Divalproex sodium in migraine prophylaxis: A dose-controlled study. *Cephalalgia, 17,* 103–108.

Klappe, J. A., Rosjo, O., Charlesworth, B., Jergensen, A. P., & Soisson, T. (2002). Treatment of mild migraine with oral zolmitriptan 2.5mg provides high pain-free response rates in patients with significant migraine-related disability. *Neurology, 58,* A416.

Klapper, J. A., & Stanton, J. (1993). Current emergency treatment of severe headaches. *Headache, 33,* 560–562.

Kors, E. E., Terwindt, G. M., Vermeulen, F. L. M. G., Fitzsimons, R. B., Jardine, P. E., Heywood, P., Love, S., van den Maagdenberg, A. M., Haan, J., Frants, R.R., & Ferrari, M. D. (2001). Delayed cerebral edema and fatal coma after minor head trauma: Role of *CACNA1A* calcium channel subunit gene and relationship with familial hemiplegic migraine. *Ann Neurol, 49,* 753–760.

Kuritzky, A., Zoldan, Y., & Melamed, E. (1992). Selegeline, a MAO B inhibitor, is not effective in the prophylaxis of migraine without aura—an open study. *Headache, 32,* 416.

Lance, J. W., Fine, R. D., & Curran, D. A. (1963). An evaluation of methysergide in the prevention of migraine and other vascular headache. *Med J Aust, 1,* 814–818.

Lane, P. L., McLellan, B. A., & Baggoley, C. J. (1989). Comparative efficacy of chlorpromazine and meperidine with dimenhydrinate in migraine headache. *Ann Emerg Med, 18,* 360–365.

Lataste, X., Taylor, P., & Notter, M. (1989). DHE nasal spray in the acute management of migraine attacks. *Cephalalgia, 9*(Suppl 10), 342–343.

Leone, M., Grazzi, L., Mantia, L. L., & Bussone, G. (1991). Flunarizine in migraine: A mini review. *Headache, 31,* 388–391.

Lewis, C. T., Molland, E. A., Marshall, V. R., Tresidder, G. C., & Blandy, J. P. (1975). Analgesic abuse, ureteric obstruction and retroperitoneal fibrosis. *BMJ, 2,* 76–78.

Lipton, R. B., & Goadsby, P. J. (2001). Acute management of migraine: Clinical trials of triptans vs other agents. In J. Olesen, M. D. Ferrari, & P. P. A. Humphrey (Eds.), *The triptans: Novel drugs in migraine* (pp. 285–296). Oxford, UK: Oxford University Press.

Lipton, R. B., Ottman, R., Ehrenberg, B. L., & Hauser, W. A. (1994). Comorbidity of migraine: The connection between migraine and epilepsy. *Neurology, 44,* 28–32.

Little, P. J., Jennings, G. L., Skews, H., & Bobik, A. (1982). Bioavailability of dihydroergotamine in man. *Br J Pharmacol, 13,* 785–790.

Liu, G. T., Schatz, N. J., Galetta, S. L., Volpe, N. J., Skobieranda, F., & Komorsky, G. S. (1995). Persistent positive visual phenomena in migraine. *Neurology, 45,* 664–668.

Loh, L., Nathan, P. W., Schott, G. D., & Zilkha, K. J. (1984). Acupuncture versus medical treatment for migraine and muscle tension headache. *J Neurol Neurosurg Psychiatry, 47,* 333–337.

Louis, P., & Spierings, E. L. H. (1982). Comparison of flunarizine (Sibelium®) and pizotifen (Sandomigran®) in migraine treatment: A double-blind study. *Cephalalgia, 2,* 197–203.

Maciewicz, R., Borsook, S., & Strassman, A. (1988). Intravenous lidocaine relieves acute vascular headache. *Headache, 28,* 309.

Magee, R. (1991). Saint Anthony's fire revisited. Vascular problems associated with migraine medication. *Med J Aust, 154,* 145–149.

Magos, A. L., Zilkha, K. J., & Studd, J. W. W. (1983). Treatment of menstrual migraine by oestradiol implants. *J Neurol Neurosurg Psychiatry, 46,* 1044–1046.

Maier, H. W. (1926). L'ergotamine inhibiteur du sympathique etudie en clinique, comme moyen d'exploration et comme agent therapeutique. *Rev Neurol (Paris), 33,* 1104–1108.

Malaquin, F., Urbun, T., Ostinelli, J., Ghedita, H., & Lacronique, J. (1989). Pleural and retroperitoneal fibrosis from dihydroergotamine. *N Engl J Med, 321,* 1760.

Markley, H. G., Cleronis, J. C. D., & Piepko, R. W. (1984). Verapamil prophylactic therapy of migraine. *Neurology, 34,* 973–976.

Masel, B. E., Chesson, A. L., Peters, B. H., Levin, H. S., & Alperin, J. B. (1980). Platelet antagonists in migraine prophylaxis. A clinical trial using aspirin and dipyridamole. *Headache, 20,* 13–18.

Massiou, H. (1996). A comparison of sumatriptan nasal spray and intranasal dihydroergotamine (DHE) in the acute treatment of migraine. *Funct Neurol, 11,* 151.

Matharu, M. S., Bartsch, T., Ward, N., Frackowiak, R. S. J., Weiner, R. L., & Goadsby, P. J. (2004). Central neuromodulation in chronic migraine patients with suboccipital stimulators: A PET study. *Brain, 127,* 220–230.

Mathew, N. T., & Ali, S. (1991). Valproate in the treatment of persistent chronic daily headache. An open label study. *Headache, 31,* 71–74.

Mathew, N. T., & Lucker, C. (1996). Gabapentin in migraine prophylaxis: A preliminary open label study. *Neurology, 46,* A169.

Mathew, N. T., Rapoport, A., Saper, J., Magnus, L., Klapper, J., Ramadan, N., Stacey, B., & Tepper, S. (2001). Efficacy of gabapentin in migraine prophylaxis. *Headache, 41,* 119–128.

Mathew, N. T., Saper, J. R., Silberstein, S. D., Rankin, L., Markley, H. G., Solomon, S., Rapoport, A. M., Silber, C. J., & Deaton, R. L. (1995). Migraine prophylaxis with divalproex. *Arch Neurol, 52,* 281–286.

Mathew, N. T., Stubits, E., & Nigam, M. (1982). Transformation of migraine into daily headache: Analysis of factors. *Headache, 22,* 66–68.

Mathew, N. T., Tiejen, G. E., & Lucker, C. (1996). Serotonin syndrome complicating migraine pharmacotherapy. *Cephalalgia, 16,* 323–327.

McDavis, H. L., & Hutchison, J. (1999). Frovatriptan Phase III Investigators. Frovatriptan—a review of overall clinical efficacy. *Cephalalgia, 19,* 363–364.

McQueen, J., Loblay, R. J., Swain, A. R., Anthony, M., & Lance, J. W. (1989). A controlled trial of dietary modification in migraine. In F. C. Rose (Ed.), *New advances in headache research* (pp. 235–242). London: Smith-Gordon.

Melchart, D., Linde, K., Fische, P., White, A., Allais, G., Vickers, A., & Berman, B. (1999). Acupuncture for recurrent headaches: A systematic review of randomized controlled trials. *Cephalalgia, 19,* 779–786.

Menken, M., Munsat, T. L., & Toole, J. F. (2000). The global burden of disease study—implications for neurology. *Arch Neurol, 57,* 418–420.

Merikangas, K. R., Merikangas, J. R. (1995). Combination monoamine oxidase inhibitor and beta-blocker treatment of migraine. *Biol Psychiatry, 37,* 1–8.

Migraine Nimodipine European Study Group (MINES). (1989). European multicenter trial of nimodipine in the prophylaxis of common migraine (migraine without aura). *Headache, 29,* 633–638.

Milton, K. A., Allen, M. J., Abel, S., Jenkins, V. C., James, G. C., Rance, D. J., & Eve, M. D. (1997). The safety, tolerability, pharmacokinetics and pharmacodynamics of oral and intravenous eletriptan, a potent and selective "5HT1D-like" receptor partial agonist. *Cephalalgia, 17,* 44.

Mitsikostas, D. D., & Polychronidis, I. (1997). Valproate versus flunarizine in migraine prophylaxis, a randomized, double-open, clinical trial. *Funct Neurol, 12,* 267–276.

Morgan, P., Rance, D., James, G., Mitchell, R., & Milton, A. (1997). Comparative absorption and elimination of eletriptan in rat, dog and human. *Cephalalgia, 17,* 414.

Muller-Schweinitzer, E., & Fanchamps, A. (1982). Effects of arterial receptors of ergot derivatives used in migraine. In M. Critchley (Ed.), *Advances in neurology* (Vol. 33, pp. 343–355). New York: Raven Press.

Murphy, J. J., Heptinstall, S., & Mitchell, J. R. A. (1988). Randomized double-blind placebo-controlled trial of feverfew in migraine prevention. *Lancet, 2,* 189–192.

Myllyla, V. V., Havanka, H., Herrala, L., Kangasniemi, P., Rautakorpi, I., Turkka, J., Vapaatalo, H., & Eskerod, O. (1998). Tolfenamic acid rapid release versus sumatriptan in the acute treatment of migraine: Comparable effect in a double-blind, randomized, controlled, parallel-group study. *Headache, 38,* 201–207.

O'Dea, J. P. K., & Davis, E. H. (1990). Tamoxifen in the treatment of menstrual migraine. *Neurology, 40,* 1470–1471.

Oldman, A. D., Smith, L. A., McQuay, H. J., & Moore, R. A. (2002). Pharmacological treatments for acute migraine: Quantitative systematic review. *Pain, 97,* 247–257.

Palevitch, D., Earon, G., & Carasso, R. (1997). Feverfew (*Tanacetum parthenium*) as a prophylactic treatment for migraine—a double-blind placebo-controlled study. *Phytother Res, 11,* 508–511.

Palmer, K. J., & Spencer, C. M. (1997). Zolmitriptan. *CNS Drugs, 7,* 468–478.

Parker, G. B., Pryor, D. S., & Tupling, H. (1980). Who does migraine improve during a clinical trial? Further results from a trial of cervical manipulation for migraine. *Aust N Z J Med, 10,* 192–198.

Parker, G. B., Tupling, H., & Pryor, D. S. (1978). A controlled trial of cervical manipulation for migraine. *Aust N Z J Med, 8,* 589–593.

Pascual, J., Bussone, G., Hernandez, J. F., Allen, C., Vrijens, F., Patel, K., & Rizatriptan-Sumatriptan Preference Study Group (2001). Comparison of preference for rizatriptan 10-mg wafer versus sumatriptan 50-mg tablet in migraine. *Eur Neurol, 45,* 275–283.

Pascual, J., & Cabarrocas, X. (2002). Within-patient early versus delayed treatment of migraine attacks with almotriptan: The sooner the better. *Headache, 42,* 28–31.

Pedersen, E., & Moller, C. E. (1966). Methysergide in migraine prophylaxis. *Clin Pharmacol Ther, 7,* 520–526.

Peikert, A., Wilimzig, C., & Kohne-Volland, R. (1996). Prophylaxis of migraine with oral magnesium: Results from a prospective, multi-center, placebo-controlled and double-blind randomized study. *Cephalalgia, 16,* 257–263.

Peroutka, S. J. (1990). The pharmacology of current anti-migraine drugs. *Headache, 30,* 5–11.

Pfaffenrath, V., Diener, H.-C., Fischer, M., Friede, M., & Henneicke-von Zepelin, H. H. (2002). The efficacy and safety of *Tanacetum parthenium* (feverfew) in migraine prophylaxis—a double-blind, multicentre, randomized placebo-controlled dose-response study. *Cephalalgia, 22,* 523–532.

Pfaffenrath, V., Wessely, P., Mener, C., Isler, H. R., Evers, S., Grotemeyer, K. H., Taneri, Z., Soyka, D., Gobel, H., & Fischer, M. (1996). Magnesium in the prophylaxis of migraine—a double-blind placebo-controlled study. *Cephalalgia, 16,* 436–440.

Potter, D. L., Hart, D. E., Calder, C. S., & Storey, J. R. (2000). A double-blind, randomized, placebo controlled, parallel study to determine the efficacy of topiramate in the prophylactic treatment of migraine. *Neurology, 54,* A15.

Prusinski, A., & Kozubski, W. (1987).Use of verapamil in the treatment of migraine. *Wiad Lek, 40,* 734–738.

Quality Standards Subcommittee of the American Academy of Neurology. (1994). The utility of neuroimaging in the evaluation of headache patients with normal neurologic examinations. *Neurology, 44,* 1353–1354.

Rance, D., Clear, N., Dallman, L., Llewellyn, E., Nuttall, J., & Verrier, H. (1997). Physicochemical comparison of eletriptan and other 5-HT1D-like agonists as a predictor of oral absorption potential. *Headache, 37,* 328.

Raskin, N. H. (1986). Repetitive intravenous dihydroergotamine as therapy for intractable migraine. *Neurology, 36,* 995–997.

Reutens, D. C., Fatovich, D. M., Stewart-Wynne, E. G., & Prentice, D. A. (1991). Is intravenous lignocaine clinically effective in acute migraine? *Cephalalgia, 11,* 245–247.

Rompel, H., & Bauermeister, P. W. (1970). Aetiology of migraine and prevention with carbamazepine (Tegretol): Results of a double-blind, cross-over study. *S Afr Med J, 44,* 75–80.

Rosenfeld, W. E. (1997). Topiramate: A review of the preclinical, pharmacokinetic, and clinical data. *Clin Ther, 19,* 1294–1308.

Rothrock, J. F. (1997). Successful treatment of persistent migraine aura with divalproex sodium. *Neurology, 48,* 261–262.

Rowbotham, G. F. (1949). *The surgical treatment of migraine. IV Congress Neurologique International* (pp. 147–152). Paris: Masson and Cie.

Sandor, P. S., Di Clemente, L., Coppola, G., Vendenheede, M., Fumal, A., & Schoenen, J. (2003). Coenzyme Q10 for migraine prophylaxis: A randomised controlled trial. *Cephalalgia, 23,* 577.

Saper, J. R., Silberstein, S. D., Lakem, A. E., & Winters, M. E. (1994). Double-blind trial of fluoxetine: Chronic daily headache and migraine. *Headache, 34,* 497–502.

Scherl, E. R., & Wilson, J. F. (1995). Comparison of dihydroergotamine with metoclopramide versus meperidine with promethazine in the treatment of acute migraine. *Headache, 35,* 256–259.

Schoenen, J., Jacquy, J., & Lenaerts, M. (1998). Effectiveness of high-dose riboflavin in migraine prophylaxis—a randomized controlled trial. *Neurology, 50,* 466–470.

Seaber, E., On, N., Phillips, S., Churchus, R., Posner, J., & Rolan, P. (1996). The tolerability and pharmacokinetics of the novel antimigraine compound 311C90 in healthy male volunteers. *Br J Clin Pharmacol, 41,* 141–147.

Selby, G., & Lance, J. W. (1960). Observations on 500 cases of migraine and allied vascular headache. *J Neurol Neurosurg Psychiatry, 23,* 23–32.

Shuaib, A., Ahmed, F., Muratoglu, M., & Kochanski, P. (1999). Topiramate in migraine prophylaxis: A pilot study. *Cephalalgia, 19,* 379–380.

Sicuteri, F., Michelacci, S., & Anselmi, B. (1964). Individuazione della proprieta vasoattive ed antiemicraniche dell' indomethacin, nuovo antiflogistico di derivazione indolica. *Settimana Medica, 52,* 335–345.

Silberstein, S., Karim, R., Kamin, M., Jordan, D., & Hulihan, J. (2002). Topiramate prophylaxis in patients suffering from migraine without aura: Results from a randomized, double-blind, placebo-controlled trial. *Eur J Neurol, 9,* 44.

Silberstein, S. D. (1996). Divalproex sodium in headache: Literature review and clinical guidelines. *Headache, 36,* 547–555.

Silberstein, S. D., & Goadsby, P. J. (2002). Migraine: Preventative treatment. *Cephalalgia, 22,* 491–512.

Silberstein, S. D., Neto, W., Schmitt, J., & Jacobs, D. (2004). Topiramate in migraine prevention: Results of a large controlled trial. *Arch Neurol, 61,* 490–495.

Silberstein SD., & Wilmore, J. (1996). Divalproex sodium: Migraine treatment and monitoring. *Headache, 36,* 239–242.

Solomon, G. D. (1986). Verapamil and propranolol in migraine prophylaxis: A double-blind crossover study. *Headache, 26,* 325.

Solomon, G. D. (1989). Verapamil in migraine prophylaxis—a five-year review. *Headache, 29,* 425–427.

Solomon, G. D., & Diamond, S. (1987). Verapamil in migraine prophylaxis—comparison of dosages. *Clin Pharmacol Ther, 1,* 202.

Solomon, G. D., Steel, J. G., & Spaccavento, L. J. (1983). Verapamil prophylaxis of migraine: A double-blind, placebo-controlled study. *JAMA, 250,* 2500–2502.

Sorensen, K. V. (1988). Valproate: A new drug in migraine prophylaxis. *Acta Neurol Scand, 78,* 346–348.

Speight, T. M., & Avery, G. S. (1972). Pizotifen (BC-105): A review of its pharmacological properties and its therapeutic efficacy in vascular headaches. *Drugs, 3,* 159–203.

Stewart, W. F., Lipton, R. B., Chee, E., Sawyer, J., & Silberstein, S. D. (2000). Menstrual cycle and headache in a population sample of migraineurs. *Neurology, 55,* 1517–1523.

Storer, R. J., & Goadsby, P. J. (2004). Topiramate inhibits trigeminovascular neurons in the cat. *Cephalalgia, 24,* in press.

Tfelt-Hansen, P. (1989). Therapy of migraine. *Curr Opin Neurol , 2,* 212–216.

Tfelt-Hansen, P., Block, G., Dahlof, C., Diener, H.-C., Ferrari, M. D., Goadsby, P. J., et al. (2000a). Guidelines for controlled trials of drugs in migraine: Second edition. *Cephalalgia, 20,* 765–786.

Tfelt-Hansen, P., De Vries, P., & Saxena, P. R. (2000b). Triptans in migraine. A comparative review of pharmacology, pharmacokinetics and efficacy of triptans in migraine. *Drugs, 6,* 1259–1287.

Tfelt-Hansen, P., Ibraheem, J. J., & Paalzow, L. (1982). *Clinical pharmacology of ergotamine studied with a high performance liquid chromatographic method.* New York: Raven Press.

Tfelt-Hansen, P., & Johnson, E. S. (1993). Ergotamine. In J. Olesen, P. Tfelt-Hansen, & K. M. A. Welch (Eds.), *The headaches* (pp. 313–322). New York: Raven Press.

Tfelt-Hansen, P., Olesen, J., Aebelholt-Krabbe, A., Melgaard, B., & Veilis, G. (1980). A double-blind study of metoclopramide in the treatment of migraine attacks. *J Neurol Neurosurg Psychiatry, 43,* 369–371.

Tfelt-Hansen, P., Saxena, P. R., Dahlof, C., Pascual, J., Lainez, M., Henry, P., Diener, H., Schoenen, J., Ferrari, M. D., & Goadsby, P. J. (2000c). Ergotamine in the acute treatment of migraine—a review and European consensus. *Brain, 123,* 9–18.

Thomas, D. R., Gittins, S. A., Collin, L. L., Middlemiss, D. N., Riley, G., Hagan, J., Gloger, I., Ellis, C. E., Forbes, I. T., & Brown, A. M. (1998). Functional characterisation of the human cloned 5-HT7 receptor (long form). Antagonist profile of SB-258719. *Br J Pharmacol, 124,* 1300–1306.

Thomsen, L. L., Dixon, R., Lassen, L. H., Gibbens, M., Langemark, M., Bendtsen, L., Daugaard, D., & Olesen, J. (1996). 311C90 (Zolmitriptan), a novel centrally and peripheral acting oral 5-hydroxytryptamine-1D agonist: A comparison of its absorption during a migraine attack and in a migraine-free period. *Cephalalgia, 16,* 270–275.

Thomsen, L. L., Ostergaard, E., Olesen, J., & Russell, M. B. (2003). Evidence for a separate type of migraine with aura: Sporadic hemiplegic migraine. *Neurology, 60,* 595–601.

Tognetto, M., Creminon, C., Amadesi, S., Trevisani, M., Giovanni, G., Piffanelli, A., et al. (2001). Neuropeptide release from slices of rat and guinea pig trigeminal ganglia: Modulation by dihydroergotamine and sumatriptan. *Journal of Headache and Pain, 2,* 83–90.

Touchon, J., Bertin, L., Pilgrim, A. J., Ashford, E., & Bes, A. (1996). A comparison of subcutaneous sumatriptan and dihydroergotamine nasal spray in the acute treatment of migraine. *Neurology, 47,* 361–365.

Treves, T. A., Streiffler, M., & Korczyn, A. D. (1992). Naproxen sodium versus ergotamine tartrate in the treatment of acute migraine attacks. *Headache, 32,* 280–282.

Vardi, Y., Rabey, I. M., Streifer, M., Schwartz, A., Lindner, H. R., & Zor, U. (1976). Migraine attacks. Alleviation by an inhibitor of prostaglandin synthesis and action. *Neurology, 26,* 447–450.

Visser, W. H., de Vriend, R. H., Jaspers, N. H., & Ferrari, M. D. (1996). Sumatriptan-nonresponders: A survey in 366 migraine patients. *Headache, 36,* 471–475.

Volans, G. N. (1974). Absorption of effervescent aspirin during migraine. *BMJ, 2,* 265–269.

Waelkens, J. (1981). Domperidone in the prevention of complete classical migraine. *BMJ, 284,* 944.

Waelkens, J. (1984). Dopamine blockade with domperidone: Bridge between prophylactic and abortive treatment of migraine? A dose-finding study. *Cephalalgia, 4,* 85–90.

Welch, K. M., & Ramadan, N. M. (1995). Mitochondria, magnesium and migraine. *J Neurol Sci, 134,* 9–14.

Welch, K. M. (1986). Naproxen sodium in the treatment of migraine. *Cephalalgia, 6,* 85–92.

White, J. C., & Sweet, W. H. (1955). *Pain: Its mechanisms and neurosurgical control.* Springfield, IL: Charles C Thomas.

Wilkinson, M. (1983). Treatment of the acute migraine attack—current status. *Cephalalgia, 3,* 61–67.

Winner, P., Mannix, L. K., Putnam, D. G., McNeal, S., Kwong, J., O'Quinn, S., & Richardson, M. S. (2003). Pain-free results with sumatriptan taken at the first sign of migraine pain. 2. Randomized, double-blind, placebo-controlled studies. *Mayo Clin Proc, 78,* 1214–1222.

Winner, P., Ricalde, O., Force, B. L., Saper, J., & Margul, B. (1996). A double-blind study of subcutaneous dihydroergotamine vs subcutaneous sumatriptan in the treatment of acute migraine. *Arch Neurol, 53,* 180–184.

Wirth, F. P., & van Buren, J. M. (1971). Referral of pain from dural stimulation in man. *J Neurosurg, 34,* 630–642.

Wober, C., Woberbingol, C., Koch, G., & Wessely, P. (1991). Long-term results of migraine prophylaxis with flunarizine and beta-blockers. *Cephalalgia, 11,* 251–256.

Ziegler, D., Ford, R., Kriegler, J., Gallagher, R. M., Peroutka, S., Hammerstad, J., et al. (1994). Dihydroergotamine nasal spray for the acute treatment of migraine. *Neurology, 44,* 447–453.

Ziegler, D. K. (1997). Opioids in headache treatment. Is there a role? In N. T. Mathew (Ed.), *Neurologic clinics of North America* (Vol. 15, pp. 199–207). Philadelphia: Saunders.

Ziegler, D. K., Hurwitz, A., Preskorn, S., Hassanein, R., & Seim, J. (1993). Propranolol and amitriptyline in prophylaxis of migraine. Pharmacokinetic and therapeutic effects. *Arch Neurol, 50,* 825–830.

Ziegler, V. E., Clayton, P. J., & Biggs, J. T. (1977). A comparative study of amitriptyline and nortriptyline with plasma levels. *Arch Gen Psychiatry, 34,* 707–712.

Chapter 10
Tension-Type Headache

Tension headache may be defined as a constant tight or pressing sensation, usually bilateral, that may initially be episodic and related to stress but that can recur almost daily in its chronic form. Such a definition amounts to saying that tension headache is a chronic headache without migrainous features (such as vomiting, blurring of vision, and focal neurologic symptoms). Thus such a definition bypasses the question of whether tension headache and migraine form a continuum, with vomiting and neurologic disturbance appearing only when headaches are acute and severe.

Ziegler and Hassanein (1982) analyzed the symptoms of 1200 patients attending a headache clinic and could not isolate any particular combination of characteristics that clearly defined migraine and tension headache as separate entities. They concluded that the most reliable features for the diagnosis of migraine were the episodicity and relative brevity of attacks. Patients who suffer from both tension headache and migraine usually distinguish the two forms of headache on the grounds of severity and associated symptoms much in the same way as a clinician taking a case history, but this does not clarify whether the two conditions share a similar pathophysiology.

Drummond and Lance (1984) analyzed the case histories of 600 patients presenting with the complaint of headache to a neurology clinic, comparing their clinical diagnosis with that made by a computer analysis that correlated the symptoms and other features of the headache. The clinical and computer diagnosis had no trouble in agreeing on the diagnosis of cluster headache and migraine with aura but had difficulty finding a dividing line between migraine and tension-type headache. For example, of episodic headaches recurring up to once per week, 55% were unilateral, and most were accompanied by the usual migrainous symptoms of nausea and photophobia. Of those headaches recurring daily, 20% were unilateral, nausea was still a feature in about 25%, and photophobia in about 50% (Figure 10.1). The explanation for this may have been the inclusion of patients whose frequency of migraine increased until it became daily, which Mathew, Reuveni, and Perez (1987) describe as "transformed migraine." We agree with Mathew (1993) and Silberstein, Lipton, and Sliwinski (1996) that this is a common cause of chronic daily headache, and we discuss this further in Chapter 11.

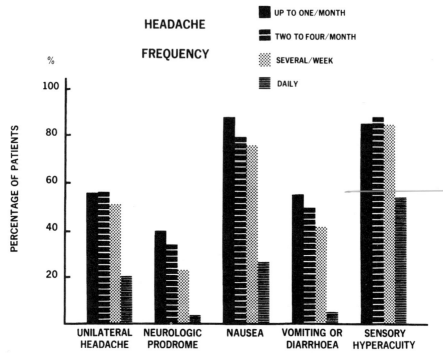

FIGURE 10.1 Relationship between the frequency of headache and migrainous characteristics. The percentage of patients with each symptom diminishes as headache frequency increases. (From Drummond & Lance, 1984, by permission of the editor of *Journal of Neurology, Neurosurgery, and Psychiatry.*)

Until the pathophysiology of headache is fully understood, tension-type headache can be recognized as an entity separate from migraine by the criteria put forward by the Headache Classification Committee of the International Headache Society (2004). The committee divided tension-type headaches into episodic (frequent and infrequent) and chronic varieties, with a subclassification for those patients with and without evidence of excessive contraction of the jaw and scalp muscles. The episodic type of tension headache is characterized by a frequency of less than 15 headache days each month, 1 to 14 days a month being classified as frequent, and less than 12 a year as infrequent. Both episodic and chronic types must have at least two of the following features:

1. Bilateral location.
2. A pressing or tight (nonpulsating) quality.
3. Mild or moderate intensity.
4. Not aggravated by routine physical activity and not accompanied by nausea and vomiting. Photophobia or phonophobia may be present, but not both. This criterion may have to be reconsidered, because quantitative testing shows sensitivity of patients to both is greater than that in controls (Vanagaite Vingen, & Stovner, 2000).

CLINICAL FEATURES OF TENSION-TYPE HEADACHE

Prevalence, Age, and Sex Distribution

Most people have probably been aware of a dull headache at some time of their lives after exposure to glare, flickering light, eye strain, noise, or a succession of harassing incidents. Of the 740 normal subjects interviewed, Rasmussen et al. (1991) found a lifetime prevalence of tension-type headache in 578 (78%), fulfilling the IHS criteria for episodic tension-type in 488 and most of those criteria in 66. The remaining 24 patients had chronic tension-type headache. The latter group are more heavily represented in medical practice, because most people with occasional mild headaches usually treat themselves with analgesics or simply put up with their discomfort.

Tension-type headache may start in childhood, affecting approximately 10% (Rasmussen, 1993) or 15% (Lance, Curran, & Anthony, 1965) by the age of 10 years (see Figure 7.1). The condition may be intractable and continue throughout life. Many patients have suffered from headaches almost every day for 10, 20, or 30 years.

Schwartz et al. (1998) studied the epidemiology of tension-type headache in 13,345 members of a Maryland community. The prevalence of episodic tension-type headache in the past year was 38.3% but only 2.2% for the chronic variety. More women than men had episodic headaches (ratio 1.6:1) but were subject to the chronic form twice as often as men. The average number of headaches for the year was 30 for the episodic group and 285 for the chronic patients. The prevalence of episodic tension-type headache increased with socioeconomic level, in contrast to chronic tension-type headache and migraine, which were more common in households with lower incomes.

Morbidity and Economic Impact

The survey of Schwartz et al. (1998) determined that 8.3% of patients with episodic tension-type headaches lost an average of 8.9 workdays each year because of their headaches, and 43.6% reported reduced effectiveness days, averaging 5 per year. Of patients with chronic tension-type headache, 11.8% had lost workdays (average 27.4 each) and reported an average of 20.4 days of lowered effectiveness.

Most patients with chronic tension-type headache continue to carry out their daily responsibilities, although 74% of the 245 patients examined by Holroyd et al. (2000) said they experienced days of disability with a mean of 7 days each in the past 6 months. Almost half the patients were anxious or depressed, which contributed to their degree of impairment as well as to the severity of the pain itself.

Family History

Approximately 18% of patients with tension headache give a family history of migraine (Lance & Anthony, 1966), which is much the same as for the general population. However, a family background of some form of headache is found in the history of 40% of patients with tension headache (Friedman, von Storch, & Merritt, 1964).

Russell et al. (1999) obtained information about family history from 122 patients with chronic tension-type headache, 35 males and 87 females, mean age 45.8 years. The mean age of onset was 26.5 years. Parents, siblings, and children had a 2.1- to 3.9-fold increased risk of chronic tension-type headache during their lifetime. There was an increased risk for spouses. Of those patients older than age 60 years, the mean duration was 22.1 years.

Past Health

There is no evidence that allergic disorders or childhood vomiting attacks are more common in patients complaining of tension headache than in the general community, but psychosomatic disorders such as irritable bowel syndrome may be associated.

Site of Headache

Headache was bilateral in 80% of the patients with chronic daily headache in the series Drummond and Lance (1984) analyzed and in almost 90% in the population-based analysis of tension-type headache by Rasmussen et al. (1991).

Quality of Headache

The pain in tension headache is usually dull and persistent and undulates in intensity during the day. It is often described as a feeling of heaviness, pressure, or weight on the head or tightness rather than pain and may extend like a band around the head. Some patients experience sudden jabs of pain on one side or at the back of the head ("ice-pick pains") superimposed on a general background of discomfort. About one quarter of patients with tension headache have headaches that become severe and assume a pulsating quality at times, forming a group intermediate between muscle contraction headache and migraine, which Lance and Curran (1964) called "tension-vascular headache." About 10% of patients with tension headache are also subject to frank migraine.

In one study, Hunter and Phillips (1981) found the intensity of headache experienced and the reaction of the patient to pain varied with the mood of the patient, the symptoms being more severe when the patient was depressed.

Time and Mode of Onset

In episodic cases, the headache develops during or after recognizable stress. In more severe cases, the headache comes on in anticipation of some unpleasant situation, such as a distasteful interview. Contemplation of the day's tasks may be enough to start a headache while traveling to work. In Lewis Carroll's *Through the Looking Glass,* Tweedledum remarked before the projected battle with Tweedledee: "I'm very brave generally, only today I happen to have a headache!"

In the chronic form, the patient either awakens with the headache or notices it shortly after getting up, and it remains throughout the day, without regard to the emotional content of the day's activities. Some 10% of patients, not necessarily those who are depressed, may be woken up by headache between 1 and 4 AM in the manner of a patient with migraine.

Frequency and Duration

Of 466 patients attending our neurologic clinic for the treatment of tension headache, the headache recurred fewer than 10 times each month in 49 patients, from 10 to 30 times each month in 64 patients, and was present every day in the remaining 354 patients (Lance & Curran, 1964). This contrasts with the population-based study in which Rasmussen et al. (1991) found that only 3% of 740 people questioned suffered from chronic tension-type headache (defined as more than 180 headache days each year). It is apparent that patients attending clinics are those who are most severely affected and that figures from clinics do not necessarily reflect the pattern of tension headache as seen by the general practitioner. The spectrum of tension headache extends from headache of half an hour's duration recurring every few months to a perpetual, unremitting ache present "all day and every day."

Associated Phenomena

Tension headache is not accompanied by any of the focal neurologic symptoms that add a distinctive character to most attacks of migraine. There is often a constant mild photophobia, not severe enough to make the patient retreat to a darkened room but often sufficient to encourage the wearing of sunglasses on all but the gloomiest day. Vanagaite Vingen, and Stovner (1998) examined 40 patients with tension-type headache, supposedly chosen by IHS criteria, but found that most patients when tested quantitatively were more sensitive to light and sound than a control group, and more so when they had a headache.

Other symptoms are those of an anxiety state. Slight nausea may be present in the early mornings, or when the headache is severe, but vomiting is rare. Giddiness or lightheadedness usually indicates a tendency to overbreathe in times of anxiety. Abdominal distension, excessive belching, and passing of flatus are commonly the result of unnoticed air swallowing. The patient often speaks of difficulty in concentrating and a lack of interest in work or hobbies. More flagrant depressive symptoms may appear, which are attributed to the presence of headache. Pain under the left breast, pain in the back or coccygeal region, and indigestion are other psychosomatic symptoms commonly associated with tension headache. The patient may awaken with a bruised sensation inside the mouth lateral to the posterior upper molar tooth, as the result of extreme mandibular movements during sleep (Every, 1960).

Underlying Precipitating, Aggravating, and Relieving Factors

It is deceptively easy to think of all patients with tension headache as having an inadequate personality. This is certainly true of some patients who are ill equipped by nature or education to cope with life's ramifications, but others have considerable achievements to their credit. It may be that the meticulous energetic personality, which has made a person prey to tension headache, has also made him or her a leader in business or industry. Men with exclusively sedentary occupations have a higher prevalence of tension-type headache (Rasmussen, 1993).

Approximately one third of patients with tension headache have symptoms of depression (Lance & Curran, 1964). Most are conscious that they are never really relaxed and are rarely elated. Many patients with tension headaches are "born two drinks down on life."

There may be obvious trigger factors for tension headache, but in many patients the headache is not limited to times of emotional overload. The headache is usually made worse by any superimposed anxiety, stress, noise, or glare. Coping with minor hassles in day-to-day living appears a more potent factor in perpetuating headache than major life events (De Benedittis & Lorenzetti, 1992). In the study by Rasmussen (1992), the pressure of working against time in women and exposure to fumes in men were found to be important precipitating causes; fatigue was a factor in both sexes. Karwautz et al. (1999) investigated 94 children and adolescents with tension-type headache and compared their social background with 151 subjects with migraine and 96 headache-free controls. The former had fewer close friends and more often came from single-parent homes, but the three groups showed no differences in other factors such as housing conditions and school problems.

Sitting in a cramped posture, such as at a school desk of the wrong height, can initiate tension-type headache in children. A related problem is "Hogwarts headaches—misery for Muggles." For those of us who are Muggles (nonwizard stock), reading the last volume of the Harry Potter series ("Harry Potter and the Order of the Phoenix" by J. K. Rowling), 870 pages in length and weighing over 1 kg, presents a challenge. For three children, concentrating on reading for long periods, the experience produced headaches that resolved when they finished the book (Bennett, 2003).

A headache that is relieved by intake of alcohol is almost invariably of the tension variety, whereas most vascular headaches become more severe. Tension-type headache is often relieved by analgesics but commonly recurs after some hours. This may lead to repeated self-medication with subsequent risk of habituation and toxicity.

PHYSICAL EXAMINATION

Formal neurologic examination is usually normal, but many patients show signs of muscular overcontraction. This is visible in the faces and foreheads of some patients, appearing as deep wrinkles. The temporal and masseter muscles may stand out and twitch, and the hands may clench the chair firmly or the fingers move restlessly during the interview. Other patients may have a bland appearance that gives no indication of the tendency to headache.

The patient may yawn, sigh, gasp, or breathe rapidly while the clinician is taking the history. These signs of overbreathing warrant management in their own right (see Appendix A).

Neck movements should be tested, the completeness of dentition and the balance of biting movements checked, and the temporomandibular joints palpated to identify any abnormalities that could initiate reflex muscle contraction and thus contribute to tension headache. The clinician should also observe the posture, because craning the neck forward can cause nuchal and occipital pain.

Pathophysiology

Psychologic Factors

The evidence from psychologic tests points to anxiety, depression, and hypochondriasis being common factors in tension-type headache, as are suppressed anger (Hatch et al., 1991) and feelings of inadequacy (Passchier et al., 1991). Nevertheless, subjects with tension-type headache did not differ from controls in any of the affective or anxiety disorders in the study reported by Merikangas et al. (1993). Rasmussen (1992) found a higher index of neurosis in patients with tension headache than in patients with migraine. Patients with chronic headache resemble those with chronic pain from other sources in that they deny having general life problems. As the headaches become more frequent and severe, the patients are more inclined to view their illness as somatic rather than psychologic in origin (Demjen & Bakal, 1981). Mitsikostas and Thomas (1999) found that 10% of patients with chronic tension headache had symptoms of frank depression.

External forces are obviously important. One of us can recall a day's consulting in which three women said that their headaches began when they were married and stopped when they separated!

Muscle Contraction and Myofascial Tenderness

Many patients describe a sensation of tension or pressure in the frontalis muscle after excessive frowning, which passes away when the forehead is relaxed. Others become aware of a similar sensation in the masseter or temporalis muscles after clenching the jaw, which is eased by ceasing muscle contraction. Every (1960) has drawn attention to nocturnal tooth grinding fang-sharpening movements of the jaw that occur during sleep as a manifestation of repressed aggression. The latter syndrome may be recognized by the association of chronic headache with pain in the temporomandibular joints and jaw muscles and a raw, tender spot on the buccal mucosa opposite the posterior part of the upper gum, which results from excessive lateral movement of the mandible during sleep. Jensen and Rasmussen (1996) reported that 87% of patients with chronic tension-type headache and 66% with the episodic form had increased pericranial muscle tenderness and/or electromyographic activity, both indications of excessive muscle contraction.

When 58 patients prone to tension-type headache clenched their jaws for 30 minutes, 69% developed a headache, compared with 17% of control subjects (Jensen & Olesen, 1996). Muscle tenderness increased in those patients who developed headache, but their tolerance to painful pressure and heat remained unchanged, whereas pain and thermal pain thresholds actually increased in those subjects who remained free of headache. This suggests that excessive muscle contraction plays some part in the genesis of tension-type headache in those subjects with defective mobilization of their endogenous pain-control system. A logical extension of this thought is that electromyogram (EMG) biofeedback would be most effective in reducing pain in patients who consistently overcontract muscles. However, Schoenen et al. (1991b) could not find any such correlation. They recorded the EMG of frontal, temporal, and trapezius muscles in 32 patients with chronic tension-type headaches and in 20 healthy volunteers and found that muscle activity was, on average, significantly higher in the patients with headache but did not correlate with headache severity, anxiety, or response to biofeedback.

Jensen (1999) has summarized the extracranial contribution to tension headache.

Vascular Factors

No evidence exists that sustained vasoconstriction causes tension headache. Lactic acid concentration and resting blood flow was normal in a tender trapezius muscle, but blood flow increased significantly less with static exercise in patients with chronic tension-type headache compared with controls (Ashina et al., 2002). Sensitivity to painful vascular dilation appears intermediate between that of patients with migraine and normal controls. Martin and Mathews (1978) reported that inhaling amyl nitrite increased the severity of tension headache on 43% of occasions and did not alter the intensity on 48% of occasions, whereas no patients reported any increase after inhaling a placebo substance. In another study, Krabbe and Olesen (1980) found that the intravenous infusion of histamine produced a pulsating headache in 14 of 25 patients with migraine, 5 out of 10 patients with tension headache, and none of 13 normal controls. Despite this apparent susceptibility to vascular pain in patients with tension headache, the xenon-133 inhalation method demonstrated no significant change in cortical or extracranial blood flow in tension headache (Sakai & Meyer, 1978). Acetazolamide increases cerebral blood flow and provokes headache in patients with migraine but not in patients with tension-type headache (Shirai et al., 1996).

The part possibly played by nitric oxide (NO) has recently been investigated. An intravenous (IV) infusion of glyceryl trinitrate, a donor of NO, caused a headache that peaked in 8 hours in patients with chronic tension headache and in 20 minutes after the start of the infusion in controls (Ashina et al., 2000). However, an IV infusion of an inhibitor of nitric oxide synthase (NOS) to reduce the formation of NO eased the pain of chronic tension-type headache by 30% (Ashina et al., 1999b) and diminished hardness but not tenderness in the trapezius muscle (Ashina et al., 1999a). This suggests that NO plays no part in myofascial input in tension-type headache but may act centrally by diminishing neuronal sensitization or vascular dilation in some patients.

Humoral Factors

In patients with tension-type headache, the platelet content of 5-hydroxytryptamine (5-HT) was reported to be low or the plasma content high by Rolf, Wiele, and Brune (1981), Anthony and Lance (1989), Shimomura and Takahashi (1990), and Jensen and Hindberg (1994), but was reported to be normal by Shukla et al. (1987), Ferrari et al. (1987), and Bendtsen et al. (1997). A possible explanation for this discrepancy is that platelet 5-HT concentration is diminished in patients with analgesic-induced headache (Srikiatkhachorn & Anthony, 1996). The low values obtained in tension-type headache are thus liable to be influenced by the consumption of analgesics. Nevertheless, Bendtsen et al. (1997) found no difference in platelet or plasma 5-HT in patients taking two or more analgesic tablets daily and those who took fewer. The only significant deviation from normal in their study was reduced platelet uptake of 5-HT in patients with chronic tension headache.

Ferrari et al. (1990) found patients with tension headache to have a low platelet content and high plasma levels of methionine-enkephalin, which may have implications for pain control mechanisms.

Central Factors

PRESSURE-PAIN THRESHOLD.   Some dispute in the past has centered on the susceptibility of patients with tension headache to painful stimuli. Drummond (1987) found that muscle tenderness increased at the site of headache but that the pain threshold to finger pressure was the same as in normal controls. Schoenen et al. (1991a) confirmed that the pain threshold in pericranial sites (forehead, temple, and occipital region) was lowered in chronic tension-type headache and also found greater sensitivity to pressure over the Achilles tendon. Langemark et al. (1989) and Jensen and Rasmussen (1996) have also reported the pain threshold to be lowered in chronic tension-type headache, suggesting that central pain mechanisms may be impaired.

Langemark et al. (1993) used measurements of the flexor withdrawal reflex in response to sural nerve stimulation as another index of pain control. The median threshold for this protective reflex was significantly lower in 36 patients with chronic tension-type headache than in 26 matched control subjects. Sicuteri (1981) compared chronic tension headache to the syndrome of abstinence from narcotics and postulated a defect in pain control pathways, possibly involving opioid receptors and serotonergic transmission. However, the intensity of headache remains unaltered by IV injection of naloxone 4 mg (Langemark, 1989).

Because muscle tenderness remains constant in episodic tension-type headaches irrespective of the presence or absence of headache (Bove & Nilsson, 1999), excessive afferent input from the pericranial musculature probably does not play a primary role in initiating headache.

INHIBITION OF JAW CLENCHING.   If one bites firmly on a hard object, jaw closure is mercifully inhibited, to protect the teeth. A similar reflex inhibition can be elicited by electrical stimulation of trigeminal innervated territory, the usual site being lateral to the lips, while the jaws are clenched. Two silent periods in the EMG of the temporalis muscle may be detected in this way, designated as exteroceptive suppressions 1 and 2 (ES1 and ES2). Schoenen et al. (1987) compared these silent periods in 25 patients with chronic tension headache, 20 suffering from migraine without aura, and 22 control subjects. The latency of ES1 was similar in all groups. The latency of ES2 was also similar in all groups, but the duration was significantly shorter in the patients with tension headache. Zwart and Sand (1995) and Bendtsen et al. (1996) could not confirm this finding, which raises questions about the duration of ES2 being a measure of diminished central pain control.

Conclusions About Pathophysiology

In some patients with tension-type headache, psychologic factors appear paramount, often associated with excessive contraction of neck, forehead, and jaw muscles. Some cases also seem to show a central deficit of pain control with lowering of the pain threshold. What part amine depletion and other central factors play in the genesis of chronic daily headache is still uncertain. Some have postulated that prolonged painful input from myofascial tissues sensitizes spinal and supraspinal structures to produce chronic tension-type headache (Jensen, 1999; Bendtsen, 2000). We think a more likely mechanism is a primary failure of modulation by the brain's endogenous pain-control system.

TREATMENT

Many patients suffering from chronic muscle-contraction headache suspect they have a cerebral tumor or other serious intracranial disorder. The first step in treatment is to listen carefully and give patients a careful examination to give them confidence that their complaint is being taken seriously and that the doctor is not jumping to a facile conclusion to prescribe an antidepressant and move on to the next patient.

The second step in treatment is to check whether the scalp and facial muscles are indeed contracting for much of the time without reason. This can be achieved partly by questions at the end of history taking: "Do your friends comment that you always look serious or worried? Do you find yourself clenching your jaw, grinding your teeth, making a tight fist with your hands?" The answers to these questions can be quite surprising. Some patients have had to seek dental attention because their teeth are tender or chipped from unremitting pressure of their jaws. We have had patients who have repeatedly broken their dentures by the same mechanism. Some state that even on awakening from sleep they notice their fingers flexed firmly or jaw clenched.

The presence of unnecessary muscular contraction can be demonstrated to the patient at the end of the physical examination. Most cannot relax the jaw muscles, so the physician cannot move the jaw freely. Patients are unable to let the head loll back when the shoulders are supported, because the neck muscles remain rigid. They cannot permit their elevated arm to fall limply to the couch when the examiner asks them to.

Correcting various physical factors may be necessary to help patients reach their goal of muscular relaxation. Correcting a refractive error or orthoptic treatment for a latent ocular imbalance may remove the factors of eye strain that encourage a pattern of wasteful muscle activity. Dental treatment may be important to open a closed bite, restore a chewing surface, or improve dentures so that the bite is evenly distributed. Cervical traction or manipulation may be useful if neck pain from degenerated intervertebral discs is triggering the tension headache. Observation by patients of their posture in sitting at a desk or driving a car can be important in correcting a tendency to overcontract muscles unnecessarily.

The management of the patient with tension headache must necessarily be psychologic, physiologic (aimed at relaxation of the facial and scalp muscles), and usually pharmacologic.

Psychologic Management

It may be argued that all patients with muscle contraction headache should be referred to a psychiatrist in the first instance. This is certainly our policy with any patient who shows signs of serious mental disturbance, but it is neither practical for every tense patient to be seen by a psychiatrist, nor would it be desirable, because many patients resent the implication of mental illness.

Most can be managed by the doctor of first contact, providing he or she has the time and interest to take a history and counsel the patient. Some patients will not admit to any problem or source of anxiety and may simply have a long-standing habit of muscle contraction in response to the ordinary pressures of everyday life. Others may have easily identifiable worries and anxieties concerned with their work or home life, which may respond to sympathetic discussion. Some tension headaches clear up as soon as the patient goes on vacation. One woman said that her symptoms mysteriously eased as soon as her husband went away on a business trip, only to return as soon as he did. The man or woman with marital or relationship problems or who is the victim of verbal or physical abuse lives with a constant provocation to headache, which may be hard to remove by any amount of psychologic counseling. Careful thought about the patient and his or her reactions to stress, combined with advice about personal problems and adjustment of work pattern and lifestyle, may help ease the patient's anxiety. The use of social agencies to provide support for those who are finding it more difficult to care for themselves is also part of the doctor's role in helping the patient to overcome the symptom of headache. Referring an individual or couple for expert sexual counseling can often be very useful, because many individuals are blighted by ignorance or feelings of inadequacy, shame, or guilt that are often eased by confiding in their medical adviser.

Our view is to combine simple counseling at the first interview with an explanation of how the patient's emotional conflicts are translated into headache by muscular activity. This is then followed by some form of relaxation therapy, considered as physiologic management.

Hyperventilation is a common accompaniment of tension headache (and migraine). Most patients can overcome this with explanation and advice (see Appendix A).

Hypnosis

Melis et al. (1991) treated 26 patients with chronic tension headache in 1-hour sessions each week for a month. They induced trances by eye fixation and then suggested that the patients transfer pain from the head to some other part of the body where it would be more easily tolerated. Headaches declined in frequency, duration, and intensity compared with a waiting-list group. No mention is made of pain being experienced in other areas to which it was supposedly transferred.

Physiologic Management: Relaxation and Biofeedback

Relaxation exercises, usually modified from those Jacobsen (1938) described, have become generally accepted as the most direct means of overcoming the habitual overcontraction of muscles in tension headache. Warner and Lance (1975) combined relaxation therapy with some of the techniques of transcendental meditation in treating 17 patients with chronic tension headache. After personal training, the patient practiced at home with the help of tape recordings of the instructor's voice. When followed up after 6 months, four patients were free of headache, seven had 1 to 4 headaches each month (instead of 12 to 30), and only 6 were unimproved. Only 3 required analgesics or tranquilizers, whereas 14 were habitual users before relaxation therapy.

Feedback techniques may guide the patient in controlling muscle activity and promoting relaxation. Feedback from the EMG of the frontal or temporal muscles has been the most popular method. The amplified EMG signal is played back to the patient through a loudspeaker or earphones, either directly or transformed into a clicking, humming, or buzzing noise, which varies in intensity in proportion to the integrated EMG activity. Controlled trials of EMG feedback have found it effective in reducing the frequency and severity of headache (Blanchard et al., 1980; Bussone et al., 1998). Arena et al. (1995) reported that EMG feedback from the upper trapezius muscles was more effective than using the frontal muscles or than relaxation therapy alone.

Feedback can be regarded as a technique to assist relaxation training in reducing the general level of anxiety and associated vascular changes, as well as any specific effect it has on muscular contraction.

Clinicians can often find many ways to make the patient aware of nervous tension and ways to relieve it. Our own practice is to explain the relaxation process to the patients as described in Appendix B. Some patients are referred to physiotherapists or psychologists who take a particular interest in relaxation therapy. This approach may occasionally be sufficient to relieve tension headache without any need for tranquilizers or antidepressant agents.

Acupuncture

Acupuncture and physiotherapy (relaxation, massage, cryotherapy, and transcutaneous nerve stimulation) were compared in the management of 62 female patients with chronic tension headache (Carlsson, Fahlcrantz, & Augustinsson, 1990). Headache was reduced in both groups, more in those undergoing physiotherapy, but even so, the headache score was reduced only from 3.7 (out of a maximum of 5) to 2.5.

Two recent controlled trials of acupuncture for tension-type headache (White et al., 2000; Karst et al., 2001) could not find any evidence of benefit from the treatment after follow-up of 3 months and 5 months, respectively.

Pharmacologic Management

Episodic tension headache often responds promptly to aspirin or paracetamol (acetaminophen). The occasional use of analgesics presents no real problem, except for epigastric pain from gastric irritation as a side effect of aspirin in some patients. When analgesic tablets are taken daily, they may lead to rebound headaches as the effect wears off and therefore predispose to chronic daily headache. The object of regular interval (prophylactic) therapy is to rid the patient of headache if possible, or at least to reduce its intensity and frequency while reserving the use of analgesics for acute episodes. Pharmacotherapy should go hand in hand with psychologic counseling and relaxation training.

The most widely used agent for the management of chronic tension headache is amitriptyline, shown to be effective in an open and a double-blind crossover trial (Lance & Curran, 1964). Improvement in this trial was not correlated with the presence or absence of pre-existing depression. Of the 98 patients treated, 58 improved substantially, only 18 of whom had symptoms of depression. Surprisingly, another trial of amitriptyline in the treatment of chronic tension-type headache (Pfaffenrath et al., 1994) did not demonstrate any advantage over placebo. A later controlled trial reaffirmed the value of amitriptyline in reducing the frequency and duration of chronic tension-type headache but could not demonstrate any benefit from the use of the specific serotonin reuptake inhibitor (SSRI) citalopram (Bendtsen, Jensen, & Olesen, 1996).

Bendtsen and Jensen (2000) treated 33 nondepressed patients with chronic tension headache with amitriptyline 75 mg daily and with citalopram 20 mg daily. Muscle tenderness declined in those patients who responded to amitriptyline without any change in pressure or pain threshold, suggesting that the effect on headache was specific and not simply a general analgesic effect.

Holroyd, O'Donnell, and Stensland (2001) compared the responses of 203 adults with chronic tension-type headache to amitriptyline or nortriptyline, relaxation/cognitive therapy ("stress therapy") plus placebo, stress therapy plus amitriptyline/nortriptyline, and placebo alone. The combined therapy reduced headaches to less than half in 64%, better than the antidepressants alone (38%), stress management (35%), or placebo (29%). Holroyd et al. (2003) found that patients who had not responded to tricyclics did not improve when subsequently treated with the SSRI paroxetine.

Blood levels of amitriptyline vary 10-fold with the same dose per kilogram body weight, so titrate the dose carefully for each patient. Our own practice is to start with 10 mg or half of a 25-mg tablet at night and to ask patients to increase the nocturnal dose slowly to 75 mg each night if they can tolerate this without morning drowsiness. Patients who respond lose their headaches or notice substantial improvement 2 to 14 days after starting treatment and are advised to continue for at least 6 months and then wean off the medication slowly over a period of 2 to 3 months. Amitriptyline may cause dryness of the mouth, tremor, and weight gain. Its use should be avoided in patients with glaucoma or prostate hypertrophy, because of its atropine-like side effects, and in patients with cardiac dysrhythmias or epilepsy. For patients unable to tolerate amitriptyline, dothiepin or imipramine is worth a trial. Protriptyline 20 mg daily has been suggested as an option for managing tension-type headache, because it is less sedative, and patients tend to lose rather than gain weight (Cohen, 1997).

Tomkins et al. (2001) performed a meta-analysis of tricyclic antidepressants, serotonin antagonists, and SSRIs in the prophylaxis of chronic headache, including 17 trial arms limited to tension headache. The six studies of SSRIs that measured effects on headache burden found no significant benefit, but the response to antidepressants overall showed the response to be twice that of patients treated with placebo in both patients with migraine and patients with tension headache.

Mathew and Ali (1991) reported that sodium valproate in doses of 1000 to 2000 mg daily for 3 months reduced the index of chronic daily headache to half or less in 18 of 30 patients, with the mean number of headache-free days each month increasing from 5.5 to 17.7. These promising results could not be replicated by Vijayan and Spillane (1995), who treated 16 patients with chronic daily headache unresponsive to other forms of treatment. Only 2 of the group improved, whereas 8 of the 16 reported side effects. The withdrawal of analgesics and ergotamine under supervision in a hospital proved beneficial for 38 patients whose chronic daily headache was attributed to excessive intake of these drugs (Schnider et al., 1996). At a 5-year follow-up, 18 patients were virtually headache free, and the frequency of headache was reduced to eight or fewer each month in another 19 patients.

For patients resistant to these measures, pizotifen (pizotyline), cyproheptadine, or beta-blockers may be used as for migraine, but clinical trials have not substantiated their effectiveness. I have found phenelzine 15 mg, given two or three times daily, with the usual warnings about foods and drugs to be avoided while on monoamine oxidase (MAO) inhibitors, useful in some cases. Benzodiazepines are also helpful, but a high risk of habituation follows continued use.

The local application of a traditional Asian remedy (Tiger Balm) proved more effective than a placebo liniment and provided relief comparable with that obtained with paracetamol (acetaminophen) when Schattner and Randerson (1996) submitted them to a controlled trial.

Botulinum Toxin

Botulinum toxin A entered into public awareness as its use expanded from the treatment of dystonia to removing wrinkles. It seems a logical extension to diminish the input from frowning or jaw-clenching muscles with the aim of reducing tension-type headache. Schmitt et al. (2001) conducted a double-blind trial of injections of botulinum toxin 20 units into the frontal and temporal muscles of patients with chronic tension-type headache. However, 8 weeks after injection, the pain intensity, the number of pain-free days, and consumption of analgesics were not less than those of a control group.

Burch et al. (2001) injected 50 units into the frontal muscles of 41 patients with chronic tension-type headaches, somewhat reducing pain intensity but not headache frequency.

Evers et al. (2002) reviewed all the relevant publications according to the criteria of evidence-based medicine. Injecting 24 to 100 units into the relevant muscles produced conflicting results. The only two studies that met Criterion 1B of evidence-based medicine (Burch et al., 2001; Schmitt et al., 2001) were negative.

Psychogenic Headache

The term *psychogenic headache* is used to describe the association of headache with florid psychiatric disturbance such as acute depression, schizophrenia, or hysteria. Headache may be incorporated into the delusional system of such patients. There is no way in which a mechanism can be postulated for such headaches incorporating peripheral pain pathways. The headache is a concept of disordered thought processes and appears or disappears with the mental state that engendered it.

CONCLUSION

Certain personality characteristics are more common in patients with tension-type headaches: anxiety, depression, suppressed anger, and a feeling of inadequacy. Activity in frontal, temporal, and nuchal muscles is often increased when the subject is at rest or under stress. Pericranial muscles are often unduly tender, and their pain threshold is diminished; in some cases, the pain threshold to pressure or thermal stimuli may also be lowered in other parts of the body.

Patients with tension headache are more susceptible to painful vascular dilation than are normal controls but less so than patients with migraine.

Tension-type headache appears to be a central disinhibitory phenomenon, probably with neurotransmitter changes underlying personality traits, defective pain control, and sensitivity to both myofascial and vascular input.

Management includes psychologic counseling, relaxation therapy, advice about hyperventilation when necessary, and the use of tricyclic antidepressants, of which amitriptyline is the most widely prescribed.

References

Anthony, M., & Lance, J. W. (1989). Plasma serotonin in patients with chronic tension headaches. *J Neurol Neurosurg Psychiatry, 52,* 182–184.

Arena, J. G., Bruno, G. M., Hannah, S. L., & Meador, K. Y. (1995). A comparison of frontal electromyographic feedback training, trapezius electromyographic feedback training and progressive muscle relaxation therapy in the treatment of tension headache. *Headache, 35,* 411–419.

Ashina, M., Bendtsen, L., Jensen, R., Lassen, L. H., Sakai, F., & Olesen, J. (1999a). Possible mechanisms of action of nitric oxide synthase inhibitors in chronic tension-type headache. *Brain, 122,* 1629–1635.

Ashina, M., Bendtsen, L., Jensen, R., & Olesen, J. (2000). Nitric oxide-induced headache in patients with chronic tension-type headache. *Brain, 123,* 1830–1837.

Ashina, M., Lassen, L. H., Bendtsen, L., Jensen, R., & Olesen, J. (1999b). Effect of inhibition of nitric oxide synthase on chronic tension-type headache: A randomised crossover trial. *Lancet, 353,* 287–289.

Ashina, M., Stallknecht, B., Bendtsen, L., Pederson, J. F. Galbo, H., Dalgaard, P., et al. (2002). In vivo evidence of altered skeletal muscle blood flow in chronic tension-type headache. *Brain, 125,* 320–326.

Bendtsen, L. (2000). Central sensitization in tension-type headache–possible pathophysiological mechanisms. *Cephalalgia, 20,* 486–508.

Bendtsen, L., & Jensen, R. (2000). Amitriptyline reduces myofascial tenderness in patients with chronic tension-type headache. *Cephalalgia, 20,* 603–610.

Bendtsen, L., Jensen, R., Brennum, J., Arendt-Nielsen, L., & Olesen, J. (1996). Exteroceptive suppression of temporal muscle activity is normal in chronic tension-type headache and not related to actual headache state. *Cephalalgia, 16,* 251–256.

Bendtsen, L., Jensen, R., Hindberg, I., Gammelroft, S., & Olesen, J. (1997). Serotonin metabolism in chronic tension-type headache. *Cephalalgia, 17*, 843–848.

Bendtsen, L., Jensen, R., & Olesen, J. (1996). A non-selective (amitriptyline), but not a selective (citalopram), serotonin reuptake inhibitor is effective in the prophylactic treatment of chronic tension-type headache. *J Neurol Neurosurg Psychiatry, 61*, 285–290.

Bennett, H. J. (2003). Hogwarts headaches—misery for Muggles. *N Engl J Med, 349*, 18.

Blanchard, E. B., Andrasik, F., Ahles, T. A., Teders, S. J., & O'Keefe, D. (1980). Migraine and tension headache: A meta-analytic review. *Behav Ther, 11*, 613–631.

Bove, G. M., & Nilsson, N. (1999). Pressure pain threshold and pain tolerance in episodic tension-type headache do not depend on the presence of headache. *Cephalalgia, 19*, 174–178.

Burch, C. M., Kokoska, M. S., Glaser, D. A., & Hollenbeak, C. S. (2001). Treatment of frontal tension headaches with botulinum toxin A. *Cephalalgia, 21*, 489.

Bussone, G., Grazzi, L., D'Amico, D., Leone, M., & Andrasik, F. (1998). Biofeedback-assisted relaxation training for young adolescents with tension-type headache: a controlled study. *Cephalalgia, 18*, 463–467.

Carlsson, J., Fahlcrantz, A., & Augustinsson, L. E. (1990). Muscle tenderness in tension headache treated with acupuncture or physiotherapy. *Cephalalgia, 10*, 131–141.

Cohen, G. L. (1997). Protriptyline, chronic tension-type headaches and weight loss in women. *Headache, 37*, 433–436.

De Benedittis, G., & Lorenzetti, A. (1992). The role of stressful life events in the persistence of primary headache: Major events vs. daily hassles. *Pain, 51*, 35–42.

Demjen, S., & Bakal, D. (1981). Illness behaviour and chronic headache. *Pain, 10*, 221–229.

Drummond, P. D. (1987). Scalp tenderness and sensitivity to pain in migraine and tension headache. *Headache, 27*, 45–50.

Drummond. P. D., & Lance, J. W. (1984). Clinical diagnosis and computer analysis of headache symptoms. *J Neurol Neurosurg Psychiatry, 47*, 128–133.

Evers, S., Rahmann, A., Vollmer-Haase, J., & Husstedt, I. W. (2002). Treatment of headache with botulinum toxin A–a review according to evidence-based medicine. *Cephalalgia, 22*, 699–710.

Every, R. G. (1960). The significance of extreme mandibular movement. *Lancet, ii*, 37.

Ferrari, M. D., Frohlich, M., Odink, J. J., Portielje, J. E., & Bruyn, G. W. (1987). Methionine-enkephalin and serotonin in migraine and tension headache. In F. Clifford Rose (Ed.), *Current problems in neurology*. Vol. 4. *Advances in headache research* (pp. 227–234). London: John Libbey.

Ferrari, M. D., Odink, J. J., Frohlich, M., Tapparelli, C., Portielje, J., & Bruyn, G. W. (1990). Methionine-enkephalin in migraine and tension headache. Differences between classic migraine, common migraine and tension headache, and changes during attacks. *Headache, 30*, 160–164.

Friedman, A., von Storch, T. J. C., & Merritt, H. H. (1964). Migraine and tension headaches. A clinical study of two thousand cases. *Neurology, 4*, 773–788.

Hatch, J. P., Schoenfeld, L. S., Boutros, N. N., Seleshi, E., Moore, D. J., & Cur-Provost, M. (1991). Anger and hostility in tension-type headache. *Headache, 31*, 302–304.

Headache Classification Subcommittee of the International Headache Society. (2004). The International Classification of Headache Disorders (2nd ed.). *Cephalalgia, 24*(Suppl. 1), 37–43.

Holroyd, K. A., Labus, J. S., O'Donnell, F. J., & Cordingley, G. E. (2003). Treating chronic tension-type headache not responding to amitriptyline hydrochloride: A pilot evaluation. *Headache, 43*, 999–1004.

Holroyd, K. A., O'Donnell, F. J., & Stensland, M. (2001). Management of chronic tension-type headache with tricyclic antidepressant medication, stress management therapy, and their combination. *JAMA, 285*, 2208–2215.

Holroyd, K. A., Stensland, M., Lipchik, G. L., Hill, K. R., O'Donnell, F. S., & Cordingley, G. (2000). Psychosocial correlates and impact of chronic tension-type headaches. *Headache, 49*, 3–16.

Hunter, M., & Philips, C. (1981). The experience of headache—an assessment of the qualities of tension headache pain. *Pain, 10*, 209–219.

Jacobsen, E. (1938). *Progressive relaxation*. Chicago: University of Chicago Press.

Jensen, R. (1999). Pathophysiological mechanisms of tension-type headache: A review of epidemiological and experimental studies. *Cephalalgia, 19*, 602–621.

Jensen, R., & Hindberg, I. (1994). Plasma serotonin increase during episodes of tension-type headache. *Cephalalgia, 14*, 219–222.

Jensen, R., & Olesen, J. (1996). Initiating mechanisms of experimentally induced tension-type headache. *Cephalalgia, 16*, 175–182.

Jensen, R., & Rasmussen, B. K. (1996). Muscular disorders in tension-type headache. *Cephalalgia, 16*, 97–103.

Karst, M., Reinhard, M., Thum, P., Wiese, B., Rollnik, J., & Fink, M. (2001). Needle acupuncture in tension-type headache: A randomized placebo-controlled study. *Cephalalgia, 21*, 637–642.

Karwautz, A., Wöber, C., Lang, T., Bock, A., Wagner-Ennsgraber, C., Veselu, C., et al. (1999). Psychosocial factors in children and adolescents with migraine and tension-type headache: A controlled study and review of the literature. *Cephalalgia, 19*, 32–43.

Krabbe, A. A., & Olesen, J. (1980). Headache provocation by continuous intravenous infusion of histamine. Clinical results and receptor mechanisms. *Pain, 8*, 253–259.

Lance, J. W., & Anthony, M. (1966). Some clinical aspects of migraine. *Arch Neurol, 15*, 356–361.

Lance, J. W., & Curran. D. A. (1964). Treatment of chronic tension headache. *Lancet, i*, 1236–1239.

Lance, J. W., Curran, D. A., & Anthony, M. (1965). Investigations into the mechanism and treatment of chronic headache. *Med J Aust, 2*(22), 909–914.

Langemark, M. (1989). Naloxone in moderate dose does not aggravate chronic tension headache. *Pain, 39*, 85–93.

Langemark, M., Bach, F. W., Jensen, T. S., & Olesen, J. (1993). Decreased nociceptive flexion reflex threshold in chronic tension-type headache. *Arch Neurol, 50*, 1061–1064.

Langemark, M., Jensen, K., Jensen, T. S., & Olesen, J. (1989). Pressure pain thresholds and thermal nociceptive thresholds in chronic tension-type headache. *Pain, 38*, 203–210.

Martin, P. R., & Mathews, A. M. (1978). Tension headaches: Psychophysiological investigation and treatment. *J Pyschosom Res, 22*, 389–399.

Mathew, N. T. (1993). Transformed migraine. *Cephalalgia, 13*(Suppl. 12), 78–83.

Mathew, N. T., & Ali, S. (1991). Valproate in the treatment of persistent chronic daily headache. An open label study. *Headache, 31*, 71–74.

Mathew, N. T., Reuveni, U., & Perez, F. (1987). Transformed or evolutive migraine. *Headache, 27*, 102–106.

Melis, P. M. L., Rooimans, W., Spierings, E. L. H., & Hoogduin, C. A. L. (1991). Treatment of chronic tension-type headache with hypnotherapy: A single-blind time controlled study. *Headache, 31*, 686–689.

Merikangas, K. R., Stevens, D. E., & Angst, J. (1993). Headache and personality: Results of a community sample of young adults. *J Psychiatr Res, 27*, 187–196.

Mitsikostas, D. D., & Thomas, A. M. (1999). Comorbidity of headache and depressive disorders. *Cephalalgia, 19*, 211–217.

Passchier, J., Schouten, J., van der Donk, J., & van Romunde, L. K. J. (1991). The association of frequent headaches with personality and life events. *Headache, 31*, 116–121.

Pfaffenrath, V., Diener, H. C., Isler, H., Meyer, C., Scholz, E., Taneri, Z., et al. (1994). Efficacy and tolerability of amitriptylinoxide in the treatment of chronic tension-type headache: A multi-centre controlled study. In F. Clifford Rose (Ed.), *New advances in headache research* (Vol. 3, pp. 265–274). London: Smith-Gordon.

Rasmussen, B. K. (1992). Migraine and tension-type headache in a general population: Psychosocial factors. *Int J Epidemiol, 21*, 1138–1143.

Rasmussen, B. K. (1993). Migraine and tension-type headache in a general population: precipitating factors, female hormones, sleep pattern and relation to lifestyle. *Pain, 53*, 65–72.

Rasmussen, B. K., Jensen, R., Schroll, M., & Olesen, J. (1991). Epidemiology of headache in a general population—a prevalence study. *J Clin Epidemiol, 44*, 1147–1157.

Rolf, L. H., Wiele, G., & Brune, G. G. (1981). 5-Hydroxytryptamine in platelets of patients with muscle contraction headache. *Headache, 21*, 10–11.

Russell, M. B., Østergaard, S., Bendtsen, L., & Olesen, J. (1999). Familial occurrence of chronic tension-type headache. *Cephalalgia, 19*, 207–210.

Sakai, F., & Meyer, J. S. (1978). Regional cerebral hemodynamics during migraine and cluster headache measured by the $_{133}$Xe inhalation method. *Headache, 18*, 122–132.

Schattner, P., & Randerson, D. (1996). Tiger balm as a treatment of tension headache. *Aust Family Physician, 25*, 216–222.

Schmitt, W. J., Slowey, E., Fravi, N., Weber, S., & Burgunder, J. M. (2001). Effect of botulinum toxin A injections in the treatment of chronic tension-type headache: A double-blind placebo-controlled trial. *Headache, 41*, 658–664.

Schnider, P., Aull, S., Baumgartner, C., Marterer, A., Wöber, C., Zeiler, K., et al. (1996). Long-term outcome of patients with headache and drug abuse after inpatient withdrawal: Five-year follow-up. *Cephalalgia, 16*, 481–485.

Schoenen, J., Bottin, D., Hardy, F., & Gerard, P. (1991a). Cephalic and extracephalic pressure pain thresholds in chronic tension-type headache. *Pain, 47*, 145–149.

Schoenen, J., Gerard, P., De Pasqua, V., & Juprelle, M. (1991b). EMG in pericranial muscles during postural variation and mental activity in healthy volunteers and patients with chronic tension-type headache. *Headache, 31*, 321–324.

Schoenen, J., Jamart, B., Gerard, P., Lenarduzzi, P., & Delwaide, P. J. (1987). Exteroceptive suppression of temporalis muscle activity in chronic headaches. *Neurology, 37*, 1834–1836.

Schwartz, B. S., Stewart, W. F., Simon, D., & Lipton, R. B. (1998). Epidemiology of tension-type headache. *JAMA, 279*, 381–383.

Shimomura, T., & Takahashi, K. (1990). Alteration of platelet serotonin in patients with chronic tension-type headache during cold pressor test. *Headache, 30*, 581–583.

Shirai, T., Meyer, J. S., Akiyama, H., Mortel, K. F., & Willis, P. M. (1996). Acetazolamide testing of cerebral vasodilator capacity provokes "vascular" but not tension headaches. *Headache, 36*, 589–594.

Shukla, R., Shanker, K., Nag, D., et al. (1987). Serotonin in tension headache. *J Neurol Neurosurg Psychiatry, 50*, 1682–1684.

Sicuteri, F. (1981). Opioid receptor impairment—underlying mechanism in "pain diseases." *Cephalalgia, 1*, 77–82.

Silberstein, S. D., Lipton, R. B., & Sliwinski, M. (1996). Classification of daily and near-daily headaches: field trial of revised IHS criteria. *Neurology, 47*, 871–875.

Srikiatkhachorn, A., & Anthony, M. (1996). Platelet serotonin in patients with analgesic-induced headache. *Cephalalgia, 16*, 423–426.

Tomkins, G. E., Jackson, J. L., O'Malley, P. G., Balden, E., & Santoro, J. E. (2001). Treatment of chronic headache with antidepressants: A meta-analysis. *Am J Med, 111*, 54–63.

Vanagaite Vingen, J., & Stovner, L. J. (1998). Photophobia and phonophobia in tension-type and cervicogenic headache. *Cephalalgia, 18*, 313–318.

Vijayan, N., & Spillane, T. (1995). Valproic acid treatment of chronic daily headache. *Headache, 35*, 540–43.

Warner, A. K., & Lance, J. W. (1975). Relaxation therapy in migraine and chronic tension headache. *Med J Aust, 1*, 298–301.

White A. R., Resch, K. L., Chan, J. C., Norris, C. D., Modi, S. K., Patel, J. N., et al. (2000). Acupuncture for episodic tension-type headache: A multicentre randomized controlled trial. *Cephalalgia, 20*, 632–637.

Zeigler, A. K., & Hassanein, R. S. (1982). Migraine muscle contraction headache dichotomy studied by statistical analysis of headache symptoms. In F. Clifford Rose (Ed.), *Advances in migraine research and therapy* (pp. 7–11). New York: Raven Press.

Zwart, J.-A., & Sand, T. (1995). Exteroceptive suppression of temporalis muscle activity: A blind study of tension-type headache, migraine and cervicogenic headache. *Headache, 35*, 338–343.

Chapter 11
Chronic Daily Headache

Chronic daily headache (CDH) often presents a diagnostic and therapeutic challenge and is a major cause of concern and sometimes despair to the caring physician. We have thus devoted a new chapter to gather together some of the issues around this group of headache disorders. Some patients have an underlying organic disease. These in a sense are the lucky ones, at least for the clinician, because once the diagnosis is established, the treatment is relatively straightforward. These conditions are listed here as secondary causes of CDH, to jog the memory of the reader, but are dealt with elsewhere in this book:

Secondary Causes of Chronic Daily Headache

- Changes in cerebrospinal fluid (CSF) pressure
- Idiopathic intracranial hypertension
- Intracranial hypotension from a CSF leak
- Systemic infections, such as Lyme disease, tuberculous or cryptococcal meningitis, and human immunodeficiency virus (HIV)
- Obstructive sleep apnea (habitual snoring is a risk factor for CDH) (Scher, Libron, & Stewart, 2003)
- Caffeine-induced headache (Check history of cola drink consumption in children.)
- Temporal arteritis in the older patient
- Post-traumatic headache

Primary Causes of Chronic Daily Headache

- Chronic migraine (or the more broadly defined transformed migraine)
- Chronic cluster headache and the other trigeminal-autonomic cephalgias (see Chapter 12)
- Hemicrania continua (a relatively rare primary headache syndrome responsive to indomethacin)
- Chronic tension-type headache
- New daily persistent headache (NDPH)
- Hypnic headache (see Chapter 13)

We deal with the chronic trigeminal-autonomic cephalalgias elsewhere (see Chapter 12) and here deal with chronic migraine, chronic tension-type headache, hemicrania continua (HC), and NDPH. (Hypnic headache is discussed in Chapter 13.) These conditions affect a difficult group of headache sufferers in whom diagnostic features may become blurred and who present a therapeutic challenge. These entities have been comprehensively reviewed in recent years (Silberstein & Lipton, 2001; Goadsby & Boes, 2002a; Gladstone, Eross, & Dodick, 2003).

CLASSIFICATION AND PREVALENCE OF CHRONIC DAILY HEADACHE

The term *chronic daily headache* is usually applied to patients who have had headaches 15 days or more in a month for more than 3 months. In practice, most such patients report headaches that have not left them day or night for many years. Population-based studies have placed the prevalence of CDH as high as 3% to 5% of the general population. Silberstein, Lipton, and Sliwinski (1996) have proposed the following classification for CDH: It consists of daily or near-daily headache lasting longer than 4 hours for more than 15 days per month. Each of the following can occur with and without medication overuse, which needs to be addressed first in the clinical management.

1. Transformed migraine
2. Chronic tension-type headache
3. NDPH
4. HC

Note the distinction between *chronic migraine,* as defined by the International Headache Society (Headache Classification Subcommittee of the International Headache Society, 2004), and *transformed migraine,* as defined by Silberstein and colleagues (2001). The IHS definition requires 15 days or more a month on which a patient's attacks fulfill criteria for migraine without aura. Silberstein and colleagues require 15 days or more of headache per month with some link to migraine, such as clear migraine without aura in the past. Saper and Winters (1982) and Mathew, Stubits, and Nigam (1982) discussed the concept of transformed migraine, although the view that some patients with migraine have frequent headache is not a 20th-century discovery (Gowers, 1888).

Bigal and associates (2002b) applied Silberstein and colleagues' criteria to 638 patients with CDH in the United States. Patients ranged in age from 11 to 88 years; 65% were female. The most common diagnosis was reported as chronic migraine (87.4%), although in effect this meant transformed migraine. NDPH accounted for 10.8%, and chronic tension-type headache accounted for only 1%. This contrasts with a report from India: Chakravarty (2003) classified 205 patients with CDH as having transformed migraine (82.4%), but chronic tension-type headache as 16.1%, and NDPH as only 1.5%. Comparable figures from Brazil were 88.1%, 8% and 17% (Krymchantowski, 2003).

Reportedly the distinction between chronic tension-type headache and migraine is harder to determine in children and adolescents, although our experience in clinical practice is that the differentiation is exceptionally straightforward, albeit often impeded by the current diagnostic systems. Abu-Arafeh (2001) reported from Glasgow that about one third of patients attending a pediatric headache clinic had CDH and that 81% of 115 children and adolescents fitted the pattern of chronic tension-type headache. About one third of these patients had suffered from migraine as well, and about half of the patients with CDH had some migrainous features (e.g., nausea or photophobia) with the more severe of their daily headaches. The Pediatric Committee of the American Headache Society (Koenig et al., 2002) surveyed 189 patients aged 18 years or younger with CDH. Baseline headache was present about 27 days in each month and became more severe with migrainous features about 5 days a month. The fundamental problem in much of this work is the differentiation between migraine and tension-type headache, which for the typical patient is obvious but for many patients seems quite unclear.

Tension-Type Headache or Migraine?

There is a long-standing controversy about the separate nature of migraine and tension-type headache. Is there a headache diathesis, with episodic severe attacks, associated with nausea, photophobia, phonophobia, and osmophobia called *migraine* and daily milder headache without specific features being diagnosed as *tension-type headache?* Are there two biologically distinct conditions: migraine and tension-type headache? Drummond and Lance (1984) showed that as the frequency of headache increased, it became more often bilateral than unilateral and was accompanied by fewer migrainous hallmarks. Why, if a patient had severe left temporal headaches once a month with vomiting and the frequency of headache increased until it recurred daily without all the usual migrainous accompaniments but remained in the left temple, would we feel constrained to rename it "chronic tension-type headache"? Mathew (1987) introduced the term *transformed migraine* to account for this change. He considered that the transformation usually resulted from depression, stress, other emotional factors, or daily consumption of analgesic tablets or ergotamine. An alternative view might be that there are two biologically distinct conditions—migraine and tension-type headache—but that people with migraine can suffer both types; that is, migraine has a spectrum of attack manifestations, whereas tension-type headache in its pure form does not (Welch & Goadsby, 2002). Without more data and tighter definitions, particularly a more restrictive definition of tension-type headache, this problem will remain for the foreseeable future.

Overuse of Medications: Cause or Consequence of Chronic Daily Headache?

The frequent use of analgesics is a factor in CDH (Scher et al., 2003b), but it appears that people with other conditions, such as arthritis (Bahra et al., 2003), can take large quantities of analgesics without becoming susceptible to headache. Zwart and associates (2003) evaluated 32,067 adults in 1984 and again 11 years later; they found that those who used analgesics habitually had a higher risk of chronic migraine (relative risk 13.3) or other headaches (relative risk 6.2) than those who did not use analgesics. This suggests that the analgesic intake has a role in inducing frequent headache but does not exclude the possibility that a baseline headache existed at the onset of the survey, prompting the use of analgesics. Limmroth and colleagues (2002), in their study of 98 patients, found that the mean critical duration of analgesic use for production of medication overdose headache was 1.7 years for triptans, 2.7 years for ergots, and 4.8 years for analgesics. The mean monthly intake of tablets was 18, 37, and 114, respectively.

In most studies, abstinence from analgesics reduces headache frequency to half or less over a follow-up period of 3 months to 3 years (Young & Silberstein, 2001), although in clinical practice this clearly does not happen to every patient. Katsarava and associates (2003) reported a 1-year relapse rate of 38% among 98 patients. Pini, Cicero, and Sandrini (2001) found that the relapse rate after 4 years was 60%. In a reply to a letter to the editor of *Cephalalgia* (Bigal et al., 2002a) concerning these disappointing long-term results, Pini and his colleagues advised that patients who cannot withdraw from analgesics and find relief from headache should remain under medical guidance without their behavior being regarded as addictive.

PATHOPHYSIOLOGY OF CHRONIC DAILY HEADACHE

Strictly speaking, there is no particular pathophysiology to CDH, because it is a grouping, not a diagnosis with distinct biology, at least as we define it here. Much discussion concerning the pathophysiology of CDH really concerns how infrequent migraine becomes frequent and how distinct frequent migraine is from infrequent migraine. Current views on the pathophysiology of CDH center on two concepts (Silberstein & Lipton, 2001; Srikiatkhachorn, 2002; Welch & Goadsby, 2002):

1. Central sensitization of pain-processing neurons in the central nervous system by repeated activation of trigeminal nociceptors
2. Depletion of serotonin and noradrenaline in the endogenous pain-control system, permitting unrestrained inflow of afferent impulses

Burstein, Cutrer, and Yarnitsky (2000) used the progressive development of allodynia, hypersensitivity of skin and underlying tissues, in a patient with migraine headache as an indication of increasing sensitivity of central neurons. In the study by Yarnitsky and colleagues (2003), blockade of parasympathetic outflow to cerebral and meningeal blood vessels by intranasal lidocaine eased the pain of migraine headache in some patients, whereas allodynia continued to worsen. This was interpreted as indicating that the inflow of nociceptive impulses from dilated vessels in the brain and dura mater during migraine headache had sensitized second-order neurons and then third-order neurons to cause allodynia. If a similar mechanism were to cause an increasing frequency of headache, one would expect that the greater the painful trigeminal input, the greater the likelihood of frequent headache developing. Yet the severe pains of cluster headache and trigeminal neuralgia are not usually associated with increasing headache frequency per se, except perhaps for patients with, for example, cluster headache who overuse medicines aimed at relieving acute attack.

Granted central sensitivity exists in patients with CDH, evidenced by the relatively common finding of allodynia, it seems to us more likely that the endogenous pain-control system has become defective, either spontaneously or as the result of anxiety, stress, infection, or constant analgesic intake. Srikiatkhachorn and Anthony (1996) demonstrated that the blood-platelet serotonin level was low in patients with chronic tension-type headache treated with analgesics. This may reflect depletion in central serotonergic pathways known to be important in pain control. Blood levels of serotonin increased once analgesics were stopped (Hering et al., 1993). The clearest evidence that there are important central nervous system changes in the brain in frequent migraine comes from the demonstration of dorsolateral pontine activation in chronic migraine use PET (Matharu et al., 2004). Moreover, there were thalamic changes, notably in pulvinar, and thus the prospect of beginning to consider chronic migraine as primarily a disorder of altered brain processing of pain and other sensory input (Figure 11.1).

Many agents other than serotonin and noradrenaline that may be implicated in central sensitivity and the role of each have yet to be worked out. Sarchielli and colleagues (2001) reported that the CSF of patients with CDH contained a high level of nerve growth factor and substance P compared with controls. Gallai and associates (2003) demonstrated a significant increase in glutamate and nitrite levels in the CSF of patients with CDH. The increase in nitrites was accompanied by a rise in cyclic guanosine monophosphate (GMP). This suggests a central disturbance of the receptors for glutamate, N-methyl-D-aspartate (NMDA) receptors. Substance P and calcitonin-gene–related peptide (CGRP) were also elevated in the CSF compared with that of control subjects. Whether these changes indicate a causative role or are a response to chronic pain remains open to conjecture.

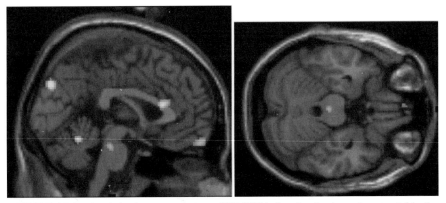

FIGURE 11.1 Statistical parametric map (SPM{F}) showing brain regions, notably the dorsal rostral pons, anterior cingulate cortex and cuneus, in which regional cerebral blood flow (rCBF) correlates with pain scores.

That the endogenous pain-control pathway is implicated in migraine has been strengthened by magnetic resonance imaging (MRI) findings of iron deposition in the periaqueductal gray matter of patients with migraine, increasing with duration of the illness (Welch et al., 2001). Could such a change underlie CDH?

TREATMENT OF CHRONIC DAILY HEADACHE

In general terms, the most effective strategy for treating frequent headache is to identify the underlying headache biology and to direct treatment at this cause. Secondary causes must be identified, and then preventive treatments must be tailored to the primary headache type. One generally agreed-on strategy is to wean patients off analgesics, ergotamine, or triptans if they have overused medication. The success rate of withdrawal therapy, often accompanied by prophylactic medication and behavioral therapy, varies from 48% to 91% in different series (Silberstein & Lipton, 2001), but a considerable proportion later experience relapse.

Many patients resist the notion that they should stop using the one instrument they see for their salvation. The weaning process can be assisted by admission to a hospital for an intravenous lignocaine (lidocaine) infusion. Williams and Stark (2003) reported the outcome of 71 patients with CDH treated by this method in hospital for a mean of 8.7 days. There was a past history of migraine in 90% of patients. Ingestion of codeine (mean: 1053 mg per week) and ergotamine (mean: 16 mg per week) were the main offenders. These agents were withdrawn successfully in 97% of patients, 70% of whom stated that their headaches had disappeared or improved 6 months after treatment. Krymchantowski and Barbosa (2000) stopped symptomatic medication suddenly in 400 patients and prescribed a short course of prednisone, tapered over 6 days, followed by preventive therapy. This significantly decreased headache frequency and has the advantage of being an outpatient treatment.

Although most clinicians have an opinion, there are no controlled trials to help decide how to choose between (1) stopping medication overuse first and (2) initiating preventive therapy at the same time as medication withdrawal. Moreover, there are no controlled data to determine whether it is better to stop acute-attack medicines abruptly or to taper them off gradually. With the exception of barbiturates and very high dosages of opiate receptor agonists, abrupt withdrawal seems safe and efficient. Abrupt withdrawal may be unpleasant for patients, and they certainly need to be made aware of this. We find clonidine a useful adjunct treatment during opiate-receptor agonist withdrawal and one or two doses of a long-acting barbiturate, such as phenobarbitone 30 mg, helpful in barbiturate withdrawal to prevent seizures.

What Is the Most Effective Preventive Treatment?

Ever since amitriptyline was shown to be effective for chronic tension-type headache in a double-blind trial in the 1960s (Lance & Curran, 1964), it has been accepted as the first line of defense in many patients with frequent headache

(Silberstein & Lipton, 2001). Dosage is best started slowly as 10 mg at night, increasing to 25 mg, 50 mg, or higher if necessary in patients who are not troubled by side effects of drowsiness, dry mouth, or constipation—all cholinergic blocking side effects. Mirtazapine is effective in chronic tension-type headache compared with placebo (Bendtsen & Jensen, 2004) and is as effective as amitriptyline, with fewer side effects (Martin-Aragus, Bustamente-Martinez, & Pedro-Pijoan, 2003).

The tricyclic antidepressants are generally more effective than the specific serotonin reuptake inhibitors (SSRIs), although SSRIs are worth a trial in refractory patients (Redillas & Solomon, 2000). Krymchantowski and colleagues (2002) found no advantage in adding fluoxetine to amitriptyline in the management of transformed migraine as diagnosed using Silberstein-Lipton criteria (Silberstein, Lipton, & Sliwinski, 1996). We are cautious of using SSRIs because they sometimes exacerbate headache. Combining tricyclic antidepressants with stress management (relaxation and coping strategies) is more effective than using the tricyclics alone to control chronic tension-type headache (Holroyd et al., 2000).

Freitagand associates (2001) found that 75% of 642 patients with CDH improved on dosage of 500 to 1000 g of valproate daily. Topiramate was reported to relieve CDH, including transformed migraine, in an open-label study (Shuaib, 2000). Gabapentin produced only a 9.1% advantage in headache-free rates over placebo in a controlled trial involving 95 patients with CDH (Spira & Beran, 2003).

Tizanidine, an α_2-adrenergic agonist that inhibits the release of noradrenaline, achieved statistical significance in reducing headache indices but not enough to be of clinical value (Saper et al., 2002).

Injection of botulinum toxin increased the number of headache-free days over a period of 3 months from 24 to 32 (Ondo, Vuong, & Derman, 2004), and more improvement occurred after a second injection. Studies directed at specific primary headache types have largely not been promising (Evers et al., 2002; Schulte-Mattler, Krack, & Bo, 2004), with one exception (Silberstein et al., 2000). However, experts whose views we value find this approach useful; thus, we conclude more work is required to understand this approach.

In chronic migraine, prophylactic agents such as propranolol, pizotifen (pizotyline), and cyproheptadine are also worth a trial. We have used monoamine oxidase inhibitors such as phenelzine in many patients refractory to other treatments.

HEMICRANIA CONTINUA

HC is an indomethacin-responsive headache classified now under Section 4 of the IHS criteria (Headache Classification Subcommittee of the International Headache Society, 2004). HC is characterized by a continuous, unilateral headache that varies in intensity, waxing and waning without disappearing completely. We discuss it here because it involves daily headache and may cause diagnostic confusion. When not identified, it represents some proportion of so-called intractable CDH.

Historical Note

HC was probably first described by Medina and Diamond (1981). Sjaastad and Spierings coined the term *hemicrania continua* in 1984, when they described two additional cases (Sjaastad & Spierings, 1984). Since then, more than 100 cases have been described in the literature.

Epidemiology

The incidence and prevalence of HC are unknown. It was once thought to be a very rare syndrome; however, headache clinics that have systematically sought out this entity have rapidly identified significant number of patients, suggesting the condition is underdiagnosed and may be more common than earlier appreciated (Peres et al., 2001; Wheeler, Allen, & Pusey, 2001). The disorder has a female preponderance, with a sex ratio of 2:1. The condition usually begins in adulthood, although the range of onset is from 5 to 67 years of age (mean: 28 years) (Peres, Siow, & Rozen, 2001).

Clinical Features

HC is a unilateral, continuous headache; in most patients the pain is exclusively unilateral, without side shift, although rare bilateral cases have been described (Pasquier, Leys, & Petit, 1987; Iordanidis & Sjaastad, 1989; Trucco, Antonaci, & Sandrini, 1992), as has a patient with unilateral, side-alternating attacks (Newman et al., 1992). The forehead, temporal, orbit, and occiput are the most common sites of pain, although any part of the head or neck can be affected (Bordini et al., 1991). The pain is typically mild to moderate in intensity. The quality of pain is described as dull, aching, or pressing. It is said to not usually be associated with photophobia, phonophobia, nausea, vomiting, or cranial autonomic symptoms (Bordini et al., 1991; Newman, Lipton, & Solomon, 1994; Peres et al., 2001), although we have seen otherwise typical indomethacin-sensitive cases with these features.

Most patients experience exacerbations of severe pain superimposed on the continuous baseline pain. These exacerbations can last from 20 minutes to several days. They occur at night and can result in a mistaken diagnosis of cluster headache or hypnic headache. The exacerbations may occur in association with cranial autonomic symptoms and migrainous features. Cranial autonomic symptoms are often present but are not as prominent as in cluster headache. Migrainous features, notably photophobia, phonophobia, and nausea, are very common during exacerbations. Patients have been described in whom a typical migrainous visual aura occurred in association with the exacerbation (Peres, Siow, & Rozen, 2002). There are few precipitating factors: Neck movements do not trigger exacerbations, although occipital tenderness is present in 68% of patients (ipsilateral 44%, bilateral 24%) (Newman et al., 1994; Peres et al., 2001). Primary stabbing headaches occur in many patients with HC and are predominantly reported during the exacerbations (Peres et al., 2001).

Although the hallmark of the condition is continuous pain, this pattern may not be clear at the beginning and some patients have periods of remission rather like cluster headache (Newman, Lipton, & Solomon, 1994). HC is chronic from onset in 53%, chronic evolved from episodic in 35%, and episodic from onset in 12% (Peres et al., 2001).

Differential Diagnosis

The status of secondary HC is unclear, with the few reports suggesting the indomethacin response is not sustained, which would prompt reinvestigation in a clinically appropriate manner. The differential diagnoses of long-lasting unilateral headache include HC (primary and secondary forms); unilateral chronic migraine or NDPH; cervicogenic headache; and the other TACs occurring in association with a constant, unilateral, interictal dull ache, particularly *paroxysmal hemicrania.* HC can be readily differentiated from chronic migraine and NDPH by the indomethacin responsiveness (Goadsby & Boes, 2002b). In addition, it is worth noting that if patients with HC overuse analgesics, they can develop a bilateral headache typical of rebound headaches. All three patients reported responded to treatment with indomethacin (Young & Silberstein, 1993). This differential diagnosis between HC and chronic paroxysmal hemicrania (CPH) is difficult when the latter involves interictal pain. There are some useful clinical pointers. First, interictal pain in CPH is usually described as mild only, whereas background pain in HC is often moderate, although it can be mild. Second, exacerbations in CPH are short lasting, typically a few minutes to an hour, whereas those in HC are longer, usually several hours. Third, the severity of pain during exacerbations is excruciating in CPH, whereas in HC it is often moderate or severe. Ultimately a biologic marker will be required to understand the difference, because in clinical practice, given that the treatment for both is indomethacin, uncertainty can be tolerated.

Investigations

The diagnosis of HC is made on the basis of clinical history, neurologic examination, and a therapeutic trial of indomethacin. An MRI scan of the brain is a reasonable screening investigation to exclude secondary causes. All patients with unilateral CDH in whom secondary causes have been excluded should have a trial of indomethacin. We suggest 25 mg three times daily for 3 days, then 50 mg three times daily for 3 days, and then 75 mg three times daily for 2 weeks. It is useful for the patient to keep a diary to aid review. The response to indomethacin treatment is usually rapid, with complete resolution of the headache occurring within 1 to 2 days of initiating the effective dosage. Injectable indomethacin 50 to 100 mg intramuscularly ("indotest") has been proposed as a diagnostic test for HC (Antonaci et al., 1998). Complete pain relief was reported to occur within 2 hours. The indotest has the advantage that the diagnosis can be rapidly established and when performed at the higher dosage (100 mg) is likely to avoid the problem of an inadequate oral indomethacin trial. One of us is currently exploring a placebo-controlled indomethacin test, and certainly there is a placebo response.

Treatment

The treatment of HC is prophylactic. As with paroxysmal hemicrania, HC has a prompt and enduring response to indomethacin. The reported effective dosage of indomethacin ranges from 25 to 300 mg daily (Newman et al., 1994; Peres et al., 2001). Skipping or delaying doses may result in the headache recurring. Concurrent treatment with gastric-mucosa–protective agents should be considered for patients who require long-term treatment. No other drug is consistently effective in HC. Other nonsteroidal anti-inflammatory drugs are generally of little or no benefit. Other drugs reported to be partially or completely effective, usually in isolated cases, include ibuprofen (Kumar & Bordiuk, 1991; Newman et al., 1994), piroxicam beta-cyclodextrin (Sjaastad & Antonaci, 1995), naproxen (Bordini et al., 1991), aspirin (Espada et al., 1999), the cyclooxygenase (COX-2) inhibitor rofecoxib (Peres & Zukerman, 2000), and paracetamol with caffeine (Bordini et al., 1991); corticosteroids may be transiently effective.

Six patients have been described who had the clinical phenotype of HC but did not respond to indomethacin (Kuritzky, 1992; Pascual, 1995). This raises the question whether there is a subset of patients with the underlying biology *and* clinical phenotype of HC who do not respond to indomethacin. If indomethacin's mode of action involves interrupting the central pathogenetic mechanism of HC, it is likely that all patients will respond to indomethacin and the indomethacin-resistant cases do not represent true HC. However, until the underlying pathophysiology of HC and the mode of action of indomethacin are better understood, this issue will remain unresolved. Diagnostic criteria have been proposed that accommodate both indomethacin-responsive and indomethacin-resistant patients who fit the clinical phenotype (Goadsby & Lipton, 1997); these criteria seem useful in clinical practice (Bigal et al., 2002c). For the moment it appears simplest to restrict the diagnosis to the indomethacin-sensitive cases as the IHS has done (Headache Classification Subcommittee of the International Headache Society, 2004) until the biologic basis for this clinically very remarkable effect is clear (Figure 11.2 and 11.3).

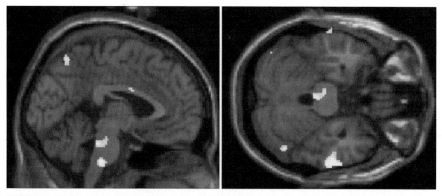

FIGURE 11.2   Statistical parametric map (SPM{t}) showing increased regional cerebral blood flow (rCBF) in the dorsal rostral pons during hemicrania continua headache compared with the pain-free state.

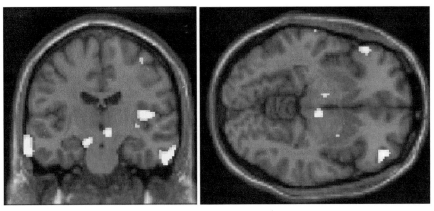

FIGURE 11.3　Statistical parametric map (SPM{t}) showing increased regional cerebral blood flow (rCBF) in the posterior hypothalamus during hemicrania continua headache compared with the pain-free state.

NEW DAILY PERSISTENT HEADACHE

In 1986 Vanast described the sudden onset of headache without apparent reason that continued as a CDH. The history can be remarkable, because patients can recall exactly what they were doing and when at the time of onset. This condition must be distinguished from those caused by some structural derangement, listed earlier as secondary causes of CDH. Patients with primary NDPH have headache either with a migrainous phenotype or completely featureless headache (Goadsby & Boes, 2002b). In our experience, the latter is extremely refractory to treatment. Some patients with NDPH attribute the onset of headache to a viral infection and could be thus classified as postviral. Others, previously headache free, describe the headache as developing at a certain time on a certain day and never relinquishing its grip thereafter. If these are postviral, the infection is not clinically apparent. Diaz-Mitoma, Vanast, and Tyrrell (1987) investigated 32 patients with this syndrome and compared the result of virus studies with those of 32 control subjects. Of the patients, 25 complained of severe fatigue, 12 had a history of infectious mononucleosis, and 20 were found to be excreting Epstein-Barr (E-B) virus in the oropharynx compared with 4 of the controls. When an early antigen titer of greater than 1:32 was taken as evidence of active E-B infection, 27 of the patients but only 8 of the controls tested positive. Although perhaps patients with NDPH are more susceptible to infection by the E-B virus, it seems more likely that E-B virus, a human herpes virus, caused the headache.

Santoni and Santoni-Williams (1993) investigated headaches that had persisted daily for about 2 weeks in 108 patients and found evidence of systemic infection, chiefly involving an adenovirus, salmonella, or urinary *Escherichia coli,* but some with E-B virus, toxoplasmosis, and herpes zoster. Li and Rozen (2002) reported that 30% of 56 patients with NDPH started with an infection or flulike illness, 12% started after surgery, and 12% started after a stressful life event. Whether lingering infection can be responsible for daily headaches lasting for months or years remains to be determined.

In Li and Rozen's series, 40 were men and 16 were women, ranging in age from 12 to 78 years. Eighty-two percent could pinpoint the exact day their headache started. The history of antecedent headache was no greater than to be expected in the general population. The headaches were bilateral in 64%, associated with nausea in 68%, and associated with photophobia in 66%.

Pain continued throughout the day in 79%. MRI and computed tomography (CT) scanning in 49 patients showed no significant abnormality. Headache had persisted from 6 months to 10 years, lasting throughout each day for 79%.

References

Abu-Arafeh, I. (2001). Chronic tension-type headache in children and adolescents. *Cephalalgia, 21,* 830–836.

Antonaci, F., Pareja, J. A., Caminero, A. B., & Sjaastad, O. (1998). Chronic paroxysmal hemicrania and hemicrania continua. Parenteral indomethacin: The "Indotest." *Headache, 38,* 122–128.

Bahra, A., Walsh, M., Menon, S., & Goadsby, P. J. (2003). Does chronic daily headache arise *de novo* in association with regular analgesic use? *Headache, 43,* 179–190.

Bendtsen, L., & Jensen, R. (2004). Mirtazapine is effective in the prophylactic treatment of chronic tension-type headache. *Neurology, 62,* 1706–1711.

Bigal, M. E., Rapoport, A. M., Sheftell, F. D., & Tepper, S. J. (2002a). Long-term follow-up of patients treated for chronic daily headache with analgesic overuse. *Cephalalgia, 22,* 327–328.

Bigal, M. E., Sheftell, F. D., Rapoport, A. M., Lipton, R. B., & Tepper, S. J. (2002b). Chronic daily headache in a tertiary care population: Correlation between the International Headache, Society diagnostic criteria and proposed revisions of criteria for chronic daily headache. *Cephalalgia, 22,* 432–438.

Bigal, M. E., Tepper, S. J., Rapoport, A. M., & Sheftell, F. D. (2002c). Hemicrania continua: Comparison between two different classification systems. *Cephalalgia, 22,* 242–245.

Bordini, C., Antonaci, F., Stovner, L. J., Schrader, H., & Sjaastad, O. (1991). "Hemicrania continua": A clinical review. *Headache, 31,* 20–26.

Burstein, R., Cutrer, M. F., & Yarnitsky, D. (2000). The development of cutaneous allodynia during a migraine attack. *Brain, 123,* 1703–1709.

Chakravarty, A. (2003). Chronic daily headaches: Clinical profile in Indian patients. *Cephalalgia, 23,* 348–353.

Diaz-Mitoma, F., Vanast, W. J., & Tyrrell, D. L. (1987). Increased frequency of Epstein-Barr virus excretion in patients with new daily persistent headaches. *Lancet, 1,* 411–415.

Drummond, P. D., & Lance, J. W. (1984). Clinical diagnosis and computer analysis of headache symptoms. *J Neurol Neurosurg Psychiatry, 47,* 128–133.

Espada, F., Escalza, I., Morales-Asin, F., Nasas, I., Inignez, C., & Mauri, J. A. (1999). Hemicrania continua: Nine new cases. *Cephalalgia, 19,* 442.

Evers, S., Rahmann, A., Vollmer-Haase, J., & Husstedt, I.-W. (2002). Treatment of headache with botulinum toxin A—a review according to evidence-based medicine criteria. *Cephalalgia, 22,* 699–710.

Freitag, F. G., Diamond, S., Diamond, M. L., & Urban, G. J. (2001). Divalproex in the long-term treatment of chronic daily headache. *Headache, 41,* 271–278.

Gallai, V., Alberti, A., Gallai, B., Coppola, F., Floridi, A., & Sarchielli, P. (2003). Glutamate and nitric oxide pathway in chronic daily headache: Evidence from cerebrospinal fluid. *Cephalalgia, 23,* 166–174.

Gladstone, J., Eross, E., & Dodick, D. (2003). Chronic daily headache: A rationale approach to a challenging problem. *Semin Neurol, 23,* 265–274.

Goadsby, P. J., & Boes, C. (2002a). Chronic daily headache. *J Neurol Neurosurg Psychiatry, 72,* ii2–ii5.

Goadsby, P. J., & Boes, C. J. (2002b). New daily persistent headache. *J Neurol Neurosurg Psychiatry, 72,* ii6–ii9.

Goadsby, P. J., & Lipton, R. B. (1997). A review of paroxysmal hemicranias, SUNCT syndrome and other short-lasting headaches with autonomic features, including new cases. *Brain, 120,* 193–209.

Gowers, W. R. (1888). *A manual of diseases of the nervous system.* Philadelphia: P. Blakiston.

Headache, Classification Subcommittee of the International Headache Society. (2004). The International Classification of Headache, Disorders (second edition). *Cephalalgia, 24,* 1–160.

Hering, R., Gardiner, I., Catarci, T., Whitmarsh, T., Steiner, T., & de Belleroche, J. (1993). Cellular adaptation in migraineurs with chronic daily headache. *Cephalalgia, 13,* 261–266.

Holroyd, K. A., O'Donnell, F. J., Lipchik, G. L., Cordingley, G. E., & Carlson, B. W. (2000). Management of chronic tension-type headache with (tricyclic) antidepressant medication, stress-management therapy and their combination: A randomized controlled trial. *JAMA, 285,* 2208–2215.

Iordanidis, T., & Sjaastad, O. (1989). Hemicrania continua: A case report. *Cephalalgia, 9,* 301–303.

Katsarava, Z., Limmroth, V., Finke, M., Diener, H.-C., & Fritsche, G. (2003). Rates and predictors for relapse in medication overuse headache: A 1-year prospective study. *Neurology, 60,* 1682–1683.

Koenig, M. A., Gladstein, J., McCarter, R. J., Hershey, A. D., Wasiewski, W., & Pediatric Committee of the American Headache Society. (2002). Chronic daily headache in children and adolescents presenting to tertiary headache clinics. *Headache, 42,* 491–500.

Krymchantowski, A. V. (2003). Primary headache diagnosis among chronic daily headache patients. *Arq Neuropsiquiatr, 61,* 364–367.

Krymchantowski, A. V., & Barbosa, J. S. (2000). Prednisone as initial treatment of analgesic-induced daily headache. *Cephalalgia, 20,* 107–113.

Krymchantowski, A. V., Silva, M. T., Barbosa, J. S., & Alves, L. A. (2002). Amitriptyline versus amitriptyline combined with fluoxetine in the preventive treatment of transformed migraine: A double-blind study. *Headache, 42,* 510–514.

Kumar, K. L., & Bordiuk, J. D. (1991). Hemicrania continua: A therapeutic dilemma. *Headache, 31,* 345.

Kuritzky, A. (1992). Indomethacin-resistant hemicrania continua. *Cephalalgia, 12,* 57–59.

Lance, J. W., & Curran, D. A. (1964). Treatment of chronic tension headache. *Lancet, i,* 1236–1239.

Li, D., & Rozen, T. D. (2002). The clinical characteristics of new daily persistent headache. *Cephalalgia, 22,* 66–69.

Limmroth, V., Katsarava, Z., Fritsche, G., Przywara, S., & Diener, H.-C. (2002). Features of medication overuse headache following overuse of different acute headache drugs. *Neurology, 59,* 1011–1014.

Martin-Aragus, A., Bustamente-Martinez, C., & Pedro-Pijoan, J. M. (2003). Treatment of chronic tension type headache with mirtazapine and amitriptyline. *Rev Neurol, 37,* 101–105.

Matharu, M. S., Bartsch, T., Ward, N., Frackowiak, R. S. J., Weiner, R. L., & Goadsby, P. J. (2004). Central neuromodulation in chronic migraine patients with suboccipital stimulators: A PET study. *Brain, 127,* 220–230.

Mathew, N. T. (1987). Transformed or evolutional migraine. *Headache, 27,* 305–306.

Mathew, N. T., Stubits, E., & Nigam, M. (1982). Transformation of migraine into daily headache: Analysis of factors. *Headache, 22,* 66–68.

Medina, J. L., & Diamond, S. (1981). Cluster headache variant: Spectrum of a new headache syndrome. *Arch Neurol, 38,* 705–709.

Newman, L. C., Lipton, R. B., Russell, M., & Solomon, S. (1992). Hemicrania continua: Attacks may alternate sides. *Headache, 32,* 237–238.

Newman, L. C., Lipton, R. B., & Solomon, S. (1994). Hemicrania continua: Ten new cases and a review of the literature. *Neurology, 44,* 2111–2114.

Ondo, W. G., Vuong, K. D., & Derman, H. S. (2004). Botulinum toxin A for chronic daily headache: A randomized, placebo-controlled, parallel design study. *Cephalalgia, 24,* 60–65.

Pascual, J. (1995). Hemicrania continua. *Neurology, 45,* 2302–2303.

Pasquier, F., Leys, D., & Petit, H. (1987). Hemicrania continua: The first bilateral case. *Cephalalgia, 7,* 169–170.

Peres, M. F. P., Silberstein, S. D., Nahmias, S., Sechter, A. L., Youssef, I., Rozen, T. D., et al. (2001). Hemicrania continua is not that rare. *Neurology, 57,* 948–951.

Peres, M. F. P., Siow, H. C., & Rozen, T. D. (2002). Hemicrania continua with aura. *Cephalalgia, 22,* 246–248.

Peres, M. F. P., & Zukerman, E. (2000). Hemicrania continua responsive to rofecoxib. *Cephalalgia, 20,* 130–131.

Pini, L. A., Cicero, A. F., & Sandrini, M. (2001). Long-term follow-up of patients treated for chronic headache with analgesic overuse. *Cephalalgia, 21,* 878–883.

Redillas, C., & Solomon, S. (2000). Prophylactic treatment of chronic daily headache. *Headache, 40,* 83–102.

Santoni, J. R., & Santoni-Williams, C. J. (1993). Headache, and painful lymphadenopathy in extracranial or systemic infection: etiology of new daily persistent headache. *Internal Med, 32,* 530–533.

Saper, J. R., Lake III, A. E., Cantrell, D. T., Winner, P. K., & White, J. R. (2002). Chronic daily headache prophylaxis with tizanidine: A double-blind, placebo-controlled multicenter outcome study. *Headache, 42,* 470–482.

Saper, J. R., & Winters, M. (1982). Chronic "mixed" headaches. Profile and analysis of 100 consecutive patients experiencing daily headaches. *Headache, 22,* 145–146.

Sarchielli, P., Alberti, A., Floridi, A., & Gallai, V. (2001). Levels of growth factor in cerebrospinal fluid of chronic daily headache patients. *Neurology, 57,* 132–134.

Scher, A. I., Lipton, R. B., & Stewart, W. F. (2003a). Habitual snoring as a risk factor for chronic daily headache. *Neurology, 60,* 1366–1368.

Scher, A. I., Stewart, W. F., Ricci, J. A., & Lipton, R. B. (2003b). Factors associated with the onset and remission of chronic daily headache in a population-based study. *Pain, 106,* 81–89.

Schulte-Mattler, W. J., Krack, P., & Bo, N. S. G. (2004). Treatment of chronic tension-type headache with botulinum toxin A: A randomized, double-blind, placebo-controlled multicenter study. *Pain, 109,* 110–114.

Shuaib, A. (2000). Efficacy of topiramate in prophylaxis of frequent severe migraines or chronic daily headaches: Experience with 68 patients over 18 months. *Cephalalgia, 20,* 423.

Silberstein, S., Mathew, N., Saper, J., Jenkins, S., & TBMCRG. (2000). Botulinum toxin type A as a migraine preventive treatment. *Headache, 40,* 445–450.

Silberstein, S. D., & Lipton, R. B. Chronic daily headache. (2001). In S. D. Silberstein, R. B. Lipto, & D. J. Dalessio (Eds.), *Wolff's Headache, and other head pain* (pp. 247–282). New York: Oxford University Press.

Silberstein, S. D., Lipton, R. B., & Sliwinski, M. (1996). Classification of daily and near-daily headaches: A field study of revised IHS criteria. *Neurology, 47,* 871–875.

Sjaastad, O., & Antonaci, F. (1995). A piroxicam derivative partly effective in chronic paroxysmal hemicrania and hemicrania continua. *Headache, 35,* 549–550.

Sjaastad, O., & Spierings, E. L. (1984). Hemicrania continua: Another headache absolutely responsive to indomethacin. *Cephalalgia, 4,* 65–70.

Spira, P. J., & Beran, R. G. (2003). Gabapentin in the prophylaxis of chronic daily headache: A randomized, placebo-controlled study. *Neurology, 61,* 1753–1759.

Srikiatkhachorn, A. (2002). Chronic daily headache: A scientist's perspective. *Headache, 42,* 532–537.

Srikiatkhachorn, A., & Anthony, M. (1996). Platelet serotonin in patients with analgesic-induced headache. *Cephalalgia, 16,* 423–426.

Trucco, M., Antonaci, F., & Sandrini, G. (1992). Hemicrania continua: A case responsive to piroxicam-beta-cyclodextrin. *Headache, 32,* 39–40.

Vanast, W. J. (1986). New daily persistent headaches: Definition of a benign syndrome. *Headache, 26,* 317.

Welch, K. M., Nagesh, V., Aurora, S., & Gelman, N. (2001). Periaqueductal grey matter dysfunction in migraine: Cause or the burden of illness? *Headache, 41,* 629–637.

Welch, K. M. A., & Goadsby, P. J. (2002). Chronic daily headache: Nosology and pathophysiology. *Curr Opin Neurol, 15,* 287–295.

Wheeler, S. D., Allen, K. F., & Pusey, T. (2001). Is hemicrania continua a migraine variant? *Cephalalgia, 21,* 508.

Williams, D. R., & Stark, R. J. (2003). Intravenous lignocaine (lidocaine) infusion for the treatment of chronic daily headache with substantial medication overuse. *Cephalalgia, 23,* 963–971.

Yarnitsky, D., Goor-Aryeh, I., Bajwa, Z. H., Ransil, B. I., Cutrer, F. M., Sottile, A., & Burnstein, R. (2003). Possible parasympathetic contributions in peripheral and central sensitization during migraine. *Headache, 43,* 704–714.

Young, W. B., & Silberstein, S. D. (1993). Hemicrania continua and symptomatic mediation overuse. *Headache, 33,* 485–487.

Young, W. B., & Silberstein, S. D. (2001). Long-term follow-up of patients treated for chronic headache with analgesic overuse. *Cephalagia, 21,* 873.

Zwart, J.-A., Dyb, G., Hagen, K., Svebak, S., & Holmen, J. (2003). Analgesic use: A predictor of chronic pain and medication overuse headache. *Neurology, 61,* 160–164.

Chapter 12
Cluster Headache and Other Trigeminal Autonomic Cephalalgias

The trigeminal autonomic cephalalgias (TACs) are characterized by episodic pain in the head or face, almost always unilateral, accompanied by discharge of the parasympathetic nervous system causing redness and watering of the eye and blockage or running of the nostril, usually confined to the painful side (Goadsby and Lipton, 1997).

The Headache Subcommittee of the International Headache Society classifies TACs as follows (Headache Classification Committee of the International Headache Society, 2004):

1. Cluster headache, episodic and chronic
2. Paroxysmal hemicrania, episodic and chronic
3. Short-lasting unilateral neuralgiform headache attacks with conjunctival injection and tearing (SUNCT)

CLUSTER HEADACHE

Definition

Episodic cluster headache can be defined as a severe unilateral head or facial pain that typically lasts from 15 minutes to 3 hours, associated commonly with ipsilateral conjunctival injection, lacrimation, and blockage of the nostril, usually recurring once or more daily for a period of weeks or months. The term *cluster headache* derives from the tendency for the pain to appear in bouts, separated by intervals of complete freedom (Kunkle et al., 1952). Researchers now recognize a chronic form, without remission, and other variations. An ocular Horner's syndrome on the symptomatic side is a common accompaniment.

195

The nature of the attack and pattern of recurrence are so characteristic that clinicians can readily distinguish cluster headache from migraine and trigeminal neuralgia. Nevertheless, they refer many patients to neurologists with the provisional diagnosis of one or another of these disorders (Bahra & Goadsby, 2004), and the British literature has referred to the condition as "migrainous neuralgia." A Dutch survey found that one third of patients had consulted a dentist and one third an ear, nose, and throat specialist before receiving the diagnosis (van Vliet et al., 2003).

Nomenclature

Dr. Hansruedi Isler of Zurich described the first convincing description of cluster headache by Van Swieten, physician to Empress Marie Theresa in Vienna, in 1745 (Isler, 1993):

> A healthy robust man of middle age [was suffering from] troublesome pain which came on every day at the same hour at the same spot above the orbit of the left eye, where the nerve emerges from the opening of the frontal bone; after a short time the left eye began to redden, and to overflow with tears; then he felt as if his eye was slowly forced out of its orbit with so much pain, that he nearly went mad. After a few hours all these evils ceased, and nothing in the eye appeared at all changed.

In 1840 Romberg described as "ciliary neuralgia" recurrent pain in the eye that was generally confined to one side and associated with photophobia (Romberg, 1840). "The pupil is contracted. The pain not infrequently extends over the head and face. The eye generally weeps and becomes red. These symptoms occur in paroxysms of a uniform or irregular character, and isolated or combined with facial neuralgia and hemicrania." Romberg considered ciliary neuralgia to be mainly caused by scrofula but thought it was also brought on by discharges, especially seminal emissions. In the English medical literature Harris first recorded this condition in 1925 as ciliary (migrainous) neuralgia, and others later elaborated on this description (Harris, 1936; Horton, MacLean, & Craig, 1939).

The uncertainty about the nature and etiology of this disorder is reflected by other names that have been used to describe similar syndromes over the past century, such as "red migraine," "erythroprosopalgia," "erythromelalgia of the head," "syndrome of hemicephalic vasodilation of sympathetic origin," "autonomic faciocephalalgia," "greater superficial petrosal neuralgia," and "histamine cephalalgia." Symonds (1956) used the noncommittal title of "a particular variety of headache." Sphenopalatine neurosis (Sluder, 1910) and Vidian neuralgia (Vail, 1932) were described as affecting mostly female patients and appear more akin to lower-half headache, now known as facial migraine, than to the syndrome under discussion. The extent to which the more peculiar syndromes were recognized that we would now call paroxysmal hemicrania or even SUNCT (see later) is not and may never be clear.

Prevalence

Cluster headache is considerably less common than migraine, but the ratio of one to the other varies from 1:6 to 1:50 in reports from different sources, depending on the interest and orientation of each clinic. The population-based survey from the Vaga study of Sjaastad and colleagues (2003) reported a population 1-year prevalence of cluster headache of 0.3%. On screening 6400 patient records in Olmsted County, Minnesota, Swanson et al. (1994) found the incidence of cluster headache was approximately 9.8 per 100,000 per year or $\frac{1}{25}$ that of migraine. Kudrow (1980) estimated that the prevalence of cluster headache in the United States was 0.4% for men and 0.08% for women. Ekbom, Ahlborg, and Schele (1978) diagnosed cluster headache in 0.09% of 18-year-olds called up for military service. D'Alessandro et al. (1986) studied the population of the Republic of San Marino (21,792 people) by reviewing medical records for the preceding 15 years and writing to every inhabitant. They found 15 cases (14 men, 1 woman), giving a prevalence of 69 cases per 100,000 population, that is, 0.07%. A recent update by personal interview reported a prevalence of 56 per 100,000 (Tonon et al., 2002).

Varieties of Cluster Headache

The International Headache Society recognizes at least two basic forms of cluster headache, an episodic form and a chronic form. The nomenclature is at best arbitrary, because any disorder that comes and goes with significant disability during bouts for half one's lifetime could be called chronic, at least in principle. The distinction in cluster headache, imperfect as it is, draws attention to two groups of patients, one in whom (the episodic form) acute attack therapy dominates, and the other whose disease burden is more persistent and who almost invariably require long-term prevention. Better terminology is probably required.

Episodic Cluster Headache

The current definition of episodic form suggests it recurs in periods lasting 7 days to 1 year, separated by pain-free periods lasting 1 month or more. Commonly, bouts last between 2 weeks and 3 months, with remissions from 3 months to 3 years.

Chronic Cluster Headache

Some patients experience recurrent cluster pains for more than 1 year with brief (shorter than 1 month) or no remissions. In some patients the pain may be unremitting from the onset (primary chronic cluster), whereas in others it may develop from episodic cluster headache (secondary chronic cluster). In a series of 494 patients, Ekbom et al. (2002) reported 10.8% had the chronic form.

Cluster-Tic Syndrome

Sudden jabs of pain resembling trigeminal neuralgia may be experienced by patients suffering from cluster headache or paroxysmal hemicrania (PH). Lance and Anthony (1971) commented on ticlike pains in three of their cluster headache patients and described an additional case where the typical lancinating pains of trigeminal neuralgia culminated in an attack of cluster headache. The stabbing pains in this case were felt in the right upper and lower jaw, and after 3 months they radiated to the right temple. Pain then started in the right temple and persisted for 30 minutes, associated with watering of the right eye and nostril. These cluster like episodes then recurred three times daily for some weeks. After 1 month, the pain spread from temple to vertex, appeared two or three times daily, and persisted for 30 to 90 minutes on each occasion. These headaches then ceased, but the jabbing pains persisted. The cluster-type headaches recurred for 5 days every 2 months for 3 years. When the ticlike pain was controlled by carbamazepine, the cluster headaches ceased.

In general the cluster headache component spans the range of typical cluster headache, attacks lasting 45 minutes with autonomic features such as lacrimation and nasal blocking, to shorter attacks of 30 seconds at a frequency of 40 a day, more suggestive of a paroxysmal hemicrania (Alberca & Ochoa, 1994). Many other reports in the literature find a similar association of cluster and tic-like pains (Diamond, Freitag, & Cohen, 1984; Solomon, Apfelbaum, & Guglielmo, 1985; Watson & Evans, 1985; Klimek, 1987; Pascual and Berciano, 1993; Mulleners and Verhagen, 1996; Monzillo et al., 2000). We agree with these authors that the relationship is more than coincidental.

Clinical Features

Sex Distribution

Cluster headache is predominantly a male disease. Of 425 patients Kudrow (1980) reported, the male-to-female ratio was 5:1, and in a series of 400 patients Kunkel (1981) described the ratio as 9:1. Most series report that about 85% of patients are male, but the recognized prevalence appears to be increasing in women, with Bahra, May, and Goadsby (2002) reporting a male-to-female ratio of 2.5:1.

Age of Onset

The illness usually starts in the second to fourth decades of life, but Kudrow (1980) described one child who developed typical symptoms at the age of 3 years, and other cases have been reported to start before the age of 12 years (Ekbom, 1970; Lance & Anthony, 1971). Kudrow (1980) and Manzoni et al. (1983) found the peak age of onset to fall between ages 20 and 29 years, but the first bout may be delayed until age 75 or 83 (Evers et al., 2002). Ekbom et al. (2002) reported that the male-to-female sex ratio was highest when the age of onset was 30 to 49 years (7.2:1) and lowest after age 50 (2.3:1).

Site of Pain

The pain of cluster headache is almost always unilateral, with perhaps 1 in 100 patients having convincing bilateral pain. It almost always affects the same side of the head in each bout, but we have seen swapping sides within and between bouts. In 32 of the 60 patients on whom Lance and Anthony (1971) reported, the attacks were exclusively right sided, in 23 left sided, and in 5 the side affected varied from bout to bout or on different days in the same bout. The pain is felt deeply in and around the eye by 60% to 90% of patients. It commonly radiates to the supraorbital region, temple, maxilla, and upper gum on the same side of the face and may occasionally be limited to those areas, not involving the upper face (Ekbom, 1975). In some patients the ipsilateral nostril aches and burns, and a few complain of aching in the roof of the mouth. In other patients, the lower gum, jaw, or chin are also involved. The pain may spread to the ear, the neck, or "the entire half of the head." Presentation with pain in the gums or jaw may be interpreted as toothache (Brooke, 1978) and in one series led to 48% of patients having an unnecessary dental procedure (Bahra & Goadsby, 2004).

Quality of Pain

The pain of cluster headache is peculiarly distressing, and we have had many patients who have had other pain experiences, such as renal colic or childbirth, report that the pain of an attack of cluster headache is much worse. It may be throbbing or pulsating on occasions, but the majority describe the pain as constant and severe. Common adjectives used to describe it are burning, boring, piercing, tearing, and screwing. A dull background pain persists in the eye, temple, or upper jaw between attacks or precedes a bout by some hours or days in some cases. Some patients experience sudden jabs of pain in the affected areas at the time of headache, most often primary stabbing headache and less often cluster-tic.

Periodicity of Bouts

About 10% of patients with the characteristic pain and accompaniments have a pattern of recurrence resembling that of migraine without any long periods of freedom (chronic cluster headache). Most patients suffer one or two bouts each year. The periodicity of bouts in our series did not depend consistently on the time of year (Lance & Anthony, 1971). Of patients who reported their bouts occurred seasonally, five said they recurred in spring, six in summer, six in autumn, and seven in winter.

Duration of Bouts

The usual length of each bout is 4 to 8 weeks, but patients vary considerably.

Daily Frequency of Attacks During a Bout

The usual number of daily attacks varies from one to three. Most patients said their attacks were liable to recur at a particular time of the day or night. Manzoni et al. (1983b) found peaks at 1 AM, 2 PM, and 9 PM.

Duration of Attacks

Each particular episode usually starts suddenly, lasts for 10 minutes to 2 hours, and may end abruptly or fade away more slowly. Occasional episodes may be sustained for 8 hours or more.

Associated Features

Associated features are outlined in Table 12.1. Lacrimation and reddening of the eye on the affected side is common and is occasionally bilateral (Bahra et al., 2002). About one third of patients report drooping of the ipsilateral eyelid and miosis, which clinicians have observed in two thirds of patients examined during attacks (Ekbom, 1970; Kudrow, 1980). Ptosis and miosis may be apparent between attacks (see Figure 5.1), and clinicians can demonstrate them on the symptomatic side by pupillography in all patients between attacks (Drummond, 1988). Flushing of the periorbital area is not often observed clinically, but an increase in skin temperature around the orbit, cheek, and nose of about 0.25°C to 1.5°C can be measured by thermography during attacks (Drummond & Lance, 1984) (Figure 12.1). The nostril is often blocked or running on one or both sides. A running nostril cannot be explained by lacrimation, because it is not always associated with a weeping eye. Autonomic symptoms sometimes start before pain, and Salvesen (2000) has described a bout of autonomic symptoms in cluster pattern without headache.

Photophobia and phonophobia certainly occur in cluster headache but are much less common than in migraine (Bahra et al., 2002). Curiously, both may be ipsilateral to the pain, and we find this generally useful when distinguishing trigeminal autonomic cephalalgias from migraine, because in migraine the photophobia and phonophobia are bilateral.

Gastrointestinal disturbances are less common than in migraine, but about half of the patients feel nauseated and may vomit. Nausea may precede the onset of facial pain. Photophobia may be intense, and patients may complain of phonophobia.

Hyperalgesia of the face and scalp is common and can be so extreme in some cases that the patient cannot bear to touch the affected areas. Two of our patients had noticed an itching sensation behind the eye, one immediately preceding pain in the eye and the other for some weeks before a bout began. Others complained of a dull, intermittent ache or jabs of pain behind the eye between severe paroxysms.

Focal neurologic symptoms or signs, of the type common in migraine, are less usual in cluster headache. One of our patients mentioned occasional "spots before the eyes," and another described "little flashing lights in front of the eyes" during the headache. Four described a feeling of dizziness, giddiness, or a "rising feeling in the head" associated with impaired balance at the time of the attack. One patient had experienced a tonic seizure of the left arm on three occasions associated with a pain in the right eye and temple. The left hand assumed the position of carpal spasm for a period of minutes (Lance & Anthony, 1971). Sutherland and Eadie (1972) reported a patient with scintillating scotomas before cluster headache, two patients with paraesthesias on the side of the body opposite to the head pain, and one patient with twitching of the contralateral foot. Recent large series have confirmed that typical aura can be seen in acute

TABLE 12.1 Associated features of cluster headache in 60 patients

Ocular		Vascular	
Lacrimation			
Unilateral	49	Flushing of face	12
		Pallor of face	2
Bilateral	3	Prominent, tender temporal artery	10
Conjunctival injection	27	Prominent veins in forehead	2
Partial Horner's syndrome	19	Puffiness around eyes	6
Photophobia	12	Lumps in mouth	2
Blurred vision	5	Cold hands and feet	1
Polyuria	4	**Neurologic**	
Nasal		Hyperalgesia of scalp and face	10
Blocked nostril			
Unilateral	28	Itching behind eye (preceding headache)	2
		Flashing lights in front of eyes	1
Bilateral	4	Spots in front of eyes	1
Running nostril			
Unilateral	9	Vertigo and mild ataxia	4
		Mental confusion	1
Bilateral	1	Unilateral carpal spasm	1
Epistaxis	1		
Gastrointestinal			
Anorexia	2		
Nausea	26		
Vomiting			
Occasionally	9		
Regularly	9		
Diarrhea	2		

From Lance and Anthony, 1971.

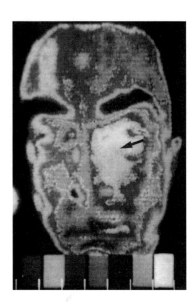

FIGURE 12.1 Thermogram demonstrating the areas of increased temperature in a patient during the pain of cluster headache. Compare with Figure 18.1, showing a similar effect after radiofrequency lesions of the trigeminal ganglion.

cluster headache, usually with, rather than before, the pain (Siberstein et al., 2000; Bahra et al., 2002).

Precipitating Factors

The trigger factor most consistently mentioned by patients is the taking of alcoholic drinks, and this is only operative during a susceptible period, that is, during a bout. Vasodilators, such as nitrates, also precipitate an attack at this time. We have found that solvents, varnish, or perfumes, as well as a warm evironment (the latter sometimes in the context of menopausal flushing), often trigger attacks.

Relieving Factors

Some patients can find ease from pain by pressing on the superficial temporal arteries, by applying heat or cold to the eye, or by pacing up and down with a hand clasped over one eye. We have not heard of a nontherapeutic factor that consistently provides relief.

Past History and Associated Disorders

Nothing very remarkable distinguishes the past health of patients with cluster headache other than an association with peptic ulcer and coronary disease, although this may be predictable given the high prevalence of smoking. No convincing association with migraine or allergic disorders appears.

Trauma

Of our original 60 patients, 8 had experienced a head injury, and in 4 the site of injury could conceivably be relevant to the ensuing cluster headache. One patient had required extensive plastic surgery for facial and scalp lacerations following a car accident, and left-sided cluster headache started 21 months after the injury. The second had gravel embedded in the right temple from a road accident at the age of 17 years, and cluster headaches involving the right temple and right side of the face began 7 years later. The third patient developed right frontotemporal cluster headache 30 years after a shotgun injury to the forehead, in which fragmented pellets were still embedded. The fourth patient experienced a blow to the forehead at the age of 22 years, following which he was subject to a dull right-sided headache for 3 years. Eight years after the injury, right-sided cluster headaches developed, involving the right forehead and right side of the face.

We have subsequently seen patients with head injury that very often involves the ophthalmic division of the trigeminal nerve and particularly the supraorbital nerve before the onset of cluster headache. Reik (1987) described four patients who developed cluster headache after head injury, two immediately and two delayed. Turkewitz et al. (1992) surveyed the literature and found reports of 78 patients, including those just mentioned. Kudrow (1980) found a history of significant head injury in 5.2% of his 495 patients. Clear reports describe the development of cluster headache after eye removal, a further form of trauma in this setting (Evers et al., 1997) or after dental extraction (Soros et al., 2001).

Genetic Background

Kudrow (1980) reported that about 3% of cluster headache patients have one relative affected by the disorder, whereas Russell, Andersson, and Iselius (1996) found a positive family history in 7%; Leone et al. (2001) found 20% positive.

Segregation analysis suggested that cluster headache is transmitted by an autosomal dominant gene with a penetration of 0.3 to 0.34 in males and 0.17 to 0.21 in females (Russell et al., 1995). There have been occasional reports of cluster headache in twins (Sjaastad et al., 1993).

No evidence exists that the migraine gene *CACNA1A* is involved in cluster headache (Haan et al., 2001; Sjöstrand et al., 2001).

The prevalence of migraine in parents and siblings (22% in our series) was not significantly greater than that of patients with tension-type headache (18%) and was much less than that of typical migraine patients (45%) (Lance & Anthony, 1966). Ekbom (1970) found a family history of migraine in 16% of patients with cluster headache compared with 65% of migraine patients.

The Cluster Headache Personality

Graham (1972) claimed that cluster headache patients had certain characteristics that he described as "leonine facies." Such patients tend to have a ruddy complexion and multifurrowed thick skin. He considered that they drank and smoked heavily, were ambitious and hard working, and tended to be the prototype aggressive executive-type male. According to Graham this appearance conceals feelings of guilt, anger, inadequacy, and dependency, which show themselves in brief outbursts of hysterical behavior during an attack of cluster headache.

Kudrow and Sutkus (1979) submitted 41 patients with cluster headaches to Minnesota Multiphasic Personality Inventory (MMPI) testing in comparison with 217 patients suffering from other forms of headache. They could not find any difference between the characteristics of migraine and cluster headache patients, but both of these groups gave significantly different results from patients with tension or post-traumatic headaches. An independent study, using the Freiburg Personality Inventory (Cuypers, Altenkirch, & Bunge, 1981) came to much the same conclusion after comparing 40 patients with cluster headache and 49 patients with migraine. Patients with cluster headache had a slightly increased score of nervousness and a slightly diminished score for traits of "masculinity," which could simply reflect the impact of a painful relapsing disorder.

It may be concluded that cluster headache patients are not unduly neurotic, despite the strange behavior of some at the height of their headaches. The concept of a cluster-headache appearance or personality seems outdated and is without good evidence. We have not experienced it in our many hundreds of patients with the disorder, and it is best considered as a historical curiosity.

Symptomatic Clusterlike Headache

The pain and autonomic symptoms of cluster headache may be simulated by intracranial, structural lesions, particularly in the vicinity of the cavernous sinus or involving the pituitary gland. The wide range of lesions apparently producing clusterlike headache is described in Table 12.2.

Pathophysiology

There are three major aspects of the pathophysiology of cluster headache that need to be accounted for to explain the syndrome:

1. The source of the pain in acute cluster headache
2. Cranial autonomic features
3. Episodic pattern of the attacks, which is in many ways the defining clinical signature of the disorder compared to migraine (Lance & Goadsby, 1998)

These features raise the classic issues of the location of the lesion and the generic terminology that should be applied to these and related headaches, such as migraine.

The Source of Pain in Cluster Headache

Patients with cluster headache often state that they can relieve pain at one site, for example, in the temple, by direct pressure over the site, but that pain felt in or behind the eye persists or may become worse. Applying heat to the eye usually relieves orbital pain temporarily. Pain does not arise in the eye itself, because cluster headache may develop or persist after enucleation of the eye (see Table 12.2). Localization of pain to the eye characterizes other disorders involving the internal carotid artery, and the frequency of involvement of the ocular sympathetic supply to produce a partial Horner's syndrome suggests that sympathetic fibers may be compromised in the pericarotid vascular plexus by dilation, engorgement, or edema of the vessel wall (Kunkle & Anderson, 1961; Nieman & Hurwitz, 1961).

TABLE 12.2   Cranial and other lesions reported to be associated with clusterlike headache

Vascular Causes

Carotid artery dissection (Rosebraugh et al., 1997) or aneurysm (Greve & Mai, 1988)

Vertebral artery dissection (Cremer et al., 1995) or aneurysm (West & Todman, 1991)

Pseudoaneurysm of intracavernous carotid artery (Koenigsberg et al., 1994)

Anterior communicating artery aneurysm (Sjaastad et al., 1976; Greve & Mai, 1988)

Occipital lobe AVM (Mani & Deeter, 1982)

Middle cerebral artery territory AVM (Munoz et al., 1996)

AVM in soft tissue of scalp above ear (Thomas, 1975)

Frontal lobe and corpus callosum AVM (Gawel et al., 1989)

Cervical cord infarction (de la Sayette et al., 1999)

Lateral medullary infarction (Cid et al., 2000)

Frontotemporal subdural hematoma (Formisano et al., 1990)

Tumors

Prolactinoma (Greve & Mai, 1988)

Pituitary adenoma (Tfelt-Hansen et al., 1982)

Parasellar meningioma (Hannerz, 1989)

Sphenoidal meningioma (Lefevre et al., 1984; Molins et al., 1989)

Epidermoid tumor in the prepontine (behind the dorsum sella turcica) (Levyman et al., 1991)

Tentorial meningioma (Taub et al., 1995)

High cervical meningioma (Kuritzky, 1984)

Nasopharyngeal carcinoma (Appelbaum & Noronha, 1989)

Infective Causes

Maxillary sinusitis (Molins et al., 1989)

Orbitosphenoidal aspergillosis (Heidegger et al., 1997)

Herpes zoster ophthalmicus (Sacquegna et al., 1982)

Post-Traumatic or Surgery

Facial trauma (Lance & Goadsby, 1998)

Following enucleation of eye (Rogado & Graham, 1979; McKinney, 1983; Prusinski et al., 1985; Evers et al., 1997)

Dental Causes

Impacted wisdom tooth (Romoli & Cudia, 1988)

Following dental extraction (Soros et al., 2001)

AVM, Arteriovenous malformation.

Localizing the lesion in the sympathetic pathway is made easier by the sparing of sweating over the face (with the exception of the medial part of the forehead), which is mediated by fibers accompanying branches of the extracranial arteries. The site of entrapment must therefore lie distal to the bifurcation of the common carotid artery and is logically in the area around the internal carotid artery or within the orbit. Ekbom and Greitz (1970) reported the angiographic appearance of localized narrowing of the lumen of the internal carotid artery, just beyond its entry into the skull, at the height of an attack of cluster headache. They attributed this to edema or spasm of the vessel wall, and the effect persisted after pain had ceased. In contrast, the ophthalmic artery was dilated during the attack.

However, there is nothing at all unique to cluster headache in finding internal carotid artery dilation in association with head pain. Pooling of tracer in the region of the carotid artery has been noted in positron emission tomography studies of both cluster headache (May et al., 1998a) and in experimental head pain (May et al., 1998b). Indeed, it is clear that the first (ophthalmic) division of trigeminal pain preferentially dilates the internal carotid artery when compared with third division or nontrigeminal pain (May et al., 2001). It is thus clear that the dilation of the internal carotid in cluster headache may be an epiphenomenon, and indeed we have seen in a patient studied after ipsilateral trigeminal nerve section that dilation is not at all necessary for pain (Matharu & Goadsby, 2002).

The trigeminal nerve is intact in patients with cluster headache who have not had surgical procedures, and corneal responses to tactile stimulation are normal (Vijayan & Watson, 1985). Sandrini et al. (1991) found the corneal pain threshold reduced ipsilaterally during attacks in 10 out of 15 patients. Of 27 patients examined carefully during cluster headache, 10 had cutaneous hyperalgesia and 12 had deep hyperalgesia in the face, arm, or whole body on the side of the pain (Procacci et al., 1989). These phenomena are presumably secondary to activation of the thalamus by trigeminothalamic pathways (Zagami & Lambert, 1990; Zagami & Goadsby, 1991). Further evidence for trigeminovascular activation in cluster headache comes from the finding that cranial levels of calcitonin gene-related peptide (CGRP) are elevated during acute spontaneous (Goadsby & Edvinsson, 1994) or nitroglycerin-triggered (Fanciullacci et al., 1995) attacks.

Input from the upper cervical spine may also play a part in the pain of cluster headache, given the overlap of sensory processing in the trigeminocervical complex (Goadsby & Hoskin, 1997; Goadsby, Hoskin, & Knight, 1997; Bartsch & Goadsby, 2002, 2003). Some patients can precipitate attacks of cluster headache by moving the neck. Injecting a local anesthetic agent and long-acting corticosteroid into the ipsilateral greater occipital nerve can alter the pattern of recurrence of cluster headache (Anthony, 1987; Peres et al., 2002). A meningioma compressing the spinal cord at the level of the first and second cervical segments caused episodic pain with lacrimation and redness of the eye indistinguishable from cluster headache (Kuritzky, 1984). In eight patients a syndrome resembling cluster headache followed whiplash injury to the neck (Hunter & Mayfield, 1949). Interestingly, stimulating the greater occipital nerve in rats produced ipsilateral conjunctival injection, lacrimation, ptosis, or pupillary changes in one third of the animals (Vincent et al., 1992), and one of us has seen a large basilar aneurysm present with cranial autonomic symptoms (Giffin & Goadsby, 2001).

We can conclude that the spinal tract and nucleus of the trigeminal nerve, descending to the C2 segment, becomes hyperactive unilaterally during cluster headache and that the main perceived source of pain is the internal carotid artery and its proximal branches. Because afferents in upper cervical roots converge with trigeminal neurons in the second cervical segment of the spinal cord, they may also contribute to the level of excitation in central pain pathways.

Vascular Changes

Dahl et al. (1990) found that regional cerebral blood flow did not increase in cluster attacks provoked by glyceryl trinitrate, 1 mg sublingually, but the velocity of blood flow in the middle cerebral arteries decreased, more so on the symptomatic side. A similar reduction in flow marked spontaneous attacks, suggesting that during cluster headache the artery dilated. These findings are broadly consistent with our recent magnetic resonance angiography (MRA) experience but are not restricted to cluster headache (May et al., 2001).

Hörven and Sjaastad (1977) reported that corneal intraocular pressure and corneal temperatures all increased on the affected side during cluster headache, indicating intraocular vasodilation. Drummond and Lance (1984) made thermographic observations on 11 patients with spontaneous attacks and 22 patients during attacks induced by nitroglycerin or alcohol. At the height of a spontaneous attack, in 7 patients the affected orbital region was 0.25°C to 1.25°C warmer than the other side (Figure 12.2), but temperature remained symmetric in 4, whereas the ipsilateral cheek became 0.25°C to 1.5°C warmer in 10 of the 11 patients. Similar changes appeared in induced attacks, but pain felt behind the eye did not always correlate with increased heat loss from the area. Increase in cutaneous blood flow usually followed the onset of pain and was considered a secondary phenomenon, a vasodilator reflex mediated by the trigeminal nerve as the afferent limb and the greater superficial petrosal (GSP) nerve as the efferent limb (Goadsby & Lance, 1988). However, antidromic discharge in trigeminal nerve fibers could not be excluded (compare thermograms taken after radiofrequency lesions of the trigeminal ganglion, in Figure 18.1).

The frequency of conjunctival injection and nasal blockage in cluster headache provides supporting evidence for dilation of capillaries in the extracranial circulation. This may be associated with edema, causing swelling of the periorbital region or buccal mucosa, described as "little lumps in the mouth."

As in migraine, certain vasoactive peptides are released in cluster headache. Levels of calcitonin gene–related peptide (CGRP), a marker for trigeminal activation, and vasoactive intestinal polypeptide, a marker of cranial parasympathetic activation, are elevated in spontaneous (Goadsby & Edvinsson, 1994) and nitroglycerin-induced cluster attacks (Fanciullacci et al., 1995). Capillaries dilate in the ipsilateral conjunctiva, nasal mucosa, and cutaneous circulation, particularly in the periorbital area.

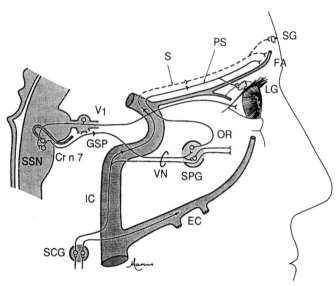

FIGURE 12.2   The mechanism of pathologic sweating during cluster headache. Sympathetic fibers (S) arising from the superior cervical ganglion (SCG) are compromised in the wall of the internal carotid artery (IC), causing their peripheral distribution to the frontal arteries (FA) and sweat glands (SG) to degenerate. Parasympathetic fibers, originating in the superior salivatory nucleus (SSN), traverse the facial nerve (Cr n 7) and the greater superficial petrosal nerve (GSP) to join the Vidian nerve (VN) and synapse in the sphenopalatine ganglion (SPG); post-ganglionic fibers then loop back as orbital rami (OR) to the cavernous sinus and internal carotid artery where they form a retro-orbital plexus with sympathetic and trigeminal fibers, before advancing to supply the lacrimal glands (LG) and cutaneous circulation of the fore-head. Conjunctival irritation stimulates afferent fibers in the first division of the trigeminal nerve (V_1), which reflexly activates parasympathetic outflow to the lacrimal glands and fore-head circulation. The dashed line represents the route taken by parasympathetic fibers that occupy the denervated sympathetic pathway and cause frontal sweating and flushing in response to the conjunctival stimulus. (From Drummond & Lance, 1992, by permission of the publishers, Oxford University Press, Oxford.)

Autonomic Changes

During cluster headache, heat loss increases from the eye and cheek on the affected side, the ipsilateral eye usually reddens or waters, and the nostril dis-charges fluid or blocks. These manifestations are usually associated, suggesting that they are produced by parasympathetic discharge through the GSP nerve (Drummond & Lance, 1984; Drummond, 1988).

Transient or permanent paralysis of the ocular sympathetic nerve supply, giv-ing rise to a partial Horner's syndrome on the symptomatic side, commonly accompanies cluster headache. Kunkle and Anderson (1961) found miosis and sometimes ptosis in 14 out of 90 patients, persisting between attacks in 7. Nieman and Hurwitz (1961) reported a permanent deficit in 10 of 50 patients. Careful investigation discloses a subtle sympathetic deficit in most patients.

Fanciullaci et al. (1982) found that the pupil on the affected side dilated less after the instillation of tyramine drops in 26 patients examined between attacks and in a further 19 examined between bouts. Because tyramine releases noradrenaline from nerve terminals, diminished pupillary dilation indicates neuronal depletion from a postganglionic sympathetic lesion. The demonstration of an excessive pupil dilation in response to a dilute solution of a sympathomimetic agent, phenylephrine, shows that there is also denervation supersensitivity of receptors (Salvesen et al., 1987). Drummond (1988) showed that the pupil on the symptomatic side dilated more slowly in darkness and constricted more rapidly in response to light than did the opposite pupil between, as well as, during attacks, and that ptosis was also present on the side of cluster headache.

Salvesen, Sand, and Sjaastad (1988) found that deficient pupillary dilation in response to hydroxyamphetamine (which, like tyramine, releases noradrenaline) and supersensitivity to phenylephrine correlated with lack of sweating on the medial aspect of the forehead and overactivity of the sweat glands in this area in response to circulating pilocarpine. Although denervation supersensitivity of the pupil may occur with central lesions, its correlation with sweating changes limited to the medial part of the forehead clearly places the lesion in the postganglionic sympathetic neuron in the region of the carotid siphon (Lance & Drummond, 1987). The reasoning behind this is that facial sweating is mediated by postganglionic fibers, which are distributed to the periphery along branches of the external carotid artery, with the exception of the medial aspect of the forehead, where the sympathetic fibers derive from the internal carotid artery, leaving the siphon to accompany the first division of the trigeminal nerve and its frontal and supraorbital branches to the skin of the medial part of the forehead (see Figure 12.2). Selective involvement of this area must implicate sympathetic fibers in the vicinity of the siphon.

Further evidence was obtained by Drummond and Lance (1992), who compared 11 cluster headache patients with another 24 patients who had a confirmed site of lesion in the cervical sympathetic pathway. Patients with a central or preganglionic lesion had a normal mydriatic response to tyramine 2% eye drops, which was diminished or absent in seven patients with a confirmed postganglionic lesion and in seven patients on the symptomatic side of cluster headache. Sweating and flushing in response to body heating was diminished on the medial aspect of the ipsilateral forehead in those patients but was excessive when lacrimation was evoked in the ipsilateral eye by the instillation of a soapy eye drop into the conjunctival sac. This can be explained by parasympathetic fibers in the vicinity of the internal carotid artery branching along the adjacent sympathetic fibers, which had degenerated as the result of a postganglionic lesion (see Figure 12.2). Irritation of the eye that causes reflex lacrimation through the greater superficial petrosal nerve and its connections therefore causes excessive flushing and sweating in the medial aspect of the forehead comparable with that observed during some attacks of cluster headache.

The most economical explanation of the partial Horner's syndrome in cluster headache is edema of the wall of the internal carotid artery compromising postganglionic sympathetic neurons in the perivascular plexus. Ekbom and Greitz (1970) have angiographically demonstrated narrowing of the lumen of this section of the internal carotid artery in one patient with cluster headache, which Dr. Fred Plum has also observed during an attack (personal communication).

Distension of the arterial wall could be caused by vasodilator peptides released from cells forming the internal carotid ganglion, lying on the ventrolateral surface of the human internal carotid artery as it enters the cranium, that are activated by the discharge along the GSP nerve, which is responsible for lacrimation and for conjunctival, nasal, and cutaneous vasodilation (Suzuki & Hardebo, 1991). The fact that salivation is reduced during the attack suggests that secretion is inhibited by intact sympathetic fibers arising from the superior cervical ganglion.

Russell and Storstein (1983) have plotted changes in cardiac rate and rhythm as an index of autonomic instability in cluster headache. Cardiac rate increases at the onset and slows during the attack. Of 27 patients monitored throughout an attack, 2 developed conduction abnormalities, 1 experienced transient atrial fibrillation, and another had an increased number of ventricular extrasystoles. Whether these changes indicate a disturbance of central autonomic innervation or are secondary to pain remains uncertain. The effect of any generalized sympathetic arousal would not be expressed in those areas supplied from fibers in the pericarotid plexus.

Section of the nervus intermedius, containing GSP fibers, does not always stop the recurrent pain of cluster headache. Indeed, even the autonomic symptoms may continue in some patients (Morgenlander & Wilkins, 1990; Rowed, 1990), possibly because the nerve is incompletely severed.

Periodicity: Circadian and Circannual Variation in Cluster Headache

BRAIN ACTIVATIONS IN CLUSTER HEADACHE.   Two biological clocks may determine the pattern of cluster headache: one to switch on the bouts of episodic cluster and to switch them off after weeks or months and the other to trigger the attacks within a bout, once or more in a 24-hour period. Given that many patients experience their attacks at a precise time of the day or night, and the timing of attacks varies if the patient moves from one time zone to another, the daily rhythm is probably set by the suprachiasmatic nucleus and hypothalamus. Demonstration of activations in the ipsilateral hypothalamus by positron-emission tomography (PET) scanning during nitroglycerin-triggered (May et al., 1998a) and spontaneous (May et al., 2000; Sprenger et al., 2004) cluster headache (Figure 12.3) supports this notion. May et al. (1999a) demonstrated structural changes (increase in hypothalamic gray matter) in the area of hypothalamic activity by an objective automated method of voxel-based morphometry. This area is not activated in comparable PET studies in migraine. Pain induced by capsaicin applied to the skin area innervated by the ophthalmic division of the trigeminal nerve did not activate the posterior hypothalamus (May et al., 1998b), indicating its specificity for cluster headache.

HORMONAL CHANGES IN CLUSTER HEADACHE.   Researchers have studied hormonal changes as indicators of hypothalamic function. Boiardi et al. (1983) found that basal growth hormone and prolactin levels were normal in cluster headache patients, and their response to insulin, levodopa, and thyrotropin-releasing hormone (TRH) was the same as control subjects. The nocturnal

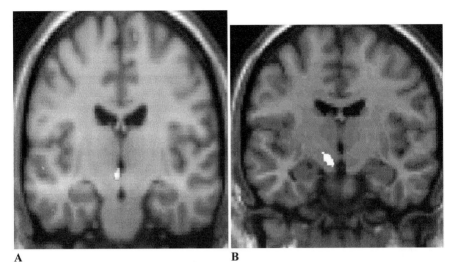

A   **B**

FIGURE 12.3   Ipsilateral activations on positron-emission tomography *(A)* and increased gray matter using voxel-based morphometry *(B)* in the posterior hypothalamic gray matter in cluster headache. (*A*, from May et al., 1998a; *B*, from May et al., 1999a.)

maximal level of melatonin is lower during cluster periods, and the cortisol level higher (Waldenlind et al., 1987). Prolactin levels rise during headache, and testosterone levels are lower in cluster periods than in remission, but not when compared with controls (Waldenlind & Gustafson, 1987). The thyrotropin response to TRH and the release of adrenocorticotropic hormone (ACTH) and cortisol during insulin-induced hypoglycemia are reduced in cluster periods (Leone et al., 1995), attributed by these authors to dysfunction of the hypothalamic paraventricular nuclei. Further studies using m-chlorophenylpiperazine (mCPP) have suggested that changes in cortisol levels in patients with cluster headache may be related to altered levels of central serotonergic activity in the central nervous system (Leone et al., 1997a). Leone and Bussone (1993) also summarized hormonal changes and the complex chronobiology of cluster headache.

Studies of humoral agents have not provided any substantial clue to the mechanism of cluster headache. Platelet 5-HT increases during pain episodes (Medina, Diamond, & Fareed, 1979) and decreases when cluster headache is successfully treated with lithium or other medication (Medina et al., 1980). Platelet noradrenaline and adrenaline are diminished in and between attacks (D'Andrea et al., 1989). Sumatriptan, a selective 5-HT$_{1B/1D}$ agonist (Goadsby, 2000), has been used to test hypothalamic function, because it stimulates the secretion of growth hormone and inhibits the release of prolactin, adrenocorticotropic hormone (ACTH), and cortisol (Pinessi et al., 2003). Responses significantly declined during cluster headache both in the active and remission period.

The mean blood level of histamine increases during cluster headache (Anthony & Lance, 1971; Medina et al., 1979), but treatment with H$_1$ and H$_2$ blocking agents has not proved helpful in management (Anthony, Lord, &

Lance, 1978; Russell, 1979). In their review of mechanisms, Ekbom, Hardebo, and Waldenlind (1988) considered the part possibly played by endorphins and vasodilator peptides.

General Conclusions About the Clinical Features and Pathophysiology of Cluster Headache

Cluster headache differs from migraine in many ways, as summarized in Table 12.3, which has been compiled from the data provided by Lance and Anthony (1966, 1971), Ekbom (1970), and Anthony and Lance (1971).

Although the recurrence of migraine depends in some instances on an internal timekeeper that sets a frequency of monthly, weekly, or sometimes even daily attacks, it is not subject to the rigid discipline that determines the pattern of cluster headache. The region of the ipsilateral hypothalamic gray matter that recent PET studies have identified to be active during acute attacks of cluster headache (Goadsby, 2002) is very likely the primary driving or permissive area for cluster headache.

Some patients become aware that an attack is about to start because they feel twinges of pain in the susceptible areas. Others detect a watering eye and stuffy nostril for half an hour or so before the pain begins. Clearly, the pain and the autonomic phenomena are independent variables, although one usually follows the other. They are compatible with paroxysmal discharge of central trigeminal, parasympathetic, and sympathetic pathways with the ocular manifestations of sympathetic activity being blocked by a postganglionic lesion in the pericarotid plexus as a result of swelling of the internal carotid arterial wall. Dilation of parts of the internal and external circulations are probably secondary to activity in vascular projections from the brainstem (the trigeminoparasympathetic reflex, Goadsby, 2002) and intensify pain by increasing input to the brainstem through trigeminal or upper cervical afferent fibers into the trigeminocervical complex. As in the case of migraine, therapy directed at the dilated arteries or at central mechanisms can ease the pain. Episodic pain may continue after surgical lesions of the trigeminal and GSP nerve, clearly indicating that the primary defect is a central disturbance.

Investigation

A picture resembling cluster headache may be symptomatic of an underlying lesion such as an arteriovenous malformation and should be excluded by CT scan of the brain. Table 12.2 is a reasonably complete list of associations with clusterlike presentations. In practice, best-available imaging of the cavernous sinus and pituitary are the highest value investigations.

Treatment

The course of cluster headache does not seem influenced by psychologic factors and does not respond to adjustment of lifestyle other than avoiding alcohol, and perhaps afternoon napping, during a bout. Management therefore focuses on rapid control of acute attacks and preventive therapy to suppress attacks.

TABLE 12.3   Differences between migraine and cluster headache

	Migraine	*Cluster Headache*
Sex distribution (%)	Female 75	Male 85
Onset in childhood (%)	25	<1
Unilateral pain (%)	65	100
Recurrence in bouts (%)	0	80
Frequency of attacks	<1–12/mo	1–8/day
Usual duration of pain	4–24 h	0.25–2 h
Associated Features		
Nausea, vomiting (%)	85	45
Blurring of vision (%)	Common	8
Lacrimation (%)	Uncommon	85
Blocked nostril (%)	Uncommon	50
Ptosis, miosis (%)	Uncommon	25
Hyperalgesia of face, scalp (%)	65	15
Teichopsia, photopsia (%)	40	<1
Polyuria (%)	30	7
Past Health		
Vomiting in childhood (%)	25	7
Family History		
Migraine (%)	50	20
Biochemical Changes		
Fall in platelet serotonin (%)	80	0
Rise in plasma histamine (%)	0	90

Percentages refer to the number of patients with the symptom or sign in relation to the total studied.

Abortive Agents

The pain of cluster headache rapidly reaches an excruciating intensity so that most oral agents are too slowly absorbed to be useful. The most efficacious abortive agents involve parenteral or pulmonary administration.

SUMATRIPTAN.   Subcutaneous sumatriptan 6 mg is the drug of choice for aborting a cluster attack. A randomized, placebo-controlled, double-blind, crossover study completed in 39 patients (Ekbom & Sumatriptan Cluster Headache Study Group, 1991) showed that sumatriptan reduced headache severity after 15 minutes in 74% of attacks, in contrast to 26% in which placebo was given. Thirty-six percent of patients were pain free within 10 minutes of taking sumatriptan, in contrast to three percent after placebo. Sumatriptan was well tolerated, and there were no serious adverse events. A double-blind, crossover, randomized study compared sumatriptan 6 mg and 12 mg with placebo in 134 patients (Ekbom et al., 1993). The 12-mg dose was no more effective than the 6-mg dose and was associated with more side effects. Two large clinical trials have assessed the effects of long-term administration of subcutaneous sumatriptan (Ekbom et al., 1995; Gobel et al., 1998). Adverse events were quantitatively similar to those seen in migraine trials and did not increase with frequent use of sumatriptan. We believe, given the devastating morbidity associated with this excruciating pain syndrome, that *it is unethical to withhold treatment for cost reasons*. Although generally well tolerated, sumatriptan is contraindicated in patients with ischemic heart disease or uncontrolled hypertension. Caution must be exercised in patients with cluster headache, because the disorder predominates in middle-aged men, who often have risk factors for cardiovascular disease, such as smoking (Manzoni, 1999).

A randomized, placebo-controlled, double-blind, crossover study completed in 86 patients showed that headache severity at 30 minutes was reduced in 56% of attacks in which sumatriptan nasal spray was administered, in contrast to 26% in which placebo was given (van Vliet et al., 2003a). Nasal sumatriptan is thus less efficacious than the subcutaneous formulation on a population basis.

ZOLMITRIPTAN.   A double-blind, placebo-controlled trial compared the efficacy of oral zolmitriptan 5 mg and 10 mg for treating acute attacks in episodic and chronic cluster headache (Bahra et al., 2000). With headache response defined as a 2-point reduction on a 5-point pain intensity scale, 30-minute response rates in episodic cluster headache were 29%, 40%, and 47% following placebo, 5 mg zolmitriptan, and 10 mg zolmitriptan, respectively. The difference reached statistical significance only for 10 mg zolmitriptan compared with placebo. In addition, significantly more episodic cluster headache patients reported mild or no pain 30 minutes after treatment with 5 and 10 mg zolmitriptan (57% and 60%, respectively) than following placebo (42%). In patients with chronic cluster headache, response rates following 5 or 10 mg zolmitriptan did not significantly differ from those seen with placebo. The efficacy of oral zolmitriptan in episodic cluster headache is modest and does not approach the efficacy or speed of subcutaneous sumatriptan or oxygen, limiting its usefulness in clinical practice. The nasal formulation is currently being tested, and initial indications are promising.

Oxygen

NORMOBARIC OXYGEN.   Oxygen inhalation is a safe and effective method for acute treatment of cluster headache. Its mechanism of action remains unclear.

Horton was the first to discover that 100% oxygen inhalation at the onset of attacks alleviates cluster headache pain (Horton, 1956). Friedman and Mikropoulos (1958) also reported on its favorable effect. Kudrow (1981) noted a significant relief from cluster pain in 75% of 52 randomly selected outpatients treated with 100% oxygen administered through a facial mask at a rate of 7 L/min for 15 minutes. Headache relief occurred in 62% of the patients within the first 7 minutes of oxygen inhalation, in 31% within 8 to 10 minutes, and in 7% within 10 to 15 minutes. The best results were obtained in episodic cluster headache patients younger than 50 years of age.

Oxygen at 6 L/min for 15 minutes was compared with air inhalation in a double-blind crossover study of 19 sufferers (Fogan, 1985). Eleven patients used both gases. Of 16 patients who used oxygen, 9 patients (56%) perceived a complete or substantial relief in 80% or more of their cluster attacks, in contrast to only 1 of 14 patients (7%) who used air. The great advantage with oxygen is that it has no established side effects, can be readily combined with other abortive and preventive treatments, and can be used several times daily, unlike subcutaneous and intranasal sumatriptan, which can only be used up to a maximum of two and three times daily, respectively. The major drawback with oxygen inhalation treatment is the practical limitation imposed by the bulky equipment, and although small portable cylinders are available, most patients find them cumbersome and inconvenient. Furthermore, the treatment forces the patient to sit still, a behavior that is usually incompatible with the excruciating pain of a cluster headache. Some patients cannot hold the mask against their face, because skin contact worsens the pain. On long-term treatment, only a few responders seem to continue using oxygen, especially chronic sufferers. Gallagher and coworkers found that 76% of patients had significant relief, but only 31% continued using oxygen for subsequent headaches (Gallagher et al., 1996). Further studies are needed to investigate patients' preferences for symptomatic treatment.

HYPERBARIC OXYGEN.   The first case report of the effectiveness of hyperbaric oxygen as an abortive agent in cluster headaches was by Weiss and colleagues (1989). Subsequently, an open trial of hyperbaric oxygen (1.3ATA) in 14 patients reported that 18 cluster attacks (12 spontaneous, 6 induced by sublingual nitroglycerin) resolved rapidly, with complete relief achieved within a mean of 6.2 minutes (range: 30 seconds to 13 minutes) (Porta et al., 1991). A small, placebo-controlled study of hyperbaric oxygen (2ATA) delivered over 30 minutes demonstrated efficacy in six of seven patients within 5 to 30 minutes (Di Sabato et al., 1993). In addition, in three of six responders the cluster bout was completely interrupted, whereas in the other three responders the cluster bout was partially interrupted for 3 to 6 days. Subsequently, hyperbaric oxygen (2.5ATA) was tested as a prophylactic treatment in cluster headache. In a double-blind, placebo-controlled, crossover study on 12 episodic and 4 chronic sufferers, no significant effect was obtained (Nilsson Remahl et al., 1997). Hyperbaric oxygen offers no advantages over normobaric oxygen.

Topical Local Anesthetics

COCAINE.   Intranasal cocaine has been reported to be effective at aborting nitroglycerin-induced cluster attacks in an open-label trial in 10 patients (Barre, 1982). The patients applied 50 mg of cocaine flakes on a cotton swab in the region of the ipsilateral pterygopalatine ganglion. Nine patients experienced 80% or more reduction in intensity of their induced cluster headache within 2 minutes. Ten percent cocaine (1 mL; 50 mg per application) was reported to be effective at aborting nitroglycerin-induced cluster attacks in a double-blind, placebo-controlled study in nine patients (Costa et al., 2000). Cocaine or saline was applied using a cotton swab in the area corresponding to the pterygopalatine fossa, under anterior rhinoscopy. All patients responded to intranasal cocaine, with pain completely ceasing after 31.3 ± 13.1 minutes, but the application method is cumbersome. Because of its addictive potential, cocaine does not have widespread medicinal uses; the drug of choice is lidocaine (lignocaine).

LIDOCAINE (LIGNOCAINE).   Kittrelle and colleagues (1985) first reported that lignocaine solution, applied topically to the region of the pterygopalatine fossa, alleviated the pain of the cluster attack. In an open-label trial of intranasal lignocaine 4% solution, four of five patients obtained rapid relief of nitroglycerin-induced cluster headaches. Lignocaine also effectively relieved spontaneous attacks. Subsequently, Hardebo and Elner (1987) reported on the use of intranasal lidocaine 4% solution in an open-label trial in 19 patients. Seven patients (37%) reported a 50% or greater response, seven patients (37%) reported a response less than 50%, and five patients (26%) reported no benefit. Robbins (1995) reported on the use of 4 to 6 sprays of lidocaine 4% in the nostril ipsilateral to the painful side in an open-label trial in 30 patients. Eight patients (27%) reported moderate relief, eight patients (27%) obtained mild relief, and fourteen patients (46%) said they had no relief from the lidocaine. No patient reported excellent relief. These findings were considerably poorer than those of Kittrelle and coworkers (1985) and of Hardebo and Elner (1987). This poorer efficacy reported by Robbins may, at least in part, be attributable to the formulation used: Robbins used a spray rather than the nose drops used in other studies (Kudrow & Kudrow, 1995). Recently, 10% lidocaine was reported to be effective at aborting nitroglycerin-induced cluster attacks in a double-blind, placebo-controlled study in nine patients (Costa et al., 2000). Lidocaine or saline was applied using a cotton swab in the area corresponding to the pterygopalatine fossa, under anterior rhinoscopy—again, a cumbersome approach.

We use lidocaine solution 20 to 60 mg, applied bilaterally as nasal drops (4 to 6% lidocaine solution) in the region of the pterygopalatine fossa. The patient needs to be instructed carefully on the self-administration of intranasal lignocaine by a nasal dropper. To ensure that the solution reaches the pterygopalatine foramen, the patient should be instructed to lie down horizontally as early as possible during an attack, with the head extending out of the bed, bent downward 30 to 45 degrees and rotated 20 to 30 degrees toward the side of the headache. The tip of the dropper is inserted above the rostral end of the inferior turbinate and pushed inward as deeply as possible before dripping. The patient should be asked to maintain the position for about 2 to 5 minutes. An alternative method of application is peg-pushing: A cotton swab on a peg is drowned in lidocaine before being applied to the region of the ipsilateral pterygopalatine foramen. However, patients often report that peg-pushing considerably worsens the pain of cluster headache, and therefore most patients cannot perform the procedure accurately. In our experience, intranasal lidocaine results in mild to moderate relief in some patients, although only a few patients obtain complete pain relief (unpublished observations). Therefore intranasal lignocaine serves as a useful adjunct to other abortive treatments but is rarely adequate on its own.

Ergot Derivatives

ERGOTAMINE.   Although Horton is usually given credit for first using ergotamine in the abortive treatment of cluster headache, it was in fact Harris who first advocated its use in 1937 (Harris, 1937; Boes et al., 2002). Horton first described the beneficial effect of intravenous ergotamine in aborting cluster headaches in a case reported in 1941 (Horton, 1941). Subsequently, Kunkle and colleagues (1952) reported the rapid termination of cluster attacks in four patients with intravenous ergotamine. Horton and coworkers (1948) reported "excellent" results in open-label use of oral Cafergot (ergotamine tartrate 1 mg and caffeine 100 mg) in 10 out of 14 patients. A subsequently published open trial of Cafergot suppositories reported a considerably lower response rate—4 of 20 patients (Magee et al., 1952). Friedman and Mikropoulos (1958) reported that oral, suppository, or intravenous preparations of ergotamine were "effective to a greater or lesser extent" in 30 of 35 patients.

Kudrow (1981) noted significant relief from cluster pain in 70% of 50 randomly selected outpatients treated with sublingual ergotamine at 15 minutes in a crossover study with 100% oxygen. The peak response to sublingual ergotamine occurred within 10 to 12 minutes of treatment. Oxygen was regarded as superior to ergotamine, especially because there were no complications and contraindications to its use.

Inhaled ergotamine, used in an open-label manner, reportedly produces an "excellent" effect in 11 of 13 patients (Speed, 1960). Another open-label study reported that inhaled ergotamine given to 12 patients relieved pain within 30 minutes in 71% of 114 attacks (Graham et al., 1960). Kudrow (1980) reported that 79 of 100 patients obtained "significant relief" from sublingual or inhaled ergotamine preparations.

There are no well-controlled trials of ergotamine in aborting cluster headaches. Inhaled, subcutaneous, intramuscular, or intravenous injections of ergotamine are now not widely available. In our experience, oral or rectal ergotamine is generally too slow in onset to provide meaningful relief in a timely manner, especially when compared with the rapid onset of action for subcutaneous sumatriptan and high-dose oxygen. Moreover, ergotamine is a potent vasoconstrictor. It is contraindicated in patients with coronary or peripheral vascular disease, arterial hypertension, and severe disease of the liver and kidney.

DIHYDROERGOTAMINE.   Parenteral dihydroergotamine (DHE) has been considered an effective abortive agent for cluster headaches for some time (Horton, 1952; Friedman & Mikropoulos, 1958). DHE is available in injectable and intranasal formulations. Although there are no controlled trials of injectable DHE, clinical experience has demonstrated that intravenous administration provides prompt and effective relief of cluster headache within 15 minutes (Dodick et al., 2000). However, given the frequency and the rapid peak intensity of cluster attacks, intravenous DHE is not a feasible long-term solution. The intramuscular and subcutaneous routes of administration provide slower relief but have the advantage that they can be self-administered.

DHE nasal spray 1 mg has been studied in a double-blind, placebo-controlled, crossover trial in 25 patients (Andersson & Jespersen, 1986). There was no difference in the headache frequency or duration, but the pain intensity was significantly reduced by DHE in contrast to placebo. The dosage used (1 mg) was lower than the recommended dosage for migraine (2 mg) and lower than the currently available preparations of DHE nasal spray (4 mg). Therefore DHE nasal spray at a dose of 2 or 4 mg may be more effective than 1 mg, although this needs to be studied in a controlled fashion.

Analgesics

Opiates, nonsteroidal anti-inflammatory drugs (NSAIDs), and combination analgesics have no routine role in acute management of cluster headache. The pain of cluster headache progresses to an excruciating intensity so rapidly that most oral agents are too slowly absorbed to act within a reasonable period of time. Furthermore, with prolonged treatment with high dosages, problems with habituation and toxicity may develop. We have certainly seen medication overuse–related headaches with opiate-receptor agonist use in patients with cluster headache. In one study of 60 patients, only 21% reported significant relief of pain with oral analgesics, but 65% continued using analgesics despite their ineffectiveness (Gallagher et al., 1996). The authors concluded that patients with cluster headache preferred to use oral analgesics for reasons not solely concerned with pain relief.

Other Drugs

SOMATOSTATIN RECEPTOR AGONISTS.   Neurons containing somatostatin are found in the regions of the central and peripheral nervous system involved in nociception, such as peripheral sensory fibers, dorsal horn of the spinal cord, trigeminal nucleus caudalis, periaqueductal gray, and the hypothalamus (Krisch, 1978; Schindler et al., 1998). Somatostatin mediates its actions by binding to high-affinity membrane receptors. Five somatostatin receptors (sst_{1-5}) have been cloned (Hoyer et al., 1995), and any antiheadache effect is, by definition, nonvascular. Intravenous somatostatin (25 µg/min for 20 minutes) was compared to treatment with ergotamine (250 µg intramuscularly) or placebo in a double-blind trial consisting of 72 attacks in 8 patients (Sicuteri et al., 1984). Infusion of somatostatin significantly reduced maximal pain intensity and pain duration in contrast to placebo, and to a degree comparable to intramuscular ergotamine. In another randomized, double-blind study, subcutaneous somatostatin was compared with ergotamine (Geppetti et al., 1985). Five patients were treated with each of the drugs for three attacks. Subcutaneous somatostatin and ergotamine were equally beneficial with regard to the effects on maximal pain intensity and the pain area, but somatostatin was less effective in reducing pain duration.

Octreotide, a more stable somatostatin analog, acts predominantly on sst_2 and sst_5 (Patel & Srikant, 1994). In a double-blind, placebo-controlled crossover study, patients were instructed to treat two attacks of cluster headache of at least moderate pain severity with at least a 24-hour break between attacks, using sub-cutaneous octreotide or matching placebo. Of 57 patients recruited, 46 provided efficacy data on attacks treated with octreotide and 45 with placebo. The headache response rate with subcutaneous octreotide was 52%, whereas that with placebo was 36% ($P < .01$). Octreotide is thus effective in the acute treatment of cluster headache (Matharu et al., 2004c). In contrast, it is not effective in acute treatment of migraine (Levy et al., 2004b).

OLANZAPINE. Olanzapine has been evaluated as a cluster headache abortive agent in an open-label trial (Rozen, 2001). Oral olanzapine at doses ranging from 2.5 to 10 mg was administered to five patients (four with chronic cluster headache, one with episodic cluster headache). It reduced the severity of cluster pain by at least 80% in four of five patients, and two patients were rendered free of pain. The only adverse effect was sleepiness. These seemingly promising results need to be replicated in a double-blind, placebo-controlled study.

Preventive Treatments

The aim of preventive therapy is to suppress attacks rapidly and to maintain remission with minimal side effects until the cluster bout is over, or for a longer period in patients with chronic cluster headache. Because very few randomized controlled clinical trials have been performed, preventive therapy in cluster headache is based partly on clinical experience.

Short-Term Prevention

Patients with either short bouts (weeks) or in whom one wishes to control the attack frequency quickly can benefit from short-term prevention. These medi-cines are distinguished by the fact that they cannot be used in the long term and thus may need to be replaced by long-term agents in many patients. Corticosteroids, methysergide, daily triptans, and nocturnal ergotamine (for patients having only predictable nocturnal headaches) are particularly useful in this setting.

Long-Term Prevention

Some patients with either long bouts of episodic cluster headache or chronic cluster headache require preventive treatment over many months, or even years.

Verapamil and lithium are particularly useful in this setting, and methysergide is used with regular breaks.

VERAPAMIL.   Meyer and Hardenberg (1983) first reported verapamil to be effective as a preventive treatment in cluster headache. In an open trial using verapamil at dosages of 160 to 720 mg daily in five chronic cluster headache patients, all patients reported a reduction in the mean monthly frequency of headaches. In a further open-label study of verapamil at dosages of 160 to 480 mg daily in 34 patients with chronic cluster headache, 79% of patients reported decreased frequency and severity of the headaches, although these improvements were not further qualified (Jonsdottir et al., 1987). In another open trial using verapamil at dosages of 240 to 600 mg daily in episodic cluster headache and 120 to 1200 mg daily in chronic cluster headache, an improvement of more than 75% was noted in 33 of 48 (69%) patients (Gabai & Spierings, 1989). A double-blind, crossover trial comparing verapamil 360 mg daily to the then-standard prophylactic drug lithium 900 mg daily, each given for 8 weeks, found equivalent effects in the 24 chronic cluster headache patients who completed the trial (Bussone et al., 1990). Verapamil and lithium were superior to placebo. Verapamil caused fewer side effects and had a shorter latency period. A double-blind, placebo-controlled trial evaluated the efficacy of verapamil 360 mg daily over a 2-week period in 26 episodic cluster headache patients (Leone, D'Amico, & Attanasio, 1999). A statistically significant reduction in headache frequency and analgesic consumption was seen in the verapamil-treated patients, with further reduction in the second week of treatment.

Verapamil is the preventive drug of choice in both episodic and chronic cluster headache in which the bout is sufficiently long to establish a suitable dose. Clinical experience has clearly demonstrated that higher dosages are needed than those used in cardiologic indications. Dosages commonly range from 240 to 960 mg daily in divided doses. Verapamil can cause heart block by slowing conduction in the atrioventricular node (Singh & Nademanee, 1987), as demonstrated by prolongation of the A–H interval (Naylor, 1988). Observing for PR interval prolongation on electrocardiography (ECG/EKG) can monitor potential development of heart block, and although this is a coarse measure, it is advisable. In our clinical experience, standard preparations of verapamil are more effective than the modified-release formulations. Constipation is the most common side effect, but dizziness, ankle swelling, nausea, fatigue, hypertension, and bradycardia may also occur. Patients should be cautioned about gum bleeding, which may predict gingival hyperplasia (Matharu et al., 2004d) and requires a dosage reduction and careful dental hygiene to avoid loss of dentition. Beta-blockers should not be given concurrently. We have not found either nimodipine or nifedipine useful in clinical practice, and the evidence for their use is scanty (Matharu et al., 2003a).

LITHIUM.   The effectiveness of lithium in psychiatric conditions of a cyclical nature, such as manic-depressive psychosis and seasonal affective disorder, led Ekbom (1974, 1977) to try this agent in cluster headache, in view of its striking circannual and circadian periodicity. Lithium was administered to five patients (three chronic and two episodic) in an open-label fashion. The lithium dosage was adjusted until a serum lithium concentration of 0.7 to 1.2 mmol/L was achieved. All three patients with chronic cluster headache had an immediate, partial remission of the headache. Withdrawal of the drug resulted in an increase in intensity and frequency of the headaches. A second period of treatment again resulted in a definite improvement. In the two patients with episodic cluster headache, lithium had only a slight or no effect on the headaches.

The effectiveness of lithium was subsequently verified in several unblinded series of cluster headache patients (Kudrow, 1977; Lieb & Zeff, 1978; Mathew, 1978; Szulc-Kuberska & Klimek, 1978; Bussone et al., 1979; Klimek et al., 1979; Savoldi, Nappi, & Bono, 1979; Wyant & Ashenhurst, 1979; Damasio & Lyon, 1980; Medina, Fareed, & Diamond, 1980; Ekbom, 1981; Manzoni et al., 1983a). Open trials have been reviewed (Ekbom, 1981; Ekbom & Solomon, 2000). Collectively, in more than 28 clinical trials involving 468 patients, good to excellent results were found in 236 (78%) of 304 patients with chronic cluster headache. The response to lithium in patients with episodic cluster headache was less robust than in chronic cluster headache, with good efficacy in 103 (63%) of a total of 164 patients treated.

Most unblinded trials used a lithium dosage ranging from 600 to 1200 mg daily. Lithium was often effective at serum concentrations (0.4 to 0.8 mEq/L) less than that usually required for treatment of bipolar disorder. Patients who improved on lithium often showed dramatic relief within the first week (Kudrow, 1977; Mathew, 1978; Ekbom, 1981). Manzoni and colleagues (1983a) assessed the long-term therapeutic efficacy of lithium in 18 patients with chronic cluster and reported that it appears durable for up to 4 years after treatment. On interruption or cessation of lithium therapy in patients with chronic cluster headache, a transition to episodic cluster headache has been recognized (Ekbom, 1981; Manzoni et al., 1983a). Some patients eventually become resistant to lithium (Ekbom, 1981).

Lithium has also been evaluated in two randomized, double-blind trials. A double-blind, crossover trial comparing verapamil 360 mg daily with lithium 900 mg daily, each given for 8 weeks, found equivalent effects in the 24 patients with chronic cluster headache who completed the trial (Bussone et al., 1990). A double-blind, placebo-controlled, randomized, parallel group trial of sustained relief with lithium 800 mg daily in 27 patients (13 on lithium, 14 on placebo) with episodic cluster headache assessed efficacy at 1 week after treatment was begun (Steiner et al., 1997). In two patients in each group, attacks ceased within 1 week, whereas substantial improvement was noted in 6 (43%) of 14 patients receiving placebo and 8 (62%) of 13 patients receiving lithium. Lithium treatment was associated with a subjective improvement rate, but this was not statistically significant in comparison with the placebo group. The authors assumed at the onset of the trial that the placebo response would be zero. This assumption turned out to be flawed, and consequently the study had inadequate power to test the proposed hypothesis. Therefore it had been assumed that placebo response in prophylactic studies of cluster headache was insubstantial. This is clearly incorrect for both acute attack and preventive treatment approaches in cluster headache (Nilsson Remahl et al., 2003).

Lithium is an effective agent for cluster headache prophylaxis, although the response is less robust in the episodic form than in the chronic form. Most patients benefit from dosages between 600 and 1200 mg daily. Lithium has the potential for many side effects and has a narrow therapeutic window. Side effects of lithium include weakness, nausea, thirst, tremor, slurred speech, and blurred vision. Toxicity is manifested by nausea; vomiting; anorexia; diarrhea; and neurologic signs of confusion, nystagmus, ataxia, extrapyramidal signs, and seizures. Hypothyroidism and polyuria (nephrogenic diabetes insipidus) can occur with long-term use. Polymorphonuclear leukocytosis may occur and be mistaken for occult infection. Renal and thyroid function tests are performed before and during treatment. We start patients at a dosage of 300 mg twice daily and thereafter titrate the dosage upward until the cluster headaches are suppressed, side effects intervene, or the serum lithium level reaches the upper part of the therapeutic range. The serum concentrations should be measured 12 hours after the last dose and should not exceed the upper level of the therapeutic range. The lithium dosage may need to be adjusted in accordance with the spontaneous, fluctuating course of this disorder. In addition, we advise drug withdrawal at least once annually to detect patients who have made a transition from chronic to episodic cluster headache. Concomitant use of NSAIDs, diuretics, and carbamazepine is contraindicated.

Serotonergic Receptor Agonists and Antagonists

METHYSERGIDE.   Methysergide is an ergot alkaloid, which is an antagonist at 5-HT_{2A}, 5-HT_{2B}, and 5-HT_{2C} receptors and an agonist at $5\text{-HT}_{1B/1D}$ receptors. Methysergide was first reported to be effective in cluster headache by Sicuteri (1959). Subsequently, several authors confirmed this observation in open-label trials of this agent (Dalsgaard-Neilsen, 1960; Friedman, 1960; Graham, 1960; Heyck, 1960; Friedman & Losin, 1961; Harris, 1961; Ekbom, 1962). The open-label trials were reviewed by Curran, Hinterberger, and Lance (1967), who noted that methysergide, used at 3 to 12 mg/day, was effective in 329 (73%) of 451 patients with episodic and chronic cluster headache.

Subsequently, Kudrow (1980) reported that in open-label use, methysergide was effective in 50 (65%) of 77 patients with episodic cluster headache and in 3 (20%) of 15 patients with chronic cluster headache, but the drug appears to lose its effectiveness with repeated use in up to 20% of patients. However, Krabbe (1989) reported a limited prophylactic benefit with methysergide, used in an open-label manner, in both episodic and chronic cluster headache. The efficacy of methysergide (used at up to 12 mg/day) was examined prospectively in 42 patients (16 episodic, 26 chronic). Of the 42 patients, 13 had good or excellent benefits, but 2 of these 13 patients had severe side effects. Thus methysergide was beneficial without side effects in 11 (26%) of 42 patients. There was no significant difference in treatment response between the episodic (25%) and chronic (27%) groups. In addition, a retrospective analysis of 164 patients treated with methysergide demonstrated a satisfactory effect in only 44 (26%).

Methysergide is indicated for treating cluster headaches, although the efficacy data from the open trials is inconsistent. Dosages up to 12 mg daily can be used if tolerated. To minimize side effects, patients can start with a low dosage and increase the dosage gradually. We start patients on 1 mg once daily and increase the daily dose by 1 mg every 3 days (in a three-times-daily regimen) until the daily dose is 5 mg; thereafter, the dose is incremented by 1 mg every 5 days. Common short-term side effects include nausea, vomiting, dizziness, muscle cramps, abdominal pain, and peripheral edema. Uncommon but troublesome side effects are caused by vasoconstriction (coronary or peripheral arterial insufficiency), which usually necessitates stopping this drug. Prolonged treatment has been associated with fibrotic reactions (retroperitoneal, pulmonary, pleural, and cardiac), although these are rare (Graham et al., 1966). Ideally, the drug should be used only in patients with short cluster bouts, preferably less than 3 to 4 months. If prolonged use is intended, the risk of fibrotic reactions can be minimized by giving the drug for 6 months followed by a monthlong holiday before starting the drug again. To avoid a sudden increase in headache frequency when methysergide is stopped, the patient should be weaned off over 1 week. We have used methysergide on a continuous basis with careful monitoring, including auscultation of the heart and yearly echocardiogram, chest radiograph, and abdominal magnetic resonance imaging (MRI) if indicated (Raskin, 1988). All patients receiving methysergide should remain under supervision of the treating physician and should be examined regularly for development of visceral fibrosis or vascular complications.

Contraindications to the use of methysergide include pregnancy, peripheral vascular disorders, severe arteriosclerosis, coronary artery disease, severe hypertension, thrombophlebitis or cellulitis of the legs, peptic ulcer disease, fibrotic disorders, lung diseases, collagen disease, liver or renal function impairment, and valvular heart disease (Silberstein, 1998).

ERGOTS, TRIPTANS, AND METHYSERGIDE.   Considerable controversy surrounds the use of ergot derivates and triptans with methysergide. This is not at all an easy subject. It is usually recommended that ergotamine or dihydroergotamine should not be taken concomitantly with methysergide, whereas other vasoconstrictive agents should be used only with caution. Methysergide is an ergot derivative (Berde & Schild, 1978), but it is a weak vasoconstrictor compared with ergotamine (Garrison, 1990). It is demethylated in vivo to methylergonovine, to which it may owe some of its activity (Saxena & De Boer, 1991). There are no reported prospective drug-interaction studies between methysergide and sumatriptan. In some early clinical studies with sumatriptan, methysergide continued to be used (Blakeborough, Fowler, & Ashford, 1993). Eighty patients were taking either of methysergide or pizotifen, both serotonin 5-HT_2 antagonists. They had used either sumatriptan injections ($n = 38$) or tablets ($n = 42$). There was insufficient power to analyze this group, but they had a similar adverse event profile (Blakeborough et al., 1993). The most worrisome case was that of a 43-year-old woman who had a myocardial infarction while taking methysergide and sumatriptan (Liston et al., 1999). She had a history of migraine without aura and atypical chest pain attributed to gastroesophageal reflux. She also had controlled hypertension. Coronary angiography revealed a

50% block of the left anterior descending coronary artery that was treated by stenting. In retrospect, sumatriptan was contraindicated in this patient because of the ischemic heart disease, although one might argue that this was a difficult diagnostic issue. For cluster headache we are unaware of any similar case. Thus the combined use of ergot derivates or sumatriptan with methysergide is not absolutely contraindicated and must remain a clinical decision based on balancing the very considerable benefit, particularly for sumatriptan and dihydroergotamine, and the concomitant use of methysergide, with each case judged on its merits.

ERGOTAMINE.   Ekbom (1947) first reported the use of ergotamine tartrate for the prophylactic treatment of cluster headaches. Of 16 patients given ergotamine at the dosage of 2 to 3 mg daily for 1 to 4 weeks, 13 patients improved considerably. Later it was reported that a rectal suppository of ergotamine 2 mg and caffeine 100 mg or intramuscular injections in doses of 0.25 to 0.5 mg at bedtime effectively prevented nocturnal attacks (Symonds, 1956). Ergotamine was widely used as the first-choice prophylaxis until the efficacy of lithium and verapamil became evident. If the patient has nocturnal attacks, 1 to 2 mg may be given at night in the form of tablets or suppositories. If the pattern of attacks is predictable, the dose can be given 30 to 60 minutes before the expected attacks. The medication needs to be monitored carefully so that the total weekly dose is not too large.

DIHYDROERGOTAMINE.   Repetitive intravenous dihydroergotamine (IV DHE) administered in an inpatient setting over a period of 3 days has been reported to be very useful in some patients with both episodic and chronic cluster headache. In a study of 54 patients with intractable cluster headache (23 episodic, 31 chronic), open-label use of repetitive IV DHE rendered all patients headache free (Mather et al., 1991). At 12 months follow-up, 83% and 39% of episodic and chronic cluster headache patients, respectively, remained free of headache. We find this approach useful in many patients.

PIZOTIFEN (PIZOTYLENE).   In 1967 Sicuteri and coworkers (1967) were the first to report the beneficial effect of pizotifen in seven cases of cluster headache. A review of seven small studies, published in 1972, reported that pizotifen has only a modest effect in cluster headache prophylaxis, being effective in 21 of 56 episodic and chronic cluster headache sufferers (38% responders) (Speight & Avery, 1972). However, in one single-blind trial of pizotifen 3 mg daily given to 28 patients with episodic cluster headache, 16 subjects had a beneficial response (57% responders) (Ekbom, 1969). Although widely used in Europe and Canada, pizotifen is not available in the United States and is generally not held to be very useful in the treatment of cluster headache.

TRIPTANS.   No controlled evidence supports the use of oral sumatriptan in cluster headache. Sumatriptan 100 mg three times daily taken before an anticipated onset of an attack or at regular times does not prevent the attack, and thus it should not be used for cluster headache prophylaxis (Monstad et al.,

1995). In open-label use, naratriptan 2.5 mg twice daily (Eekers & Koehler, 2001; Loder, 2002) and eletriptan (Zebenholzer et al., 2004) have been reported to suppress cluster headache completely. A double-blind, placebo-controlled study is needed to confirm this possible use. Because we and others (Rossi et al., 2004) have seen regular use of triptans increase cluster headache frequency, we do not readily use this approach.

Corticosteroids

The use of corticosteroids in cluster headache was first reported by Horton (1952), who found that cortisone at dosages of 100 mg daily was effective in only 4 of 21 patients. The effectiveness of prednisolone (prednisone) in stopping bouts of cluster headache was established in a double-blind trial by Jammes (1975). Couch and Ziegler (1978) reported that prednisolone (prednisone) 10 to 80 mg/day sed to treat 19 cluster headache patients (9 episodic, 10 chronic) provided greater than 50% relief in 14 patients (73%) and complete relief in 11 patients (58%). Recurrence of headaches was reported in 79% of patients when the prednisolone (prednisone) dosage was tapered. Kudrow (1980) reported that of 77 episodic cluster patients unresponsive to methysergide, prednisolone (prednisone) relieved 77% and partially improved 12%. Prednisolone (prednisone) was also found to provide marked relief in 40% of patients with chronic cluster headache and was more effective than methysergide in this patient group. Dexamethasone at a dosage of 4 mg twice daily for 2 weeks followed by 4 mg daily for 1 week has also been shown to be effective (Anthony & Draher, 1992).

Corticosteroids (prednisolone/prednisone and dexamethasone) are highly efficacious and the most rapid-acting of the prophylactic agents. As in other disorders, use of corticosteroids is contraindicated by a history of tuberculosis or psychotic disturbance. Furthermore, caution must be exercised because of the potential for serious side effects. In this regard, bony problems with steroid use have been reviewed, and the shortest course of prednisolone (prednisone) reported to be associated with osteonecrosis of the femoral head is a 30-day course. Furthermore, courses of adrenocorticotropic hormone have produced osteonecrosis after 16 days, and dexamethasone after 7 days (Mirzai et al., 1999). Thus a tapering course of prednisolone (prednisone) for 21 days is prudent, with an excess risk for bony problems if more than two courses are administered per year (Mirzai et al., 1999). We start patients on oral prednisolone (prednisone) 1 mg/kg, to a maximum of 60 mg, daily for 5 days and thereafter decrease the dose by 10 mg every 3 days. Unfortunately, relapse almost invariably occurs as the dose is tapered. For this reason, steroids are used as an initial therapy in conjunction with preventives, until the latter are effective.

Other Agents

VALPROIC ACID.   Hering and Kuritzky (1989) evaluated the effectiveness of sodium valproate as preventive therapy in 15 patients with cluster headache in an open-label clinical trial. Thirteen patients with episodic cluster headache received sodium valproate between 600 and 2000 mg daily for up to 6 months, and the two patients with the chronic subtype received 600 to 1200 mg daily. Sodium valproate was effective in 11 of the 15 patients (73%). El Amrani and colleagues (2002) reported the results of a double-blind, placebo-controlled, parallel group study of sodium valproate (1000 to 2000 mg/day) in prophylaxis of cluster headache. The study included 96 patients, 50 in the sodium valproate group (37 episodic, 11 chronic, 2 unspecified) and 46 in the placebo group (36 episodic, 6 chronic, 3 unspecified). No significant difference was noted between the two groups, with improvement in 50% of the active treatment group and 62% in the placebo group. However, the two groups were imbalanced in that the mean duration of previous cluster bouts in the patients with episodic cluster headache was shorter in the placebo group (62.4 days) than in the treatment group (78.3 days). No valid conclusion about the efficacy of sodium valproate in prophylaxis of cluster headache could be drawn because of this imbalance. We do not find this treatment a particularly useful strategy.

TOPIRAMATE.   Several open-label studies have suggested that topiramate is useful as a prophylaxis for cluster headache (Wheeler & Carrazana, 1999; Forderreuther, Mayer, & Straube, 2003; Lainez et al., 2003; Leone et al., 2003; Rapoport et al., 2003). We have used dosages from 50 to 400 mg daily with some success. Somnolence, dizziness, cognitive symptoms, and ataxia are commonly reported. Mood changes, psychosis, weight loss, and glaucoma have been reported. Paresthesias and nephrolithiasis can occur because of the weak carbonic anhydrase inhibition of the drug. We start topiramate at low dosages (15 to 25 mg daily) and increase 25 to 50 mg every 10 days to minimize both the total daily dosage and the potential for side effects.

MELATONIN.   Melatonin is a sensitive surrogate marker of circadian rhythm in humans and is under the control of the suprachiasmatic nucleus (Brzezinski, 1997). Serum melatonin levels are lowered in patients with cluster headache, particularly during a cluster bout (Waldenlind et al., 1987; Leone et al., 1995).

   Leone and coworkers (1996) performed a double-blind pilot study of melatonin versus placebo in the prophylaxis of cluster headache. After a run-in period of 1 week without prophylactic treatment, patients were randomized to receive 10-mg melatonin or placebo for 2 weeks. The authors found that, compared with the run-in period, there was a reduction in the mean number of daily attacks and a strong trend toward reduced analgesic consumption in the melatonin group but not in the placebo group. Peres and Rozen (2001) reported two patients with chronic cluster headache who were inadequately managed with verapamil 640 mg daily and then rendered pain free with add-on therapy of melatonin 9 mg daily. The authors concluded that melatonin could be an adjunct treatment for cluster headache prophylaxis, although double-blind, placebo-controlled trials are necessary to confirm this assumption.

LEUPROLIDE.   The usefulness of leuprolide (a synthetic slow-release gonadotropin-releasing hormone analog) as a prophylactic agent in cluster headache was investigated in a single-blind, placebo-controlled, randomized, parallel study in 60 men with chronic cluster headache (Nicolodi, Sicuteri, &

Poggioni, 1993). Thirty patients were administered a single dose of leuprolide 3.75 mg intramuscularly, and the remaining thirty patients were administered placebo. Leuprolide was found to induce a significant decrease of pain intensity and attack duration and frequency. The maximum effect induced by leuprolide was a 63% decrease of the pain intensity, and the mean duration of the attacks decreased from 94 minutes/day to 9.4 minutes/day. The main side effect of active treatment was decrease in libido in 6 (20%) of 30 patients. Endocrinologic measurements during treatment demonstrated an initial increase followed by a marked decrease of testosterone and luteinizing hormone.

INTRANASAL CAPSAICIN AND CIVAMIDE.   Intranasal capsaicin was first reported to be beneficial as a prophylactic agent in cluster headache by Sicuteri, Fusco, and Marabini (1989). In a double-blind, placebo-controlled study in 13 patients, 7 patients were treated with capsaicin 0.025% twice daily for 7 days in the nostril ipsilateral to the pain and the 6 control patients received camphor 3% to simulate the painful irritation associated with topical capsaicin (Marks, Rapoport, & Padla, 1993). The capsaicin-treated group experienced significantly less severe headaches over the 8 days following treatment compared with the 7 days during treatment. This improvement was not observed in the placebo-treated group. In an attempted single-blind study designed to verify the difference in efficacy of treatment with nasal capsaicin, depending on the side of application, 26 patients with episodic cluster headache received capsaicin on the symptomatic side and 26 patients were treated on the nonsymptomatic side (Fusco et al., 1994). Seventy percent of the episodic patients, treated on the ipsilateral side, experienced a significant decrease in the number of attacks for 50 to 60 days after treatment compared with the attack frequency before treatment and compared with the patients treated on the nonsymptomatic side. In a multicenter, vehicle-controlled study, patients with episodic cluster headache were treated for 7 days with either civamide 0.025% (25 g) or placebo in a volume of 100 μL (Saper et al., 2002). Although the number of headaches was reduced in the first 7 days (–60% versus –26%), the overall effect at day 20 was not significant. Nasal burning was common in the civamide group.

CHLORPROMAZINE.   Caviness and O'Brien (1980) administered chlorpromazine in 13 patients with cluster headache (11 episodic, 2 chronic) in an open-label fashion. In 12 of 13 patients the cluster headaches ceased completely within 2 weeks. Three patients had sustained relief from cluster headaches over 6 to 8 months of follow-up. The use of chlorpromazine for cluster headache needs to be balanced against the potential side effects. Tardive dyskinesia can be permanent even after a few doses, although this has been reported only occasionally. Dystonic reactions and akathisias can also occur, occasionally developing into a severe sense of restlessness or even agitation. Drowsiness occurs in many patients.

TRANSDERMAL CLONIDINE.   Clonidine, an α_2-adrenergic presynaptic agonist, has been evaluated in a study by Leone and colleagues (1997b). Transdermal clonidine 5 to 7.5 mg was administered for 2 weeks to 16 patients with episodic cluster headache. There were no significant changes in the frequency, intensity, and duration of attacks.

Greater Occipital Nerve Blockade

Anthony (1985) described the use of local anesthetic and corticosteroid injections around the greater occipital nerve (GON) homolateral to the pain. This procedure has been widely used but not subject to systematic evaluation. Recently, it was reported that of 14 patients treated with GON injection, 4 had a good response, 5 had a moderate response, and 5 no response (Peres et al., 2002). We find it a variable but sometimes effective strategy that in experienced hands has almost no morbidity save occasional small patches of alopecia because of fat atrophy (Shields, Levy, & Goadsby, 2004).

Surgery

Surgery is a last-resort measure for patients who have not responded to treatment and should be considered only when the pharmacologic options have been exploited to the fullest. Patients must be selected carefully. There is an emerging distinction between destructive procedures, which historically have been the only option, and neuromodulatory procedures. This area is moving fast, and interested readers will need to keep watching the literature.

Only patients whose headaches are exclusively unilateral should be considered for destructive surgery, because patients whose attacks have alternated sides are at risk of a contralateral recurrence after surgery. A number of procedures that interrupt either the trigeminal sensory or autonomic (cranial parasympathetic) pathways can be performed, although few are associated with long-lasting results and the side effects can be devastating. The procedures that have been reported to show some success include trigeminal sensory rhizotomy via a posterior fossa approach (Kirkpatrick, O'Brien, & MacCabe, 1993), radiofrequency trigeminal gangliorhizolysis (Mathew & Hurt, 1988), gamma knife radiotherapy (Ford et al., 1998), and microvascular decompression of the trigeminal nerve with or without microvascular decompression of the nervus intermedius (Lovely, Kotsiakis, & Jannetta, 1998). Complete trigeminal analgesia may be required for the best results. Complications include diplopia, hyperacusis, jaw deviation, corneal anesthesia, and anesthesia dolorosa. Aggressive long-term ophthalmic follow-up is essential.

The long-term follow-up from destructive procedures is relatively small. The Mayo Clinic series reported two striking findings. First, trigeminal sensory root section has a mortality (Jarrar et al., 2003). Although many cluster headache sufferers consider suicide an option, their physicians can never accept such an outcome, and thus all proposals for new therapies must be measured by that yardstick. Second, in both the Mayo Clinic series (Jarrar et al., 2003) and our own (Matharu & Goadsby, 2002), there are clearly defined patients whose attacks persist after trigeminal root section. We have three under our care at present. They respond to sumatriptan injections and require other approaches to preventive management.

Recently, Leone, Franzini, and Bussone (2001a) reported use of posterior hypothalamic neurostimulation for the treatment of intractable chronic cluster headache. The results are impressive: All patients treated thus far are responding (Franzini et al., 2003). Results from the Belgian group (Vandenheede et al.,

2004) are less encouraging: One patient has died, but clearly deep brain stimulation for intractable chronic cluster headache works for many patients who are suffering intolerably, and to some extent fit very neatly into the results of the brain-imaging studies mentioned earlier.

Following the use of greater occipital nerve injection for cluster headache and from reports of the successful suboccipital nerve stimulation in other primary headaches (Weiner & Reed, 1999; Matharu et al., 2004a), this approach is now being evaluated. It is promising and offers a much less invasive path forward in managing intractable chronic cluster headache.

PAROXYSMAL HEMICRANIA

Paroxysmal hemicrania, like cluster headache, is characterized by strictly unilateral, brief, excruciating headaches that occur in association with cranial autonomic features. Paroxysmal hemicrania differs from cluster headache mainly in the high frequency and shorter duration of individual attacks, although there is a considerable overlap in these characteristics. However, paroxysmal hemicrania responds in a dramatic and absolute fashion to indomethacin, underlining the importance of distinguishing it from cluster headache, which is not responsive to indomethacin (Headache Classification Committee of the International Headache Society, 2004).

Historical Note

Chronic paroxysmal hemicrania (CPH) was first described by Sjaastad and Dale in 1974, when they reported a case they rather aptly named "a new treatable headache entity." They consequently coined the term *chronic paroxysmal hemicrania* to describe this disorder (Sjaastad & Dale, 1976). The initial cases described were characterized by daily headaches for years without remission. Later it became clear that not all patients experienced a chronic, unremitting course; in some patients, discrete headache bouts were separated by prolonged pain-free remissions (Kudrow, Esperanca, & Vijayan, 1987; Blau & Engel, 1990; Newman et al., 1992a; Goadsby & Lipton, 1997). This remitting pattern was named *episodic paroxysmal hemicrania (EPH)* (Kudrow et al., 1987).

Epidemiology

Paroxysmal hemicrania is a rare syndrome. The prevalence of paroxysmal hemicrania is unknown, but the relationship compared with cluster headache is reported to be approximately 1% to 3% (Antonaci & Sjaastad, 1989). This is in line with our experience. Because cluster headache occurs in approximately 1 in 1000, the estimated prevalence of paroxysmal hemicrania is 1 in 50,000. The disorder has been reported in various parts of the world (Rapoport et al., 1981; Tehindrazanarivelo, Visy, & Bousser, 1992) and affects different races (Joubert, Powell, & Djikowski, 1987). In contrast to cluster headache, paroxysmal hemicrania predominates in females by a sex ratio of approximately 2:1 (Antonaci &

Sjaastad, 1989; Newman & Goadsby, 2001). The condition usually begins in adulthood at the mean age of 34 years and can last 6 to 81 years (Newman & Goadsby, 2001). We have seen a typical case begin at age 4 years.

Classification

Paroxysmal hemicrania is classified depending on the presence of a remission period. About 20% of patients have episodic paroxysmal hemicrania (EPH), which is diagnosed when there are clear remission periods between bouts of attacks, mandated as 1 month by the International Headache Society (Headache Classification Committee of the International Headache Society, 2004). The remaining 80% of patients have chronic paroxysmal hemicrania (CPH), which is diagnosed when the patients have daily attacks without a remission of at least 1 month. Notably, in paroxysmal hemicrania the chronic form dominates the clinical presentation, in contrast to cluster headache, in which the episodic form prevails.

Clinical Features

The attack profile of paroxysmal hemicrania is highly characteristic (Antonaci & Sjaastad, 1989; Goadsby & Lipton, 1997; Russell, 1999; Newman & Goadsby, 2001). The headache is strictly unilateral and without side shift in most patients. However, in four reported cases the headache demonstrated side shift (Pelz & Merskey, 1982; Bogucki, Pradalier, & Dry, 1984; Szymanska & Braciak, 1984; Pareja, 1995), and in one patient the pain was bilateral (Pollmann & Pfaffenrath, 1986). The maximum pain is most often centered on the ocular, temporal, maxillary, and frontal regions; less often, the pain involves the neck, occiput, and the retro-orbital regions. The pain is typically excruciating in severity and is described as a "claw-like," throbbing, aching, or boring sensation. The headache usually lasts 2 to 30 minutes, although it can persist for up to 2 hours. In a prospective study of 105 attacks, the mean duration was found to be 13 minutes, with a range of 3 to 46 minutes (Russell, 1984). It has an abrupt onset and cessation.

Attacks of paroxysmal hemicrania invariably occur in association with ipsilateral cranial autonomic features. Lacrimation, conjunctival injection, nasal congestion, or rhinorrhea frequently accompanies the headache; eyelid edema, ptosis, miosis, and facial sweating are less commonly reported. Interestingly, there is a case description of a patient with otherwise typical paroxysmal hemicrania, including a good indomethacin response, with no autonomic features (Bogucki et al., 1984). Photophobia and nausea may accompany some attacks, although vomiting and phonophobia are rare. It is our impression that, as in cluster headache, photophobia is more often ipsilateral on the headache side in paroxysmal hemicrania. One case of a typical migrainous aura occurring in association with paroxysmal hemicrania attacks has been reported (Matharu & Goadsby, 2001). During episodes of pain, approximately half the sufferers prefer to sit or lie still, whereas the other half take up the pacing activity usually seen with cluster headaches (Antonaci & Sjaastad, 1989).

In paroxysmal hemicrania the attacks occur at a high frequency, usually from 2 to 40 attacks daily. In a prospective study of 105 attacks in five patients, the mean attack frequency was 14 per day (range: 4 to 38) (Russell, 1984). The attacks occur regularly throughout the 24-hour period, without a preponderance of nocturnal attacks as in cluster headache. However, nocturnal attacks associated with the rapid eye movement (REM) phase of sleep have been described (Kayed, Godtlibsen, & Sjaastad, 1978).

Although most attacks are spontaneous, approximately 10% of attacks may be precipitated mechanically, either by bending or rotating the head. Attacks may also be provoked by external pressure against the transverse processes of C_{4-5}, C_2 root, or the greater occipital nerve. Alcohol ingestion triggers headaches in only 7% of patients (Antonaci & Sjaastad, 1989).

Symptomatic Paroxysmal Hemicrania and Associations

Secondary paroxysmal hemicrania has been reported to be caused by a diverse range of pathologic processes (Table 12.4). Investigation of these patients, which is driven by this list, should include at least the best available brain imaging.

The therapeutic trial of oral indomethacin should be initiated at 25 mg three times daily. If there is no or a partial response after 10 days, the dosage should be increased to 50 mg three times daily for 10 days. If the index of suspicion is high, then the dosage should be further increased to 75 mg three times daily for 14 days. Complete resolution of the headache is prompt, usually occurring within 1 to 2 days of initiating the effective dosage, although we have come across a patient who took 10 days to respond to indomethacin (unpublished observation). Injectable indomethacin 50 to 100 mg intramuscularly ("indotest") has been proposed as a diagnostic test for paroxysmal hemicrania (Antonaci et al., 1998). Complete pain relief was reported to occur for 8.2 ± 4.2 hours with intramuscular indomethacin 50 mg and 11.1 ± 3.5 hours with intramuscular indomethacin 100 mg. The indotest has the advantage that the diagnosis can be rapidly established. In patients who do not respond to indomethacin, the diagnosis should be reconsidered.

Management

Treatment of paroxysmal hemicrania is prophylactic. Indomethacin is the treatment of choice. Complete resolution of the headache is prompt, usually occurring within 1 to 2 days of initiating the effective dosage. The typical maintenance dosage ranges from 25 to 100 mg daily, but dosages of up to 300 mg daily are occasionally required. Dosage adjustments may be necessary to address the clinical fluctuations seen in paroxysmal hemicrania. During active headache cycles, skipping or even delaying doses may result in the prompt recurrence of the headache. In patients with EPH, indomethacin should be given for slightly longer than the typical headache bout and then gradually tapered. In patients with CPH, long-term treatment is usually necessary; however, long-lasting remissions have been reported in rare patients after cessation of indomethacin, and therefore drug withdrawal should be advised at least once every 6 months. Gastrointestinal side effects secondary to indomethacin may be treated with

TABLE 12.4   Lesions reported to cause paroxysmal hemicrania

Vascular Causes

Aneurysms within the circle of Willis (Medina, 1992)

Parietal arteriovenous malformation (Newman et al., 1992b)

Stroke

Middle cerebral artery (MCA) infarct (Newman et al., 1992b)

Occipital infarction (Broeske et al., 1993)

Tumors

Frontal lobe tumor (Medina, 1992)

Gangliocytoma of the sella turcica (Vijayan, 1992)

Cavernous sinus meningioma (Sjaastad et al., 1995)

Pituitary microadenoma (Gatzonis et al., 1996)

Cerebral metastases of parotid epidermoid carcinoma (Mariano et al., 1999)

Pancoast tumor (Delreux et al., 1989)

Miscellaneous

Maxillary cyst (Gatzonis et al., 1996)

Intracranial hypertension (Hannerz & Jogestrand, 1993)

Essential thrombocythaemia (MacMillan & Nukada, 1989)

Collagen vascular disease (Medina, 1992)

antacids, misoprostol, histamine H_2 receptor antagonists, or proton pump inhibitors and should always be considered for patients who require long-term treatment.

The mechanism behind the absolute responsiveness to indomethacin is unknown. It appears to be independent of indomethacin's effect on prostaglandin synthesis, because other NSAIDs have little or no effect on paroxysmal hemicrania.

In patients who do not respond to indomethacin, the diagnosis should be reconsidered. Patients who need escalating doses of indomethacin to suppress the symptoms, become refractory to treatment with indomethacin, or require continuous high-dose indomethacin may have an underlying pathologic condition and need careful diagnostic evaluation for symptomatic causes. Recall that indomethacin can temporarily lower cerebrospinal fluid (CSF) pressure (Harrigan et al., 1997; Forderreuther & Straube, 2000), so brain imaging is indicated when the clinical course is atypical.

Patients who cannot tolerate indomethacin face a difficult challenge. No other drug is consistently effective. Drugs other than indomethacin reported to be partially or completely effective, mainly in isolated cases, include other NSAIDs, such as aspirin (Antonaci & Sjaastad, 1989; Kudrow & Kudrow, 1989), naproxen (Durko & Klimek, 1987), and piroxicam beta-cyclodextrin (Sjaastad & Antonaci, 1995), the COX-2 inhibitor celecoxib (Mathew, Kailasam, &

Fischer, 2000), calcium channel antagonists (verapamil [Shabbir & McAbee, 1994; Evers & Husstedt, 1996] and flunarizine [Coria et al., 1992]), acetazolamide (Warner, Wamil, & Mclean, 1994), and steroids (Hannerz, Ericson, & Bergstrand, 1987). We have had limited success with COX-2 inhibitors and verapamil.

Natural History and Prognosis

Because paroxysmal hemicrania is a relatively recently described syndrome, there is a paucity of literature on its natural history and long-term prognosis. The available evidence suggests that it is a lifelong condition. Patients can expect sustained efficacy of indomethacin treatment without developing tachyphylaxis, although about one fourth develop gastrointestinal side effects (Pareja et al., 2001). Indomethacin does not seem to alter the condition long term, although a significant proportion of patients can decrease the dosage of indomethacin required to maintain a pain-free state. One of us has now for 4 years followed a patient who was 10 years old when she was brought in; patients remain on indomethacin with an excellent response and with headache returning after skipping only two doses.

SHORT-LASTING UNILATERAL NEURALGIFORM HEADACHE ATTACKS WITH CONJUNCTIVAL INJECTION AND TEARING (SUNCT SYNDROME)

SUNCT syndrome, like the other trigeminal autonomic cephalgias (TACs), manifests as a unilateral headache that occurs in association with cranial autonomic features. It is distinguished from the other TACs by (1) the very brief duration of attacks that can occur very frequently and (2) the presence of *prominent* conjunctival injection and lacrimation, both of which are present in most patients. Because some patients with the same clinical problem may not have conjunctival injection or tearing, we believe the syndrome should be renamed *SUNA*: short-lasting unilateral neuralgiform headache attacks with cranial autonomic features. Diagnostic criteria for this entity are available in the second edition of the IHS classification (Headache Classification Committee of the International Headache Society, 2004).

Historical Note

SUNCT syndrome was first described in 1978 (Sjaastad et al., 1978) and more fully characterized in 1989 (Sjaastad et al., 1989).

Epidemiology

The prevalence and incidence of SUNCT syndrome are unknown, although the extremely low number of reported cases suggests that it is a rare syndrome. We found only 58 complete case descriptions in the English language literature at the time of this writing (De Benedittis, 1996; Goadsby & Lipton, 1997; Pareja &

Sjaastad, 1997; Benoliel & Sharav, 1998; Raimondi & Gardella, 1998; D'Andrea, Granella, & Cadaldini, 1999; May et al., 1999b; Ertsey et al., 2000; Graff-Radford, 2000; Lain, Caminero, & Pareja, 2000; Leone et al., 2000; Morales-Asin et al., 2000; Montes et al., 2001; Moris et al., 2001; D'Andrea & Granella, 2001; D'Andrea et al., 2001; Penart, Firth & Bowen, 2001; Sabatowski et al., 2001; Sesso, 2001; ter Berg & Goadsby, 2001; Black & Dodick, 2002; Hannerz & Linderoth, 2002; Matharu, Boes, & Goadsby, 2002; Porta-Etessam et al., 2002; Chakravarty & Mukherjee, 2003; Empl, Goadsby, & Kaube, 2003; Matharu, Boes, & Goadsby, 2003b; Piovesan et al., 2003; Cohen, Matharu, & Goadsby, 2004). The disorder has a male predominance (36 males, 16 females), with a sex ratio of approximately 2:1. The typical age of onset is between 40 and 70 years, although it ranges from 10 to 82 years of age (mean: 52 years).

Pathophysiology

In pathophysiologic terms, SUNCT shares much with cluster headache (Goadsby & Lipton, 1997). Both have trigeminal and cranial autonomic activation with largely first (ophthalmic) division of trigeminal pain and prominent symptoms such as lacrimation and conjunctival injection. A single fMRI study has demonstrated activations in the posterior hypothalamic gray matter (Figure 12.4) in a comparable site to that reported in cluster headache (May et al., 1999b). It seems likely that SUNCT, like cluster headache, is a disorder of the central nervous system.

Clinical Features

The pain is usually maximal in the ophthalmic distribution of the trigeminal nerve, especially the orbital or periorbital regions, forehead, and temple, although it may radiate to the other ipsilateral trigeminal divisions. Attacks are typically unilateral; however, three patients simultaneously experienced the pain on the opposite side (Pareja & Sjaastad, 1997). The severity of pain is generally moderate to severe. The pain is usually described as stabbing, burning, pricking, or electric shocklike in character. The individual attacks last only 5 to 250 seconds (mean duration: 49 seconds) (Pareja et al., 1996b), although attacks lasting up to 2 hours each have been described (Pareja et al., 1996a; Raimondi & Gardella, 1998; Matharu et al., 2002). The paroxysms begin abruptly, reaching the maximum intensity within 2 to 3 seconds; the pain maintains at the maximum intensity before abating rapidly (Pareja & Sjaastad, 1997). The temporal pattern is quite variable, with the symptomatic periods erratically alternating with remissions. Symptomatic periods last from a few days to several months and occur once or twice annually. Remissions typically last a few months, although they can range from 1 week to 7 years. Symptomatic periods seem to increase in frequency and duration over time (Pareja & Sjaastad, 1997). The attack frequency during the symptomatic phase varies immensely among sufferers and within an individual sufferer. Attacks may be as infrequent as once a day or less to more than 30 attacks an hour. Rarely, patients report attacks that recur in a repetitive and overlapping fashion for 1 to 3 hours at a time (Pareja et al., 1994). Most

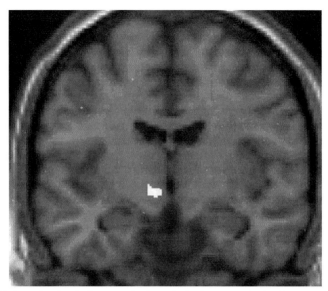

FIGURE 12.4 Activation in the posterior hypothalamic gray mater in short-lasting unilateral neuralgiform headache attacks with conjunctival injection and tearing (SUNCT). (From May et al., 1999b.)

SUNCT attacks occur during the daytime, tending to show a bimodal distribution with morning and afternoon/evening predominance. Nocturnal attacks are seldom reported (Pareja et al., 1996b).

Acute headache episodes in SUNCT syndrome are virtually always accompanied by both ipsilateral conjunctival injection and lacrimation, which are characteristically prominent. Ipsilateral nasal congestion, rhinorrhoea, eyelid edema, ptosis, miosis, and facial redness or sweating are less commonly reported. The associated conjunctival injection and tearing usually begin 1 to 2 seconds after onset of the pain and may outlast the pain by a few seconds. Nausea, vomiting, photophobia, and phonophobia are not normally associated with SUNCT syndrome, but when present, photophobia is again usually ipsilateral to the pain. Restlessness is not a feature of SUNCT syndrome (Pareja & Sjaastad, 1997).

Most patients can precipitate attacks by touching certain trigger zones within trigeminal innervated distribution and, occasionally, even from an extratrigeminal territory. Precipitants include touching the face or scalp, washing, shaving, eating, chewing, brushing teeth, talking, and coughing (Pareja & Sjaastad, 1997). Neck movements can also precipitate attacks, although some patients can reduce or abort attacks by continuously rotating their neck (Sjaastad et al., 1989; Pareja & Sjaastad, 1997). Unlike in trigeminal neuralgia, most patients have no refractory period.

Secondary SUNCT

Secondary SUNCT has been reported, and remarkably, all cases have had posterior fossa abnormalities. The secondary causes include homolateral cerebellopontine-angle arteriovenous malformations in two patients (Bussone et al., 1991; Morales et al., 1994), a brainstem cavernous hemangioma (De Benedittis, 1996), a posterior fossa lesion in a patient with human immunodeficiency virus/acquired immunodeficiency syndrome (HIV/AIDS) (Goadsby & Lipton, 1997), severe basilar impression causing pontomedullary compression in a patient with osteogenesis imperfecta (ter Berg & Goadsby, 2001), craniosynostosis resulting in a foreshortened posterior fossa (Moris et al., 2001), and ischemic brainstem infarction (Penart et al., 2001; van Vliet et al., 2003c). These posterior fossa abnormalities emphasize the absolute need for a cranial MRI in any suspected case of SUNCT. Our experience (Levy et al., 2003) and other reported cases (Ferrari, Haan, & van Seters, 1988; Massiou et al., 2002) suggest that a SUNCT-like syndrome may be seen with pituitary adenomas and that this is not related to tumor size (Levy et al., 2004a).

Differential Diagnosis

The differential diagnosis of very brief headaches includes SUNCT (primary and secondary forms), trigeminal neuralgia, primary stabbing headache, and to a lesser extent, paroxysmal hemicrania. Differentiating SUNCT from trigeminal neuralgia can be challenging in some cases, because the clinical phenotypes of the two syndromes overlap considerably. Both types of headaches are short lasting, can have a high frequency of attacks, and display clustering of attacks. Both are principally unilateral headaches, and the trigger zones behave similarly. The usual onset for both types is during middle or old age. However, these two syndromes differ in a number of striking ways (Table 12.5), awareness of which can aid in their differentiation (Sjaastad & Kruszewski, 1992; Goadsby et al., 2001). Primary stabbing headache (also known as *idiopathic stabbing headache*) refers to brief, sharp, or jabbing pain in the head that occurs either as a single episode or in brief, repeated volleys. The pain is usually over the ophthalmic trigeminal distribution, whereas the face is generally spared. The pain usually lasts a fraction of a second but can persist for up to 1 minute, overlapping with the SUNCT phenotype, and recurs at irregular intervals (hours to days). Generally these headaches are easily distinguishable clinically because they differ in several respects: In primary stabbing headache there is a female preponderance, the site and radiation of pain often varies between attacks, most attacks tend to be spontaneous, cranial autonomic features are absent, and the attacks commonly subside after administration of indomethacin (Pareja et al., 1996c; Pareja, Kruszewski, & Caminero, 1999).

SUNCT syndrome also must be differentiated from short-lasting paroxysmal hemicrania. Paroxysmal hemicrania prevails in females, the attacks have a uniform distribution through day and night, the triggers differ from those in SUNCT, and the attacks are exquisitely responsive to indomethacin. If there is any diagnostic uncertainty, a trial of indomethacin is warranted.

TABLE 12.5 Differentiating features of typical SUNCT and trigeminal neuralgia

Feature	SUNCT	Trigeminal neuralgia
Gender ratio (male: female)	2.1:1	1:2
Site of pain	V1	V2/3
Severity of pain	Moderate to severe	Very severe
Duration (seconds)	5–250	<5
Autonomic features	Prominent	Sparse or none
Refractory period	Absent	Present
Response to carbamazepine	Partial	Complete

Treatment

Until recently, SUNCT was thought to be highly refractory to treatment (Pareja et al., 1995). Several categories of drugs used in other headache syndromes, that is, nonsteroidal anti-inflammatory drugs (including indomethacin), paracetamol (acetaminophen), 5-hydroxytryptamine agonists (triptans, ergotamine, and dihydroergotamine), beta-blockers, tricyclic antidepressants, calcium channel antagonists (verapamil and nifedipine), methysergide, lithium, prednisolone (prednisone), phenytoin, baclofen, and intravenous lignocaine have proved to be ineffectual (Pareja et al., 1995). Partial improvement with carbamazepine has been observed in several patients (Pareja, Kruzewski, & Sjaastad, 1995; Peatfield, Bahra, & Goadsby, 1998; Raimondi & Gardella, 1998; Ertsey et al., 2000; Matharu et al., 2002).

Our experience with intravenous lidocaine is very different from that of Pareja and associates (1995). Lidocaine by infusion can suppress SUNCT very effectively (Matharu, Cohen, & Goadsby, 2004b). In most patients, attacks return when the dosage is lowered but, in about one fourth of patients, it seems capable of inducing a remission that lasts 6 to 9 months. We have noted a remarkably high rate of neuropsychiatric side effects, with 6 of 10 patients who had had intravenous lidocaine in the last 2 years being affected (Gil-Gouveia & Goadsby, submitted for publication). It is always reversible.

Recently, lamotrigine has been reported to be highly efficacious in a number of patients (D'Andrea et al., 1999; Leone et al., 2000; D'Andrea et al., 2001; Gutierrez-Garcia, 2002; Chakravarty & Mukherjee, 2003; Piovesan et al., 2003). Lamotrigine, 100 to 300 mg daily, induced a complete remission in seven patients and produced about an 80% improvement in the other two patients. Although the ultimate confirmation of the usefulness of lamotrigine in treating this debilitating syndrome should come from a randomized double-blind, placebo-controlled clinical trial, for now we regard it as the treatment of choice.

A number of reported cases of SUNCT patients responded completely to gabapentin (Graff-Radford, 2000; Hunt, Dodick, & Bosch, 2002; Porta-Etessam et al., 2002), typically 900 to 2700 mg daily. We have recently reported a patient who responded completely to topiramate 50 mg daily (Matharu et al., 2002). These observations clearly need to be confirmed in other cases. Nonetheless, given the debilitating nature of this headache, gabapentin and topiramate are reasonable second-line agents in patients who do not respond to a trial of lamotrigine.

Several surgical approaches have been tried in SUNCT syndrome. Anesthetic blockades of pericranial nerves have been reported to be ineffective (Pareja et al., 1995). There are six case reports of apparently successful treatment of SUNCT syndrome with surgical procedures. Two patients were treated with the Jannetta procedure (Lenaerts, Diederich, & Phuoe, 1997; Gardella et al., 2001), and one was treated with percutaneous trigeminal ganglion compression. Three patients were treated with retrogasserian glycerol rhizolysis, two of whom were treated twice. All five treatments provided complete pain relief, although the duration of the benefit ranged from 2 to 4.5 years. One of these patients went on to have a trigeminal nerve balloon compression with a good result (Hannerz & Linderoth, 2002). In addition, there is one report of a partial response with local opioid blockade of the superior cervical ganglion (Sabatowski et al., 2001). However, follow-up in some of these patients was limited to less than 18 months, which makes it difficult to assess the actual effectiveness of the procedures given the episodic nature of the syndrome. Black and Dodick reported on two SUNCT cases refractory to various surgical procedures (Black & Dodick, 2002).The first patient underwent a glycerol rhizotomy, gamma knife radiosurgery, and microvascular decompression of the trigeminal nerve, and the second patient underwent gamma knife radiosurgery of the trigeminal root exit zone and two microvascular decompressions of the trigeminal nerve. Neither patient benefited from these procedures. In addition, the first patient suffered from anesthesia dolorosa, and the second patient experienced unilateral deafness, chronic vertigo, and dysequilibrium as a result of surgery. Hannerz and Linderoth (2002) made a brief reference to a patient who had not benefited from trigeminal vascular decompression and two gamma knife radiosurgeries of the trigeminal root. We have seen two patients who failed to demonstrate a persistent response following trigeminal thermocoagulation and microvascular decompression (unpublished observations). It has been reported (in abstract form) that one patient has had deep brain stimulation in the region of the posterior hypothalamic gray matter and has achieved control of attacks (Leone et al., 2004). This is consistent with the known pathophysiology, and further observations are important. All things considered, destructive surgical procedures should be avoided.

Natural History

The natural history of SUNCT syndrome is poorly understood. In a series of 21 patients, the average duration of symptoms was 11.8 years. In 10 of these patients the duration of SUNCT exceeded 10 years. The longest reported duration of SUNCT is 48 years (Pareja & Sjaastad, 1997). It appears to be a lifelong disorder once it starts, although more prospective data are needed. The syndrome itself is not fatal and does not cause any long-term neurologic sequelae.

OTHER SYNDROMES POSSIBLY RELATED TO CLUSTER HEADACHE

Kudrow (1980), in his comprehensive monograph on cluster headache, recognizes "cluster-migraine" as an entity in which migraine patients have some of the characteristics of cluster headache, and "cluster-vertigo" for recurrent attacks of giddiness associated with bouts of cluster headache. The latter term has been criticized by Vijayan (1990), who pointed out that, when Ménière's disease and cluster headache affect the same patient, the conditions recur independently. The term *cluster-migraine* seems unhelpful and probably reflects either migraine patients who have cranial autonomic activation (Barbanti et al., 2002) or cluster headache patients who have migrainous features, such as photophobia or phonophobia (Bahra et al., 2002). Diamond, Mogabgab, and Diamond (1982) put forward the concept of "cluster headache variant," a combination of constant vascular headache with episodic exacerbations and sudden stabs of pain, mostly controlled by indomethacin. In retrospect, this is almost certainly hemicrania continua. Does the response to indomethacin of chronic paroxysmal hemicrania, exertional headache, and jabbing "ice-pick" head pains imply a common underlying factor? Until the pathophysiology of headache is more clearly understood, it is difficult to classify many of the variations seen in clinical practice.

OVERVIEW

Cluster headache must surely be mediated by paroxysmal discharge of central neurons that in turn permit trigeminal and parasympathetic nervous overactivity. Given the recent PET data, the hypothalamic gray matter, which contains the circadian or clock areas, is the most likely candidate for the fundamental driving or permissive area of the brain. The pain and autonomic phenomena usually develop together, but one may precede the other or occur in isolation, as is particularly evident after section of the trigeminal root or nervus intermedius as described earlier. That the pain of cluster headache may continue or recur after one or both of these surgical procedures further indicates its central origin. This does not deny the important contribution to pain made by the cerebral arteries or the efficacy of vasoconstrictor agents such as ergotamine in breaking the interaction between trigeminal nerves and blood vessels to relieve the pain. The ocular Horner's syndrome on the painful side is most readily explained as a postganglionic lesion of the cervical sympathetic nerves in the pericarotid plexus, which masks the effects of general sympathetic activation during the attack.

The distinctive clinical picture of cluster headache leaves no excuse for any delay in diagnosis or in applying the appropriate treatment. Most individual attacks respond well to oxygen inhalation or subcutaneous sumatriptan, if they have not already been helped by ergotamine. Most bouts of cluster headache can be brought under control by a course of steroids or prophylactic medication with verapamil, lithium, or methysergide. Rarely does one have to consider surgical intervention, but the response of otherwise intractable chronic cluster headache to neuromodulation is most encouraging.

The challenge for future research is to understand the mechanism by which hypothalamic activation translates into pain and at what level in the central nervous system preventive drugs have their actions.

References

Alberca, R., & Ochoa, J. J. (1994). Cluster tic syndrome. *Neurology, 44,* 996–999.

Andersson, P. G., & Jespersen, L. T. (1986). Dihydroergotamine nasal spray in the treatment of attacks of cluster headache. *Cephalalgia, 6,* 51–54.

Anthony, M. (1985). Arrest of attacks of cluster headache by local steroid injection of the occipital nerve. In F. C. Rose (Ed.), *Migraine: Clinical and Research Advance* (pp. 169–173). London: Karger.

Anthony, M., & Draher, B. N. (1992). Mechanism of action of steroids in cluster headache. In F. C. Rose (Ed.), *New Advances in Headache Research* (Vol. 2, pp. 271–274). London: Smith-Gordon.

Anthony, M., & Lance, J. W. (1971). Histamine and serotonin in cluster headache. *Arch Neurol, 25,* 225 229.

Anthony, M., Lord, G. D. A., & Lance, J. W. (1978). Controlled trials of cimetidine in migraine and cluster headache. *Headache, 18,* 261–264.

Antonaci, F., Pareja, J. A., Caminero, A. B., & Sjaastad, O. (1998). Chronic paroxysmal hemicrania and hemicrania continua. Parenteral indomethacin: The "indotest." *Headache, 38,* 122–128.

Antonaci, F., & Sjaastad, O. (1989). Chronic paroxysmal hemicrania (CPH): A review of the clinical manifestations. *Headache, 29,* 648–656.

Appelbaum, J., & Noronha, A. (1989). Pericarotid cluster headache. *J Neurol, 236,* 430–431.

Bahra, A., Gawel, M. J., Hardebo, J.-E., Millson, D., Brean, S. A., & Goadsby, P. J. (2000). Oral zolmitriptan is effective in the acute treatment of cluster headache. *Neurology, 54,* 1832–1839.

Bahra, A., & Goadsby, P. J. (2004). Diagnostic delays and mis-management in cluster headache. *Acta Neurol Scand, 109,* 175–179.

Bahra, A., May, A., & Goadsby, P. J. (2002). Cluster headache: A prospective clinical study in 230 patients with diagnostic implications. *Neurology, 58,* 354–361.

Barbanti, P., Fabbrini, G., Pesare, M., Vanacore, N., & Cerbo, R. (2002). Unilateral cranial autonomic symptoms in migraine. *Cephalalgia, 22,* 256–259.

Barre, F. (1982). Cocaine as an abortive agent in cluster headache. *Headache, 22,* 69–73.

Bartsch, T., & Goadsby, P. J. (2002). Stimulation of the greater occipital nerve induces increased central excitability of dural afferent input. *Brain, 125,* 1496–1509.

Bartsch, T., & Goadsby, P. J. (2003). Increased responses in trigeminocervical nociceptive neurones to cervical input after stimulation of the dura mater. *Brain, 126,* 1801–1813.

Benoliel, R., & Sharav, Y. (1998). SUNCT syndrome—case report and literature review. *Oral Surg Oral Med Oral Pathol Oral Radiol Endod, 85,* 158–161.

Berde, B., & Schild, H. O. (1978). *Ergot alkaloids and related compounds* (Vol. 49). Berlin: Springer.

Black, D. F., & Dodick, D. W. (2002). Two cases of medically and surgically intractable SUNCT: A reason for caution and an argument for a central mechanism. *Cephalalgia, 22,* 201–204.

Blakeborough, P., Fowler, P. A., & Ashford, E. A. (1993). The use of sumatriptan in patients taking migraine prophylactic agents. *Cephalalgia, 13,* 163.

Blau, J. N., & Engel, H. (1990). Episodic paroxysmal hemicrania: A further case and review of the literature. *J Neurol Neurosurg Psychiatry, 53,* 343–344.

Boes, C. J., Capobioanco, D. J., Matharu, M. S., & Goadsby, P. J. (2002). Wilfred Harris' early description of cluster headache. *Cephalalgia, 22,* 320–326.

Bogucki, A., Szymanska, R., & Braciak, W. (1984). Chronic paroxysmal hemicrania: Lack of a pre-chronic stage. *Cephalalgia, 4,* 187–189.

Boiardi, A., Bussone, E., Martini, M., Di Giulio, A. M., Tansini, E., Merati, B., & Panerai, A. E. (1983). Endocrinological responses in cluster headache. *J Neurol Neurosurg Psychiatry, 46,* 956–958.

Broeske, D., Lenn, N. J., & Cantos, E. (1993). Chronic paroxysmal hemicrania in a young child: Possible relation to ipsilateral occipital infarction. *J Child Neurol, 8,* 235–236.

Brooke, R. I. (1978). Periodic migrainous neuralgia: A cause of dental pain. *Oral Surg Oral Med Oral Pathol Oral Radiol Endod, 46,* 511–516.

Brzezinski, A. (1997). Melatonin in humans. *N Engl J Med, 336,* 186–195.

Bussone, G., Boiardi, A., Merati, B., Crenna, P., & Picco, A. (1979). Chronic cluster headache: Response to lithium treatment. *J Neurol, 221,* 181–185.

Bussone, G., Leone, M., Peccarisi, C., Micieli, G., Granella, F., Magri, M., Manzoni, G. C., & Nappi, G. (1990). Double blind comparison of lithium and verapamil in cluster headache prophylaxis. *Headache, 30,* 411–417.

Bussone, G., Leone, M., Volta, G. D., Strada, L., & Gasparotti, R. (1991). Short-lasting unilateral neuralgiform headache attacks with tearing and conjunctival injection: The first symptomatic case. *Cephalalgia, 11,* 123–127.

Caviness, V. S., & O'Brien, P. (1980). Cluster headache: Response to chlorpromazine. *Headache, 20,* 128–131.

Chakravarty, A., & Mukherjee, A. (2003). SUNCT syndrome responsive to lamotrigine: Documentation of the first Indian case. *Cephalalgia, 23,* 474–475.

Cid, C., Berciano, J., & Pascual, J. (2000). Retro-ocular headache with autonomic features resembling "continuous" cluster headache in a lateral medullary infarction. *J Neurol Neurosurg Psychiatry, 69,* 134–141.

Cohen, A. S., Matharu, M. S., & Goadsby, P. J. (2004). SUNCT syndrome in the elderly. *Cephalalgia, 24,* 508–509.

Coria, F., Claveria, L. E., Jimenez-Jimenez, F. J., & Seijas, E. V. (1992). Episodic paroxysmal hemicrania responsive to calcium channel blockers. *J Neurol Neurosurg Psychiatry, 55,* 166.

Costa, A., Pucci, E., Antonaci, F., Sances, G., Granella, F., Broich, G., & Nappi, G. (2000). The effect of intranasal cocaine and lidocaine on nitroglycerin-induced attacks in cluster headache. *Cephalalgia, 20,* 85–91.

Couch, J. R., & Ziegler, D. K. (1978). Prednisone therapy for cluster headache. *Headache, 18,* 219–221.

Cremer, P., Halmagyi, G. M., & Goadsby, P. J. (1995). Secondary cluster headache responsive to sumatriptan. *J Neurol Neurosurg Psychiatry, 59,* 633–634.

Curran, D. A., Hinterberger, H., & Lance, J. W. (1967). Methysergide. *Res Clin Stud Headache, 1,* 74–122.

Cuypers, J., Altenkirch, H., & Bunge, S. (1981). Personality profiles in cluster headache and migraine. *Headache, 21,* 21–24.

Dahl, A., Russell, D., Nyberg-Hansen, R., & Rootwelt, K. (1990). Cluster headache: Transcranial Doppler ultrasound and rCBF studies. *Cephalalgia, 10,* 87–94.

D'Alessandro, R., Gamberini, G., Benassi, G., Morganti, G., Cortelli, P., & Lugaresi, E. (1986). Cluster headache in the Republic of San Marino. *Cephalalgia, 6,* 159–162.

Dalsgaard-Neilsen, T. (1960). Über die prophylaktische Behandlung der Migraine mit Deseril. *Praxis, 49,* 867–868.

Damasio, H., & Lyon, L. (1980). Lithium carbonate in the treatment of cluster headache. *J Neurol, 224,* 1–8.

D'Andrea, G., & Granella, F. (2001). SUNCT syndrome: The first case in childhood. *Cephalalgia, 21,* 701–702.

D'Andrea, G., Granella, F., & Cadaldini, M. (1999). Possible usefulness of lamotrigine in the treatment of SUNCT syndrome. *Neurology, 53,* 1609.

D'Andrea, G., Granella, F., Ghiotto, N., & Nappi, G. (2001). Lamotrigine in the treatment of SUNCT syndrome. *Neurology, 57,* 1723–1725.

De Benedittis, G. (1996). SUNCT syndrome associated with cavernous angioma of the brain stem. *Cephalalgia, 16,* 503–506.

de la Sayette, V., Schaeffer, S., Coskun, O., Leproux, F., & Defer, G. (1999). Cluster headache-like attack as an opening symptom of a unilateral infarction of the cervical cord: Persistent anaesthesia and dysaesthesia to cold stimuli. *J Neurol Neurosurg Psychiatry, 66,* 397–400.

Delreux, V., Kevers, L., & Callewaert, A. (1989). Hemicranie paroxystique inaugurant un syndrome de Pancoast. *Rev Neurol (Paris), 145,* 151–152.

Di Sabato, F., Fusco, B. M., Pelaia, P., & Giacovazzo, M. (1993). Hyperbaric oxygen therapy in cluster headache. *Pain, 52,* 243–245.

Diamond, S., & Freitag, F. G., & Cohen, J. S. (1984). Cluster headache with trigeminal neuralgia. An uncommon association that may be more than coincidental. *Postgrad Med J, 75,* 165–172.

Diamond, S., Mogabgab, E. R., & Diamond, M. (1982). Cluster headache variant: Spectrum of a new headache syndrome responsive to indomethacin. In F. C. Rose (Ed.), *Advances in Migraine Research and Therapy* (pp. 57–65). New York: Raven Press.

Dodick, D. W., Rozen, T. D., Goadsby, P. J., & Silberstein, S. D. (2000). Cluster headache. *Cephalalgia, 20,* 787–803.

Drummond, P. D. (1988). Autonomic disturbance in cluster headache. *Brain, 111,* 1199–1209.

Drummond, P. D., & Lance, J. W. (1984). Thermographic changes in cluster headache. *Neurology, 34,* 1292–1298.

Drummond, P. D., & Lance, J. W. (1992). Pathological sweating and flushing accompanying the trigeminal lacrimation reflex in patients with cluster headache and in patients with a confirmed site of cervical sympathetic deficit. Evidence for parasympathetic cross-innervation. *Brain, 115,* 1429–1445.

Durko, A., & Klimek, A. (1987). Naproxen in the treatment of chronic paroxysmal hemicrania. *Cephalalgia, 7,* 361–362.

Eekers, P. J. E., & Koehler, P. J. (2001). Naratriptan prophylactic treatment in cluster headache. *Cephalalgia, 21,* 75–76.

Ekbom, K. (1947). Ergotamine tartrate orally in Horton's "histaminic cephalalgia" (also called Harris's ciliary neuralgia). *Acta Psychiatr Scand, 46,* 106–113.

Ekbom, K. (1969). Prophylactic treatment of cluster headache with the new serotonin agonist, BC–105. *Acta Neurol Scand, 45,* 601–610.

Ekbom, K. (1970). A clinical comparison of cluster headache and migraine. *Acta Neurol Scand, 46*(Suppl. 41), 1–48.

Ekbom, K. (1974). Litium rid kroniska symptom av cluster headache. *Opusc Med, 19,* 148–156.

Ekbom, K. (1975). Some observations on pain in cluster headache. *Headache, 14,* 219–225.

Ekbom, K. (1977). Lithium in the treatment of chronic cluster headache. *Headache, 17,* 39–40.

Ekbom, K. (1981). Lithium for cluster headache: Review of the literature and preliminary results of long-term treatment. *Headache, 21,* 132–139.

Ekbom, K., Ahlborg, B., & Schele, R. (1978). Prevalence of migraine and cluster headache in Swedish men of 18. *Headache, 18,* 9–19.

Ekbom, K., & Greitz, T. (1970). Carotid angiography in cluster headache. *Acta Radiol, 10,* 177–186.

Ekbom, K., Krabbe, A., Micelli, G., Prusinski, A., Cole, J. A., Pilgrim, A. J., Noronha, D., & Miceli, G. (1995). Cluster headache attacks treated for up to three months with subcutaneous sumatriptan (6 mg). *Cephalalgia, 15,* 230–236.

Ekbom, K., Monstad, I., Prusinski, A., Cole, J. A., Pilgrim, A. J., & Noronha, D. (1993). Subcutaneous sumatriptan in the acute treatment of cluster headache: A dose comparison study. *Acta Neurol Scand, 88,* 63–69.

Ekbom, K., & Solomon, S. (2000). Management of cluster headache. In J. Olesen, P. Tfelt-Hansen, & K. M. A. Welch (Eds.), *The Headaches* (pp. 731–740). Philadelphia: Lippincott, Williams & Wilkins.

Ekbom, K., Svensson, D. A., & Waldenlind, E. (2002). Age at onset and sex ratio in cluster headache: Observations over three decades. *Cephalalgia, 22,* 94–100.

Ekbom, K., & The Sumatriptan Cluster Headache Study Group. (1991). Treatment of acute cluster headache with sumatriptan. *N Engl J Med, 325,* 322–326.

Ekbom, K. A. (1962). Treatment of migraine, Horton's syndrome and restless legs with Deseril (UML-491). *Acta Neurol Scand, 38,* 313–318.

El Amrani, M., Massiou, H., & Bousser, M.-G. (2002). A negative trial of sodium valproate in cluster headache: Methodological issues. *Cephalalgia, 22,* 205–208.

Empl, M., Goadsby, P. J., & Kaube, H. (2003). Migraine with aura, episodic cluster headache, and SUNCT syndrome consecutively in a patient: Trigemino-vascular trinity. *Cephalalgia, 23,* 584.

Ertsey, C., Bozsik, G., Afra, J., & Jelencsik, I. (2000). A case of SUNCT syndrome with neurovascular compression. *Cephalalgia, 20,* 325.

Evers, S., Frese, A., Majewski, A., Albrecht, O., & Husstedt, I. W. (2002). Age of onset in cluster headache: The clinical spectrum (three case reports). *Cephalalgia, 22,* 160–162.

Evers, S., & Husstedt, I.-W. (1996). Alternatives in drug treatment of chronic paroxysmal hemicrania. *Headache, 36,* 429–432.

Evers, S., Soros, P., Brilla, R., Gerding, H., & Husstedt, I.-W. (1997). Cluster headache after orbital exenteration. *Cephalalgia, 17,* 680–682.

Fanciullacci, M., Alessandri, M., Figini, M., Geppetti, P., & Michelacci, S. (1995). Increase in plasma calcitonin gene–related peptide from extracerebral circulation during nitroglycerin-induced cluster headache attack. *Pain, 60,* 119–123.

Fanciullacci, M., Pietrini, U., Gatto, G., Boccuni, M., & Sicuteri, F. (1982). Latent dysautonomic pupillary lateralization in cluster headache: A pupillometric study. *Cephalalgia, 2,* 135–144.

Ferrari, M. D., Haan, J., & van Seters, A. P. (1988). Bromocriptine-induced trigeminal neuralgia attacks in a patient with pituitary tumor. *Neurology, 38,* 1482–1484.

Fogan, L. (1985). Treatment of cluster headache: A double blind comparison of oxygen vs air inhalation. *Arch Neurol, 42,* 362–363.

Ford, R. G., Ford, K. T., Swaid, S., Young, P., & Jennelle, R. (1998). Gamma knife treatment of refractory cluster headache. *Headache, 38,* 3–9.

Forderreuther, S., Mayer, M., & Straube, A. (2003). Treatment of cluster headache with topiramate: Effects and side-effects in five patients. *Cephalalgia, 23,* 69–70.

Forderreuther, S., & Straube, A. (2000). Indomethacin reduces CSF pressure in intracranial hypertension. *Neurology, 55,* 1043–1045.

Formisano, R., Angelini, A., De Vuono, G., Calisse, P., Fiacco, F., Catarci, T., Bozzao, L., & Cerbo, R. (1990). Cluster-like headache and head injury: Case report. *Ital J Neurol Sci, 11,* 303–305.

Franzini, A., Ferroli, P., Leone, M., & Broggi, G. (2003). Stimulation of the posterior hypothalamus for treatment of chronic intractable cluster headaches. The first reported series. *Neurosurgery, 52,* 1095–1101.

Friedman, A. P. (1960). Clinical observations with 1-methyl-lysergic acid butanolamide (UML-491) in vascular headache. *Angiology, 11,* 364–366.

Friedman, A. P., & Losin, S. (1961). Evaluation of UML-491 in the treatment of vascular headache. *Arch Neurol, 4,* 241–245.

Friedman, A. P., & Mikropoulos, H. E. (1958). Cluster headache. *Neurology (Minneapolis), 8,* 653–663.

Fusco, B. M., Marabini, S., Magg, C. A., Fiore, G., & Geppetti, P. (1994). Preventative effect of repeated nasal applications of capsaicin in cluster headache. *Pain, 59,* 321–325.

Gabai, I. J., & Spierings, E. L. H. (1989). Prophylactic treatment of cluster headache with verapamil. *Headache, 129,* 167–168.

Gallagher, R. M., Mueller, L., & Ciervo, C. A. (1996). Analgesic use in cluster headache. *Headache, 36,* 105–107.

Gardella, L., Viruega, A., Rojas, H., & Nagel, J. (2001). A case of a patient with SUNCT syndrome treated with Jannetta procedure. *Cephalalgia, 21,* 996–999.

Garrison, J. C. (1990). Histamine, bradykinin, 5-hydroxytryptamine and their antagonists. In A. G. Gilman, T. W. Rall, A. S. Niles, & P. Taylor (Eds.), *The Pharmacological Basis of Therapeutics* (p. 595). New York: Pergamon.

Gatzonis, S., Mitsikostas, D. D., Ilias, A., Zournas, C. H., & Papageorgiou, C. (1996). Two more secondary headaches mimicking chronic paroxysmal hemicrania. Is this the exception or the rule? *Headache, 36,* 511–513.

Gawel, M. J., Willinsky, R. A., & Krajewski, A. (1989). Reversal of cluster headache side following treatment of arteriovenous malformation. *Headache, 29,* 453–454.

Geppetti, P., Brocchi, A., Caleri, D., Marabini, S., Raino, L., & Renzi, D. (1985, Spring). Somatostatin for cluster headache attack. In V. Pfaffenrath, P. O. Lundberg, & O. Sjaastad (Eds.), *Updating in Headache* (pp. 302–305). Berlin-Heidelberg-New York-Tokyo.

Giffin, N., & Goadsby, P. J. (2001). Basilar artery aneurysm with autonomic features: An interesting pathophysiological problem. *J Neurol Neurosurg Psychiatry, 71,* 805–808.

Goadsby, P. J. (2000). The pharmacology of headache. *Prog Neurobiol, 62,* 509–525.

Goadsby, P. J. (2002). Pathophysiology of cluster headache: A trigeminal autonomic cephalgia. *Lancet Neurol, 1,* 37–43.

Goadsby, P. J., & Edvinsson, L. (1994). Human *in vivo* evidence for trigeminovascular activation in cluster headache. *Brain, 117,* 427–434.

Goadsby, P. J., & Hoskin, K. L. (1997). The distribution of trigeminovascular afferents in the nonhuman primate brain *Macaca nemestrina:* A c-fos immunocytochemical study. *J Anat, 190,* 367–375.

Goadsby, P. J., Hoskin, K. L., & Knight, Y. E. (1997). Stimulation of the greater occipital nerve increases metabolic activity in the trigeminal nucleus caudalis and cervical dorsal horn of the cat. *Pain, 73,* 23–28.

Goadsby, P. J., & Lance, J. W. (1988). Brainstem effects on intra- and extracerebral circulations. Relation to migraine and cluster headache. In J. Olesen & L. Edvinsson (Eds.), *Basic Mechanisms of Headache* (pp. 413–427). Amsterdam: Elsevier.

Goadsby, P. J., & Lipton, R. B. (1997). A review of paroxysmal hemicranias, SUNCT syndrome and other short-lasting headaches with autonomic features, including new cases. *Brain, 120,* 193–209.

Goadsby, P. J., Matharu, M. S., & Boes, C. J. (2001). SUNCT syndrome or trigeminal neuralgia with lacrimation. *Cephalalgia, 21,* 82–83.

Gobel, H., Lindner, A., Heinze, A., Ribbat, M., & Deuschl, G. (1998). Acute therapy for cluster headache with sumatriptan: Findings of a one year long-term study. *Neurology, 51,* 908–911.

Graff-Radford, S. B. (2000). SUNCT syndrome responsive to gabapentin. *Cephalalgia, 20,* 515–517.

Graham, J. R. (1960). Use of a new compound, UML-491 (1-methyl-D-lysergic acid butanolamide), in the prevention of various types of headache. *N Engl J Med, 263,* 1273–1277.

Graham, J. R. (1972). Cluster headache. *Headache, 11,* 175–185.

Graham, J. R., Malvea, B. P., & Graham, H. F. (1960). Aerosol ergotamine tartrate for migraine and Horton's syndrome. *N Engl J Med, 263,* 802–804.

Graham, J. R., Suby, H. I., LeCompte, P. R., & Sadowsky, N. L. (1966). Fibrotic disorders associated with methysergide therapy for headache. *N Engl J Med, 274,* 360–368.

Greve, E., & Mai, J. (1988). Cluster headache-like headaches: A symptomatic feature? A report of three patients with intracranial pathologic findings. *Cephalalgia, 8,* 79–82.

Gutierrez-Garcia, J. M. (2002). SUNCT syndrome responsive to lamotrigine. *Headache, 42,* 823–825.

Haan, J., van Vliet, J. A., Kors, E. E., Terwindt, G. M., Vermeulen, F. L. M. G., van den Maagdenberg, A. M., Frants, R. R., & Ferrari, M. D. (2001). No involvement of calcium channel gene (*CACNA1A*) in a family with cluster headache. *Cephalalgia, 21,* 959–962.

Hannerz, J. (1989). A case of parasellar meningioma mimicking cluster headache. *Cephalalgia, 9,* 265–269.

Hannerz, J., Ericson, K., & Bergstrand, G. (1987). Chronic paroxysmal hemicrania: Orbital phlebography and steroid treatment. A case report. *Cephalalgia, 7,* 189–192.

Hannerz, J., & Jogestrand, T. (1993). Intracranial hypertension and sumatriptan efficacy in a case of chronic paroxysmal hemicrania which became bilateral. (The mechanism of indomethacin in CPH.) *Headache, 33,* 320–323.

Hannerz, J., & Linderoth, B. (2002). Neurosurgical treatment of short-lasting, unilateral, neuralgiform hemicrania with conjunctival injection and tearing. *Br J Neurosurg, 16,* 55–58.

Hardebo, J. E., & Elner, A. (1987). Nerves and vessels in the pterygopalatine fossa and symptoms of cluster headache. *Headache, 27,* 528–532.

Harrigan, M. R., Tuteja, S., & Neudeck, B. L. (1997). Indomethacin in the management of elevated intracranial pressure: A review. *J Neurotrauma, 14,* 637–650.

Harris, M. C. (1961). Prophylactic treatment of migraine and histamine cephalgia with a serotonin antagonist (methysergide). *Ann Allergy, 19,* 500–504.

Harris, W. (1936). Ciliary (migrainous) neuralgia and its treatment. *BMJ, 1,* 457–460.

Harris, W. (1937). *The Facial Neuralgias.* London: Humphrey Milford/Oxford University Press.

Headache Classification Committee of the International Headache Society. (2004). The International Classification of Headache Disorders (second edition). *Cephalalgia, 24,* 1–160.

Heidegger, S., Mattfeldt, T., Rieber, A., Wikstroem, M., Kern, P., Kern, W., & Schreiber, H. (1997). Orbito-sphenoidal aspergillus infection mimicking cluster headache: A case report. *Cephalalgia, 17,* 676–679.

Hering, R., & Kuritzky, A. (1989). Sodium valproate in the treatment of cluster headache: An open clinical trial. *Cephalalgia, 9,* 195–198.

Heyck, H. (1960). Serotoninantagonisten in der Behandlung der Migraine und der erythroprosopalgic bings oder des Horton-syndroms. *Schweiz Med Wochenschr, 90,* 203–209.

Horton, B. T. (1941). The use of histamine in the treatment of specific types of headache. *JAMA, 116,* 377–383.

Horton, B. T. (1952). Histaminic cephalgia. *Journal-Lancet, 72,* 92–98.

Horton, B. T. (1956). Histaminic cephalalgia: Differential diagnosis and treatment. *Mayo Clin Proc, 31,* 325–333.

Horton, B. T., MacLean, A. R., & Craig, W. M. (1939). A new syndrome of vascular headache, results of treatment with histamine, a preliminary report. *Mayo Clin Proc, 14,* 250–257.

Horton, B. T., Ryan, R., & Reynolds, J. L. (1948). Clinical observations of the use of EC110, a new agent for the treatment of headache. *Mayo Clinic Proc, 23,* 105–108.

Horven, I., & Sjaastad, O. (1977). Cluster headache syndrome and migraine: Ophthalmological support for a two entity theory. *Acta Ophthalmol (Copenhagen), 55,* 35–51.

Hoyer, D., Bell, G. I., Berelowitz, M., Epelbaum, J., Feniuk, W., Humphrey, P. P., O'Carroll, A. M., Patel, Y. C., Schonbrunn, A., Taylor, J. E., et al. (1995). Classification and nomenclature of somatostatin receptors. *Trends Pharmacol Sci, 16,* 86–88.

Hunt, C. H., Dodick, D. W., & Bosch, P. (2002). SUNCT responsive to gabapentin. *Headache, 42,* 525–526.

Hunter, C. R., & Mayfield, F. H. (1949). Role of the upper cervical roots in the production of pain in the head. *Am J Surg, 78,* 743–749.

Isler, H. (1993). Episodic cluster headache from a textbook of 1745: Van Swieten's classic description. *Cephalalgia, 13,* 172–174.

Jammes, J. L. (1975). The treatment of cluster headaches with prednisone. *Dis Nerv Syst, 36,* 375–376.

Jarrar, R. G., Black, D. F., Dodick, D. W., & Davis, D. H. (2003). Outcome of trigeminal nerve section in the treatment of chronic cluster headache. *Neurology, 60,* 1360–1362.

Jonsdottir, M., Meyer, J. S., & Rogers, R. L. (1987). Efficacy, side effects and tolerance compared during headache treatment with three different calcium blockers. *Headache, 27,* 364–369.

Joubert, J., Powell, D., & Djikowski, J. (1987). Chronic paroxysmal hemicrania in a South African black. A case report. *Cephalalgia, 7,* 193–196.

Kayed, K., Godtlibsen, O. B., & Sjaastad, O. (1978). Chronic paroxysmal hemicrania. 4. "REM sleep locked" nocturnal headache attacks. *Sleep, 1,* 91–95.

Kirkpatrick, P. J., O'Brien, M., & MacCabe, J. J. (1993). Trigeminal nerve section for chronic migrainous neuralgia. *Br J Neurosurg, 7,* 483–90.

Kitrelle, J. P., Grouse, D. S., & Seybold, M. E. (1985). Cluster headache: Local anesthetic abortive agents. *Arch Neurol, 42,* 496–498.

Klimek, A. (1987). Cluster-tic syndrome. *Cephalalgia, 7,* 161–162.

Klimek, K., Szulc-Kuberska, J., & Kawiorski, S. (1979). Lithium therapy in cluster headache. *Eur Neurol, 18,* 267–268.

Koenigsberg, A. D., Solomon, G. D., & Kosmorsky, D. O. (1994). Pseudoaneurysm within the cavernous sinus presenting as cluster headache. *Headache, 34,* 111–113.

Krabbe, A. (1989). Limited efficacy of methysergide in cluster headache. A clinical experience. *Cephalalgia, 9,* 404–405.

Krisch, B. (1978). Hypothalamic and extrahypothalamic distribution of somatostatin-immunoreactive elements in the rat brain. *Cell Tissue Res, 195,* 499–513.

Kudrow, D. B., & Kudrow, L. (1989). Successful aspirin prophylaxis in a child with chronic paroxysmal hemicrania. *Headache, 29,* 280–281.

Kudrow, L. (1977). Lithium prophylaxis for chronic cluster headache. *Headache, 17,* 15–18.

Kudrow, L. (1980). *Cluster Headache: Mechanisms and Management.* Oxford, UK: Oxford University Press,

Kudrow, L. (1981). Response of cluster headache attacks to oxygen inhalation. *Headache, 21,* 1–4.

Kudrow, L., Esperanca, P., & Vijayan, N. (1987). Episodic paroxysmal hemicrania? *Cephalalgia, 7,* 197–201.

Kudrow, L., & Kudrow, D. B. (1995). Intranasal lidocaine. *Headache, 35,* 565–566.

Kudrow, L., & Sutkus, B. J. (1979). MMPI pattern specificity in primary headache disorders. *Headache, 19,* 18–24.

Kunkel, R. S. (1981, September). Eleven clues to cluster headache—and tips on drug therapy. *Modern Medicine Australia,* 14–21.

Kunkle, E. C., & Anderson, W. B. (1961). Significance of minor eye signs in headache of migraine type. *Arch Ophthalmol (Chicago), 65,* 504–508.

Kunkle, E. C., Pfieffer J. B., Jr., Wilhoit, W. M., & Hamrick, L. W., Jr. (1952). Recurrent brief headache in cluster pattern. *Trans Am Neurol Assoc, 27,* 240–243.

Kuritzky, A. (1984). Cluster headache–like pain caused by an upper cervical meningioma. *Cephalalgia, 4,* 185–186.

Lain, A. H., Caminero, A. B., & Pareja, J. A. (2000). SUNCT syndrome, absence of refractory periods and modulation of attack duration by lengthening of the trigger stimuli. *Cephalalgia, 20,* 671–673.

Lainez, M. J., Pascual, J., Pascual, A. M., Santonja, J. M., Ponz, A., & Salvador, A. (2003). Topiramate in the prophylactic treatment of cluster headache. *Headache, 43,* 784–749.

Lance, J. W., & Anthony, M. (1966). Some clinical aspects of migraine: A prospective survey of 500 patients. *Arch Neurol, 15,* 356–361.

Lance, J. W., & Anthony, M. (1971). Migrainous neuralgia or cluster headache? *J Neurol Sci, 13,* 401–414.

Lance, J. W., & Drummond, P. D. (1987). Horner's syndrome in cluster headache. In F. Clifford Rose (Ed.), *Current problems in neurology: Advances in Headache Research,* (pp. 169–174). London: John Libbey.

Lance, J. W., & Goadsby, P. J. (1998). *Mechanism and Management of Headache.* London: Butterworth-Heinemann.

Lefevre, J. P., Simmat, G., Bataille, B., Salles, M., Gil, R., Boissonnot, L., & Roulades, G. (1984). [Cluster headache due to meningioma. 2 cases (letter)]. *Presse Med, 13,* 2323.

Lenaerts, M., Diederich, N., & Phuoe, D. (1997). A patient with SUNCT cured by the Jannetta procedure. *Cephalalgia, 17,* 460.

Leone, M., Attanasio, A., Croci, D., Libro, G., Grazzi, L., D'Amico, D., Nespolo, A., & Bussone, G. (1997a). The *m*-chlorophenylpiperazine test in cluster headache: A study on central serotoninergic activity. *Cephalalgia, 17,* 666–672.

Leone, M., Attanasio, A., Grazzi, L., Libro, G., D'Amico, D., Moschiano, F., & Bussone, G. (1997b). Transdermal clonidine in the prophylaxis of episodic cluster headache: An open study. *Headache, 37,* 559–560.

Leone, M., & Bussone, G. (1993). A review of hormonal findings in cluster headache. Evidence for hypothalamic involvement. *Cephalalgia, 13,* 309–317.

Leone, M., D'Amico, D., & Attanasio, A. (1999). Verapamil is an effective prophylactic for cluster headache: Results of a double-blind multicentre study versus placebo. In J. Olesen & P. J. Goadsby (Eds.), *Cluster Headache & Related Conditions* (pp. 296–299). Oxford, UK: Oxford University Press.

Leone, M., D'Amico, D., Moschiano, F., Fraschini, F., & Bussone, G. (1996). Melatonin versus placebo in the prophylaxis of cluster headache: A double-blind pilot study with parallel groups. *Cephalalgia, 16,* 494–496.

Leone, M., Dodick, D., Rigamonti, A., D'Amico, D., Grazzi, L., Mea, E., & Bussone, G. (2003). Topiramate in cluster headache prophylaxis: An open trial. *Cephalalgia, 23,* 1001–1002.

Leone, M., Franzini, A., & Bussone, G. (2001a). Stereotatic stimulation of the posterior hypothalamic gray matter in a patient with intractable cluster headache. *N Engl J Med, 345,* 1428–1429.

Leone, M., Franzini, A., D'Amico, D., Bizzi, A., Blasi, V., D'Andrea, G., et al. (2004). Hypothalamic deep brain stimulation to relieve intractable chronic SUNCT: The first case. *Neurology, 62,* A356.

Leone, M., Lucini, V., D'Amico, D., Moschiano, F., Maltempo, C., Fraschini, F., & Bussone, G. (1995). Twenty-four-hour melatonin and cortisol plasma levels in relation to timing of cluster headache. *Cephalalgia, 15,* 224–229.

Leone, M., Rigamonti, A., Usai, S., D'Amico, D., Grazzi, L., & Bussone, G. (2000). Two new SUNCT cases responsive to lamotrigine. *Cephalalgia, 20,* 845–847.

Leone, M., Russell, M. B., Rigamonti, A., Attanasio, A., Grazzi, L., D'Amico, D., Usai, S., & Bussone, G. (2001b). Increased familial risk of cluster headache. *Neurology, 56,* 1233–1236.

Levy, M., Jager, H. R., Powell, M. P., Matharu, M. S., Meeran, K., Goadsby, P. J. (2004a). Pituitary volume and headache: Size is not everything. *Arch Neurol, 61,* 721–725.

Levy, M. J., Matharu, M. S., Bhola, R., Meeran, K., & Goadsby, P. J. (2004b, in press). Octreotide is not effective in the acute treatment of migraine. *Cephalalgia, 24.*

Levy, M. J., Matharu, M. S., & Goadsby, P. J. (2003). Prolactinomas, dopamine agonist and headache: Two case reports. *Eur J Neurol, 10,* 169–174.

Levyman, C., Dagua Filho Ados, S., Volpato, M. M., Settanni, F. A. P., & Lima, W. C. (1991). Epidermoid tumour of the posterior fossa causing multiple facial pain—a case report. *Cephalalgia, 11,* 33–36.

Lieb, J., & Zeff, A. (1978). Lithium treatment of chronic cluster headaches. *Br J Psychiatry, 133,* 556–558.

Liston, H., Bennett, L., Usher, B., & Nappi, J. (1999). The association of the combination of sumatriptan and methysergide in myocardial infarction in a premenopausal woman. *Arch Intern Med, 159,* 511–513.

Loder, E. (2002). Naratriptan in the prophylaxis of cluster headache. *Headache, 42,* 56–57.

Lovely, T. J., Kotsiakis, X., & Jannetta, P. J. (1998). The surgical management of chronic cluster headache. *Headache, 38,* 590–594.

MacMillan, J. C., & Nukada, H. (1989). Chronic paroxysmal hemicrania. *N Z Med J, 102,* 251–252.

Magee, K. R., Westerberg, M. R., & DeJong, R. M. (1952). Treatment of headache with ergotamine-caffeine suppositories. *Neurology, 2,* 477–480.

Mani, S., & Deeter, J. (1982). Arteriovenous malformation of the brain presenting as a cluster headache—a case report. *Headache, 22,* 184–185.

Manzoni, G. (1999). Cluster headache and lifestyle: Remarks on a population of 374 male patients. *Cephalalgia, 19,* 88–94.

Manzoni, G. C., Bono, G., Lanfranchi, M., Micieli, G., Terzano, M. G., & Nappi, G. (1983a). Lithium carbonate in cluster headache: Assessment of its short- and long-term therapeutic efficacy. *Cephalalgia, 3,* 109–114.

Manzoni, G. C., Terzano, M. G., Bono, G., Micieli, G., Martucci, N., & Nappi, G. (1983b). Cluster headache—clinical findings in 180 patients. *Cephalalgia, 3,* 21–30.

Mariano, H. S., Bigal, M. E., Bordini, C. A., & Speciali, J. G. (1999). Chronic paroxysmal hemicrania (CPH)-like syndrome as a first manifestation of cerebral metastasis of parotid epidermoid carcinoma: A case report. *Cephalalgia, 19,* 442–442.

Marks, D. R., Rapoport, A., & Padla, D. (1993). A double-blind placebo-controlled trial of intra-nasal capsaicin for cluster headache. *Cephalalgia, 13,* 114–116.

Massiou, H., Launay, J. M., Levy, C., El Amran, M., Emperauger, B., & Bousser, M.-G. (2002). SUNCT syndrome in two patients with prolactinomas and bromocriptine-induced attacks. *Neurology, 58,* 1698–1699.

Matharu, M. S., Bartsch, T., Ward, N., Frackowiak, R. S., Weiner, R. L., & Goadsby, P. J. (2004a). Central neuromodulation in chronic migraine patients with suboccipital stimulators: A PET study. *Brain, 127,* 220–230.

Matharu, M. S., Boes, C. J., & Goadsby, P. J. (2002). SUNCT syndrome: Prolonged attacks, refractoriness and response to topiramate. *Neurology, 58,* 1307.

Matharu, M. S., Boes, C. J., & Goadsby, P. J. (2003a). Management of trigeminal autonomic cephalalgias and hemicrania continua. *Drugs, 63,* 1637–1677.

Matharu, M. S., Cohenm, A. S., & Goadsby, P. J. (2004b). SUNCT syndrome responsive to intravenous lidocaine. *Cephalalgia, 24,* (in press).

Matharu, M. S., & Goadsby, P. J. (2001). Post-traumatic chronic paroxysmal hemicrania (CPH) with aura. *Neurology, 56,* 273–275.

Matharu, M. S., & Goadsby, P. J. (2002). Persistence of attacks of cluster headache after trigeminal nerve root section. *Brain, 175,* 976–984.

Matharu, M. S., Levy, M. J., Meeran, K., & Goadsby, P. J. (2004c). Subcutaneous octreotide in cluster headache-randomized placebo-controlled double-blind cross-over study. *Ann Neurol,* (in press).

Matharu, M. S., Levy, M. J., Merry, R. T., & Goadsby, P. J. (2003b). SUNCT syndrome secondary to prolactinoma. *J Neurol Neurosurg Psychiatry, 74,* 1590–1592.

Matharu, M. S., van Vliet, J. A., Ferrari, M. D., & Goadsby, P. J. (2004d). Verapamil-induced gingival enlargement in cluster headache. *J Neurol Neurosurg Psychiatry,* (in press).

Mather, P., Silberstein, S. D., Schulman, E., & Hopkins, M. M. (1991). The treatment of cluster headache with repetitive intravenous dihydroergotamine. *Headache, 31,* 525–532.

Mathew, N. T. (1978). Clinical subtypes of cluster headache and response to lithium therapy. *Headache, 18,* 26–30.

Mathew, N. T., & Hurt, W. (1988). Percutaneous radiofrequency trigeminal gangliorhizolysis in intractable cluster headache. *Headache, 28,* 328–331.

Mathew, N. T., Kailasam, J., & Fischer, A. (2000). Responsiveness to celecoxib in chronic paroxysmal hemicrania. *Neurology, 55,* 316.

May, A., Ashburner, J., Buchel, C., McGonigle, D. J., Friston, K. J., Frackowiak, R. S. J., & Goadsby, P. J. (1999a). Correlation between structural and functional changes in brain in an idiopathic headache syndrome. *Nat Med, 5,* 836–838.

May, A., Bahra, A., Buchel, C., Frackowiak, R. S. J., & Goadsby, P. J. (1998a). Hypothalamic activation in cluster headache attacks. *Lancet, 352,* 275–278.

May, A., Bahra, A., Buchel, C., Frackowiak, R. S. J., & Goadsby, P. J. (2000). PET and MRA findings in cluster headache and MRA in experimental pain. *Neurology, 55,* 1328–1335.

May, A., Bahra, A., Buchel, C., Turner, R., & Goadsby, P. J. (1999b). Functional MRI in spontaneous attacks of SUNCT: Short-lasting neuralgiform headache with conjunctival injection and tearing. *Ann Neurol, 46,* 791–793.

May, A., Buchel, C., Turner, R., & Goadsby, P. J. (2001). MR-angiography in facial and other pain: Neurovascular mechanisms of trigeminal sensation. *J Cereb Blood Flow Metabol, 21,* 1171–1176.

May, A., Kaube, H., Buchel, C., Eichten, C., Rijntjes, M., Jueptner, M., Weiller, C., & Diener, H. C. (1998b). Experimental cranial pain elicited by capsaicin: A PET-study. *Pain, 74,* 61–66.

McKinney, A. S. (1983). Cluster headache developing following ipsilateral orbital exenteration. *Headache, 23,* 305–306.

Medina, J. L. (1992). Organic headaches mimicking chronic paroxysmal hemicrania. *Headache, 32,* 73–74.

Medina, J. L., Fareed, J., & Diamond, S. (1980). Lithium carbonate therapy for cluster headache. Changes in number of platelets and serotonin and histamine levels. *Arch Neurol, 37,* 559–563.

Meyer, J. S., & Hardenberg, J. (1983). Clinical effectiveness of calcium entry blockers in prophylactic treatment of migraine and cluster headache. *Headache, 23,* 266–277.

Mirzai, R., Chang, C., Greenspan, A., & Gershwin, M. E. (1999). The pathogenesis of osteonecrosis and the relationships to corticosteroids. *J Asthma, 36,* 77–95.

Molins, A., Lopez, M., Codina, A., & Titus, F. (1989). [Symptomatic cluster headache? Apropos of 4 case reports]. *Med Clin (Barc), 92,* 181–183.

Monstad, I., Krabbe, A., Micieli, G., Prusinski, A., Cole, J., Pilgrim, A., et al. (1995). Preemptive oral treatment with sumatriptan during a cluster period. *Headache, 35,* 607–613.

Montes, E., Alberca, R., Lozano, P., Franco, E., Martinez-Fernandez, E., & Mir, P. (2001). Statuslike SUNCT in two young women. *Headache, 41,* 826–829.

Monzillo, P. H., Sanvito, W. L., & Da Costa, A. R. (2000). Cluster-tic syndrome, report of five new cases. *Arq Neuropsiquiatr, 58,* 518–521.

Morales, F., Mostacero, E., Marta, J., & Sanchez, S. (1994). Vascular malformation of the cerebellopontine angle associated with SUNCT syndrome. *Cephalalgia, 14,* 301–302.

Morales-Asin, F., Espada, F., Lopez-Obarrio, L. A., Navas, I., Escalza, I., & Iniguez, C. A. (2000). A SUNCT case with response to surgical treatment. *Cephalalgia, 20,* 67–68.

Morgenlander, J. C., & Wilkins, R. H. (1990). Surgical treatment of cluster headache. *J Neurosurg, 72,* 866–871.

Moris, G., Ribacoba, R., Solar, D. N., & Vidal, J. A. (2001). SUNCT syndrome and seborrheic dermatitis associated with craneosynostosis. *Cephalalgia, 21,* 157–159.

Mulleners, W. M., & Verhagen, W. I. M. (1996). Cluster-tic syndrome. *Neurology, 47,* 302.

Munoz, C., Diez-Tejedor, E., Frank, A., & Barreiro, P. (1996). Cluster headache syndrome associated with middle cerebral artery arteriovenous malformation. *Cephalalgia, 16,* 202–205.

Naylor, W. G. (1988). *Calcium Antagonists.* London: Academic Press.

Newman, L. C., & Goadsby, P. J. (2001). The paroxysmal hemicranias, SUNCT syndrome, and hypnic headache. In S. D. Silberstein, R. B. Lipton, & D. J. Dalessio (Eds.), *Wolff's Headache and Other Head Pain* (pp. 310–324). Oxford, UK: Oxford University Press,

Newman, L. C., Gordon, M. L., Lipton, R. B., Kanner, R., & Solomon, S. (1992a). Episodic paroxysmal hemicrania: Two new cases and a literature review. *Neurology, 42,* 964–966.

Newman, L. C., Herskovitz, S., Lipton, R., & Solomon, S. (1992b). Chronic paroxysmal headache: Two cases with cerebrovascular disease. *Headache, 32,* 75–76.

Nicolodi, M., Sicuteri, F., & Poggioni, M. (1993). Hypothalamic modulation of nociception and reproduction in cluster headache. I. Therapeutic trials of leuprolide. *Cephalalgia, 13,* 253–257.

Nieman, E. A., & Hurwitz, L. J. (1961). Ocular sympathetic palsy in periodic migrainous neuralgia. *J Neurol Neurosurg Psychiatry, 24,* 269–373.

Nilsson Remahl, A. I. M., Ansjon, R., Lind, F., & Waldenlind, E. (1997). No prophylactic effect of hyperbaric oxygen during active cluster headache: A double-blind placebo-controlled cross-over study. *Cephalalgia, 17,* 456.

Nilsson Remahl, A. I. M., Laudon Meyer, E., Cordonnier, C. S., & Goadsby, P. J. (2003). Placebo response rates in cluster headache trials. A review. *Cephalalgia, 23,* 504–510.

Pareja, J. A. (1995). Chronic paroxysmal hemicrania: Dissociation of the pain and autonomic features. *Headache, 35,* 111–113.

Pareja, J. A., Caminero, A. B., Franco, E., Casado, J. L., Pascual, J., & Sanchez del Rio, M. (2001). Dose, efficacy and tolerability of long-term indomethacin treatment of chronic paroxysmal hemicrania and hemicrania continua. *Cephalalgia, 21,* 869–878.

Pareja, J. A., Joubert, J., & Sjaastad, O. (1996a). SUNCT syndrome. Atypical temporal patterns. *Headache, 36,* 108–110.

Pareja, J.A., Kruszewski, P., & Caminero, A. B. (1999). SUNCT syndrome versus idiopathic stabbing headache (jabs and jolts syndrome). *Cephalalgia, 19,* 46–48.

Pareja, J. A., Kruszewski, P., & Sjaastad, O. (1995). SUNCT syndrome: Trials of drugs and anesthetic blockades. *Headache, 35,* 138–142.

Pareja, J. A., Ming, J. M., Kruszewski, P., Caballero, V., Pamo, M., & Sjaastad, O. (1996b). SUNCT syndrome: Duration, frequency and temporal distribution of attacks. *Headache, 36,* 161–165.

Pareja, J. A., Pareja, J., Palomo, T., Caballero, V., & Pamo, M. (1994). SUNCT syndrome: Repetitive and overlapping attacks. *Headache, 34,* 114–116.

Pareja, J. A., Ruiz, J., Deisla, C., Alsabbah, H., & Espejo, J. (1996c). Idiopathic stabbing headache (jabs and jolts syndrome). *Cephalalgia, 16,* 93–96.

Pareja, J. A., & Sjaastad, O. (1997). SUNCT syndrome. A clinical review. *Headache, 37,* 195–202.

Patel, Y. C., & Srikant, C. B. (1994). Subtype selectivity of peptide analogs for all five cloned human somatostatin receptors (hsstr 1–5). *Endocrinology, 135,* 2814–2817.

Peatfield, R., Bahra, A., & Goadsby, P. J. (1998). Trigeminal-autonomic cephalgias (TACs). *Cephalalgia, 18,* 358–361.

Pelz, M., & Merskey, H. (1982). A case of pre-chronic paroxysmal hemicrania. *Cephalalgia, 2,* 47–50.

Penart, A., Firth, M., & Bowen, J. R. C. (2001). Short-lasting unilateral neuralgiform headache with conjunctival injection and tearing (SUNCT) following presumed dorsolateral brainstem infarction. *Cephalalgia, 21,* 236–239.

Peres, M. F. P., & Rozen, T. D. (2001). Melatonin in the preventative treatment of chronic cluster headache. *Cephalalgia, 21,* 993–995.

Peres, M. F. P., Stiles, M. A., Siow, H. C., Rozen, T. D., Young, W. B., & Silberstein, S. D. (2002). Greater occipital nerve blockade for cluster headache. *Cephalalgia, 22,* 520–522.

Pinessi, L., Rainero, I., Valfre, W., Lo Giudice, R., Ferrero, M., Rivoiro, C., Arvat, E., Gianotti, L., Del Rizzo, P., & Limone, P. (2003). Abnormal 5-HT1D receptor function in cluster headache: A neuroendocrine study with sumatriptan. *Cephalalgia, 23,* 354–360.

Piovesan, E. J., Siow, C., Kowacs, P. A., & Werneck, L. C. (2003). Influence of lamotrigine over the SUNCT syndrome: One patient follow-up for two years. *Arq Neuropsiquiatr, 61,* 691–694.

Pollmann, W., & Pfaffenrath, V. (1986). Chronic paroxysmal hemicrania: The first possible bilateral case. *Cephalalgia, 6,* 55–57.

Porta, M., Granella, F., Coppola, A., Longoni, C., & Manzoni, G. C. (1991). Treatment of cluster headaches with hyperbaric oxygen. *Cephalalgia, 11,* 236–237.

Porta-Etessam, J., Martinez-Salio, A., Berbel, A., & Benito-Leon, J. (2002). Gabapentin (Neurontin) in the treatment of SUNCT syndrome. *Cephalalgia, 22,* 249.

Pradalier, A., & Dry, J. (1984). [Chronic paroxysmal hemicrania. Treatment with indomethacin and diclofenac]. *Therapie, 39,* 185–188.

Procacci, P., Zoppi, M., Maresca, M., Zamponi, A., Fanciullacci, M., & Sicuteri, F. (1989). Lateralisation of pain in cluster headache. *Pain, 38,* 275–278.

Prusinski, A., Liberski, P. P., & Szulc-Kuberska, J. (1985). Cluster headache in a patient without an ipsilateral eye. *Headache, 25,* 134–135.

Raimondi, E., & Gardella, L. (1998). SUNCT syndrome. Two cases in Argentina. *Headache, 38,* 369–371.

Rapoport, A. M., Bigal, M. E., Tepper, S. J., & Sheftell, F. D. (2003). Treatment of cluster headache with topiramate: Effects and side-effects in five patients. *Cephalalgia, 23,* 69–70.

Rapoport, A. M., Sheftell, F. D., & Baskin, S. M. (1981). Chronic paroxysmal hemicrania: Case report of the second known definite occurrence in a male. *Cephalalgia, 1,* 67–70.

Raskin, N. H. (1988). *Headache.* New York: Churchill-Livingstone.

Reik, L. (1987). Cluster headache after head injury. *Headache, 27,* 508–510.

Robbins, L. (1995). Intranasal lidocaine for cluster headache. *Headache, 35,* 83–84.

Roberge, C., Bouchard, J. P., Simard, D., & Gagne, R. (1992). Cluster headache in twins. *Neurology, 42,* 1255–1256.

Rogado, A. Z., & Graham, J. R. (1979). Through a glass darkly. *Headache, 19,* 58–62.

Romberg, M. H. (1840). *Lehrbuch der Nervenkrankheiten des Menschen* (Vol. 1). Berlin: Dunker.

Romoli, M., & Cudia, G. (1988). Cluster headache due to an impacted superior wisdom tooth: Case report. *Headache, 28,* 135–136.

Rosebraugh, C. J., Griebel, D. J., & DiPette, D. J. (1997). A case report of carotid artery dissection presenting as cluster headache. *Am J Med, 102,* 418–419.

Rossi, P., Lorenzo, G. D., Formisano, R., & Buzzi, M. G. (2004). Subcutaneous sumatriptan induces changes in frequency pattern in cluster headache patients. *Headache, 44,* 713–718.

Rowed, D. W. (1990). Chronic cluster headache managed by nervus intermedius section. *Headache, 30,* 401–406.

Rozen, T. D. (2001). Olanzapine as an abortive agent for cluster headache. *Headache, 41,* 813–816.

Russell, D. (1979). Cluster headache: Trial of a combined histamine H1 and H2 treatment. *J Neurol Neurosurg Psychiatry, 42,* 668–669.

Russell, D. (1984). Chronic paroxysmal hemicrania: Severity, duration and time of occurrence of attacks. *Cephalalgia, 4,* 53–56.

Russell, D. (1999). Paroxysmal hemicrania. In J. Olesen & P. J. Goadsby (Eds.), *Cluster Headache & Related Conditions* (pp. 27–36). Oxford, UK: Oxford University Press.

Russell, D., & Storstein, L. (1983). Cluster headache: A computerized analysis of 24h Holter ECG recordings and description of ECG rhythm disturbances. *Cephalalgia, 3,* 83–107.

Russell, M. B., Andersson, P. G., & Iselius, L. (1996). Cluster headache is an inherited disorder in some families. *Headache, 36,* 608–612.

Russell, M. B., Andersson, P. G., Thomsen, L. L., & Iselius, L. (1995). Cluster headache is an autosomal dominantly inherited disorder in some families: A complex segregation analysis. *J Med Genet, 32,* 954–956.

Sabatowski, R., Huber, M., Meuser, T., & Radbruch, L. (2001). SUNCT syndrome: A treatment option with local opioid blockade of the superior cervical ganglion? A case report. *Cephalalgia, 21,* 154–156.

Sacquegna, T., D'Alessandro, R., Cortelli, P., De Carolis, P., & Baldrati, A. (1982). Cluster headache after herpes zoster ophthalmicus. *Arch Neurol, 39,* 384.

Salvesen, R. (2000). Cluster headache sine headache: Case report. *Neurology, 55,* 451.

Salvesen, R., Bogucki, A., Wysocka-Bakowska, M. M., Antonaci, F., Fredriksen, T. A., & Sjaastad, O. (1987). Cluster headache pathogenesis: A pupillometric study. *Cephalalgia, 7,* 273–284.

Salvesen, R., Sand, T., & Sjaastad, O. (1988). Cluster headache: Combined assessment with pupillometry and evaporimetry. *Cephalalgia, 8,* 211–218.

Sandrini, G., Alfonso, E., Ruiz, L., Pavesi, G., Micieli, G., Manzoni, G. C., Nancia, D., & Nappi, G. (1991). Impairment of corneal pain perception in cluster headache. *Pain, 47,* 299–304.

Saper, J. R., Klapper, J., Mathew, N. T., Rapoport, A., Phillips, S. B., & Bernstein, J. E. (2002). Intranasal civamide for the treatment of episodic cluster headaches. *Arch Neurol, 59,* 990–994.

Savoldi, F., Nappi, G., & Bono, G. (1979). [Lithium salts in the treatment of cluster headache]. *Rivista di Neurologia, 49,* 128–139.

Saxena, P. R., & De Boer, M. O. (1991). Pharmacology of antimigraine drugs. *J Neurol, 238,* S28–S35.

Schindler, M., Holloway, S., Hathway, G., Woolf, C. J., Humphrey, P. P., Emson, P. C. (1998). Identification of somatostatin sst2(a) receptor expressing neurones in central regions involved in nociception. *Brain Res, 798,* 25–35.

Sesso, R. M. (2001). SUNCT syndrome or trigeminal neuralgia with lacrimation and conjunctival injection? *Cephalalgia, 21,* 151–153.

Shabbir, N., & McAbee, G. (1994). Adolescent chronic paroxysmal hemicrania responsive to verapamil monotherapy. *Headache, 34,* 209–210.

Shields, K. G., Levy, M. J., & Goadsby, P. J. (2004). Alopecia and cutaneous atrophy following greater occipital nerve infiltration. *Neurology,* (in press).

Sicuteri, F. (1959). Prophylactic and therapeutic properties of *l*-methylysergic acid butanolamide in migraine: Preliminary report. *Int Arch Allergy, 15,* 300–307.

Sicuteri, F., Franchi, G., & Del Bianco, P. L. (1967). An antaminic drug, BC 105, in the prophylaxis of migraine. *Int Arch Allergy, 31,* 78–93.

Sicuteri, F., Fusco, B. M., & Marabini, S. (1989). Beneficial effect of capsaicin application to the nasal mucosa in cluster headache. *Clin J Pain, 5,* 49–53.

Sicuteri, F., Geppetti, P., Marabini, S., & Lembeck, F. (1984). Pain relief by somatostatin in attacks of cluster headache. *Pain, 18,* 359–365.

Silberstein, S. D. (1998). Methysergide. *Cephalalgia, 18,* 421–435.

Silberstein, S. D., Niknam, R., Rozen, T. D., & Young, W. B. (2000). Cluster headache with aura. *Neurology, 54,* 219–221.

Singh, B. N., & Nademanee, K. (1987). Use of calcium antagonists for cardiac arrhythmias. *Am J Cardiol, 59,* 153B–162B.

Sjaastad, O., & Antonaci, F. (1995). A piroxicam derivative partly effective in chronic paroxysmal hemicrania and hemicrania continua. *Headache, 35,* 549–550.

Sjaastad, O., & Bakketeig, L. S. (2003). Cluster headache prevalence. Vaga study of headache epidemiology. *Cephalalgia, 23,* 528–533.

Sjaastad, O., & Dale, I. (1974). Evidence for a new (?) treatable headache entity. *Headache, 14,* 105–108.

Sjaastad, O., & Dale, I. (1976). A new (?) clinical headache entity "chronic paroxysmal hemicrania." *Acta Neurol Scand, 54,* 140–159.

Sjaastad, O., Horven, I., & Vennerod, A. M. (1976). A new headache syndrome? Headache resembling cluster headache, with recurring bouts of homolateral retrobulbar partial factor XII deficiency, bleeding tendency and a convulsive episode. *Headache, 16,* 4–10.

Sjaastad, O., & Kruszewski, P. (1992). Trigeminal neuralgia and "SUNCT" syndrome: Similarities and differences in the clinical picture. An overview. *Funct Neurol, 7,* 103–107.

Sjaastad, O., Russell, D., Horven, I., & Bunnaes, U. (1978). Multiple neuralgiform unilateral headache attacks associated with conjunctival injection and appearing in clusters. A nosological problem. Proceedings of the Scandinavian Migraine Society. Vol. 31. Arhus, 31.

Sjaastad, O., Saunte, C., Salvesen, R., Fredriksen, T. A., Seim, A., Roe, O. D., Fostad, K., Lobben, O. P., & Zhao, J. M. (1989). Shortlasting unilateral neuralgiform headache attacks with conjunctival injection, tearing, sweating, and rhinorrhea. *Cephalalgia, 9,* 147–156.

Sjaastad, O., Shen, J. M., Stovner, L. J., & Elsas, T. (1993). Cluster headache in identical twins. *Headache, 33,* 214–217.

Sjaastad, O., Stovner, L. J., Stolt-Nielsen, A., Antonaci, F., & Fredriksen, T. A. (1995). CPH and hemicrania continua: Requirements of high dose indomethacin dosages—an ominous sign? *Headache, 35,* 363–367.

Sjostrand, C., Giedratis, V., Ekbom, K., Waldenlind, E., & Hillert, J. (2001). *CACNA1A* gene polymorphisms in cluster headache. *Cephalalgia, 21,* 953–958.

Sluder, G. (1910). The syndrome of sphenopalatine ganglion neurosis. *Am J Med, 140,* 868–878.

Solomon, S., Apfelbaum, R. I., & Guglielmo, K. M. (1985). The cluster-tic syndrome and its surgical therapy. *Cephalalgia, 5,* 83–89.

Soros, P., Frese, A., Husstedt, I. W., & Evers, S. (2001). Cluster headache after dental extraction: Implications for the pathogenesis of cluster headache? *Cephalalgia, 21,* 619–622.

Speed, W. G. (1960). Ergotamine tartrate inhalation: A new approach to the management of recurrent vascular headaches. *Am J Med Sci, 240,* 327–331.

Speight, T. M., & Avery, G. S. (1972). Pizotifen (BC-105): A review of its pharmacological properties and its therapeutic efficacy in vascular headaches. *Drugs, 3,* 159–203.

Sprenger, T., Boecker, H., Tolle, T. R., Bussone, G., May, A., & Leone, M. (2004). Specific hypothalamic activation during a spontaneous cluster headache attack. *Neurology, 62,* 516–517.

Steiner, T. J., Hering, R., Couturier, E. G. M., Davies, P. T. G., & Whitmarsh, T. E. (1997). Double-blind placebo controlled trial of lithium in episodic cluster headache. *Cephalalgia, 17,* 673–675.

Sutherland, I. M., & Eadie, M. J. (1972). Cluster headache. *Res Clin Stud Headache, 3,* 92–125.

Suzuki, N., & Hardebo, J. E. (1991). Anatomical basis for a parasympathetic and sensory innervation of the intracranial segment of the internal carotid artery in man. Possible implications for vascular headache. *J Neurol Sci, 104,* 19–31.

Swanson, J. W., Yanagihara, T., Stang, P. E., O'Fallon, W. M., Beard, C. M., Melton, L. J., III, & Guess, H. A. (1994). Incidence of cluster headaches: A population-based study in Olmsted County, Minnesota. *Neurology, 44,* 433–437.

Symonds, C. P. (1956). A particular variety of headache. *Brain, 79,* 217–232.

Szulc-Kuberska, J., & Klimek, A. (1978). [Lithium treatment of chronic Horton's headaches]. *Neurol Neurochir Pol, 12,* 409–411.

Taub, E., Argoff, C. E., Winterkorn, J. M., & Milhorat, T. H. (1995). Resolution of chronic cluster headache after resection of a tentorial meningioma: Case report. *Neurosurgery, 37,* 319–321.

Tehindrazanarivelo, A. D., Visy, J. M., & Bousser, M. G. (1992). Ipsilateral cluster headache and chronic paroxysmal hemicrania: Two case reports. *Cephalalgia, 12,* 318–320.

ter Berg, H. W. M., & Goadsby, P. J. (2001). Significance of atypical presentation of symptomatic SUNCT: A case report. *J Neurol Neurosurg Psychiatry, 70,* 244–246.

Tfelt-Hansen, P., Paulson, O. B., & Krabbe, A. E. (1982). Invasive adenoma of the pituitary gland and chronic migrainous neuralgia. A rare coincidence or a causal relationship? *Cephalalgia, 2,* 25–28.

Thomas, A. L. (1975). Periodic migrainous neuralgia associated with an arteriovenous malformation. *Postgrad Med J, 51,* 460–462.

Tonon, C., Guttmann, S., Volpini, M., Naccarato, S., Cortelli, P., & D'Alessandro, R. (2002). Prevalence and incidence of cluster headache in the Republic of San Marino. *Neurology, 58,* 1407–1409.

Turkewitz, L. J., Wirth, O., Dawson, G. A., & Casaly, J. S. (1992). Cluster headache following head injury: A case report and review of the literature. *Headache, 32,* 504–506.

Vail, H. H. (1932). Vidian neuralgia. *Ann Otol Rhinol Laryngol, 41,* 837–856.

van Vliet, J. A., Bahra, A., Martin, V., Aurora, S. K., Mathew, N. T., Ferrari, M. D., & Goadsby, P. J. (2003a). Intranasal sumatriptan in cluster headache-randomized placebo-controlled double-blind study. *Neurology, 60,* 630–633.

van Vliet, J. A., Eekers, P. J., Haan, J., & Ferrari, M. D. (2003b). Features involved in the diagnostic delay of cluster headache. *J Neurol Neurosurg Psychiatry, 74,* 1123–1125.

van Vliet, J. A., Ferrari, M. D., & Haan, J. (2003c). SUNCT syndrome resolving after contralateral hemispheric ischaemic stroke. *Cephalalgia, 23,* 235–237.

Vandenheede, M., Maertens de Noordhout, A. S., Remacle, J. M., & Schoenen, J. (2004). Deep brain stimulation of posterior hypothalamus in chronic cluster headache. *Neurology, 62,* A356.

Vijayan, N. (1990). Cluster headache and vertigo. *Cephalalgia, 10,* 67–76.

Vijayan, N. (1992). Symptomatic chronic paroxysmal hemicrania. *Cephalalgia, 12,* 111–113.

Vijayan, N., & Watson, C. (1985). Corneal sensitivity in cluster headache. *Headache, 25,* 104–106.

Vincent, M. B., Ekman, R., Edvinsson, L., Sand, T., & Sjaastad, O. (1992). Reduction of calcitonin gene–related peptide in the jugular blood following electrical stimulation of rat greater occipital nerve. *Cephalalgia, 12,* 275–279.

Waldenlind, E., & Gustafsson, S. A. (1987). Prolactin in cluster headache: Diurnal secretion, response to thyrotropin-releasing hormone, and relation to sex steroids and gonadotropins. *Cephalalgia, 7,* 43–54.

Waldenlind, E., Gustafsson, S. A., Ekbom, K., & Wetterberg, L. (1987). Circadian secretion of cortisol and melatonin in cluster headache during active cluster periods and remission. *J Neurol Neurosurg Psychiatry, 50,* 207–213.

Warner, J. S., Wamil, A. W., & McLean, M. J. (1994). Acetazolamide for the treatment of chronic paroxysmal hemicrania. *Headache, 34,* 597–599.

Watson, P., & Evans, R. (1985). Cluster-tic syndrome. *Headache, 25,* 123–126.

Weiner, R. L., & Reed, K. L. (1999). Peripheral neurostimulation for control of intractable occipital neuralgia. *Neuromodulation, 2,* 217–222.

Weiss, L. D. (1989). Treatment of a cluster headache patient in a hyperbaric chamber. *Headache, 29,* 109–110.

West, P., & Todman, D. (1991). Chronic cluster headache associated with a vertebral artery aneurysm. *Headache, 31,* 210–212.

Wheeler, S. D., & Carrazana, E. J. (1999). Topiramate-treated cluster headache. *Neurology, 53,* 234–236.

Wyant, G. M., & Ashenhurst, E. M. (1979). Chronic pain syndromes and their treatment. I. Cluster headache. *Can Anaesth Soc J, 26,* 38–41.

Zagami, A. S., & Goadsby, P. J. (1991). Stimulation of the superior sagittal sinus increases metabolic activity in cat thalamus. In F. C. Rose (Ed.), *New Advances in Headache Research* (Vol. 2, pp. 169–171). London: Smith-Gordon.

Zagami, A. S., & , Lambert, G. A. (1990). Stimulation of cranial vessels excites nociceptive neurones in several thalamic nuclei of the cat. *Exp Brain Res, 81,* 552–566.

Zebenholzer, K., Wober, C., Vigl, M., & Wessely, P. (2004). Eletriptan for the short-term prophylaxis of cluster headache. *Headache, 44,* 361–364.

Chapter 13
Other Primary Headaches and Distinction from Those with Structural Cause

Many otherwise normal people get a headache when challenged by some sudden change in their internal or external environment or exposure to vasodilator agents. Others experience transient jabs of pain in the head without apparent reason. Headache can be a symptom of an epileptic discharge and can follow complex partial seizures as well as tonic-clonic attacks. This miscellaneous group of headaches can be mediated by peripheral nerve irritability, dilation of cranial blood vessels, or discharge of central pain pathways, without any pathologic change being demonstrable in these structures.

Rasmussen and Olesen (1992) assessed the lifetime prevalence of headache in 1000 people between the ages of 25 and 64 years. In this survey, 2% reported idiopathic (primary) stabbing headache; 72% had experienced hangover headache; 63% had had fever headache; and 1% each reported benign (primary) cough headache, benign (primary) exertional headache, and headaches associated with sexual activity.

THE EXPLODING HEAD SYNDROME

Pearce (1988) coined the term *exploding head syndrome* to describe the night startle that may awaken healthy individuals from sleep with the sensation of a loud bang in the head, like an explosion, sometimes associated with the perception of a flash of light. Patients may at first describe this inaccurately as a headache. It is probably a quasiepileptic experience like the nocturnal myoclonic jerk that occurs in normal people on drifting off to sleep.

PRIMARY STABBING HEADACHE

Researchers have described three varieties of stabbing headache: "ice-pick pains," "jabs and jolts syndrome," and ophthalmodynia. There is no obvious clinical or physiological reason to distinguish these now, but we will outline them separately to illustrate these similarities.

Ice-Pick Pains

Raskin and Schwartz (1980) described sharp jabbing pains in the head resembling a stab from an ice-pick, nail, or needle. They compared the prevalence of such pains in 100 patients with migraine (20 men, 80 women) and 100 headache-free controls (53 men, 47 women). Only 3 of the control subjects had experienced ice-pick pains compared with 42 of the patients with migraine, of whom 60% had more than one attack each month. The pains affected the temple or orbit more often than the parietal and occipital areas and often occurred before or during migraine headaches. Drummond and Lance (1984) noted a history of ice-pick pains in 200 of 530 patients with recurrent headache (migraine and tension headache). The site of the ice-pick pains, recorded for 92 patients, coincided with the site of the patient's habitual headache in 37 (19 unilateral and 18 bilateral). This was most apparent when the ice-pick pains were restricted to one eye or temple.

Ice-pick pains have also been described in conjunction with cluster headaches, experienced in the same area as the cluster pain. Three out of sixty patients Lance and Anthony (1971) studied and eleven of thirty three patients Ekbom (1975) examined described ice-pick pains during the cluster attack, becoming more frequent as the attack abated. Raskin and Schwartz (1980) reported similar lancinating pains with temporal arteritis, but we have not encountered this.

Pareja, Kruszewski, and Caminero (1999) considered the differential diagnosis of idiopathic (primary) stabbing headache (PSH) from trigeminal neuralgia affecting the first division and short-lasting unilateral neuralgiform headache attacks with conjunctival injection and tearing (SUNCT) syndrome. SUNCT is confined to one periocular area and is associated with autonomic features not present in PSH, which is multifocal and variable in location. SUNCT lasts more than 5 seconds and commonly continues for a minute or more. SUNCT is often triggerable without a refractory period to re-triggering, whereas PSH is not triggerable. It affects men more than women, in contrast to PSH, which mainly affects women.

Sjaastad, Pettersen, and Bakketeig (2001) conducted a large-scale study of headache epidemiology in 1838 adults living in Vaga, Norway, and found that 35.2% reported primary stabbing headaches, a much higher proportion than in previous studies. The female-to-male ratio was about 1:5; earlier, in Spain, Pareja et al. (1996) had reported 1:6.6. The mean age of onset was 28 in the Norwegian series, and 47 in the Spanish series. Pareja et al. (1996) reported that in half of the patients the primary stabbing headaches were associated with another form of headache. Stabbing pains may also affect the face, neck, or other parts of the body (Sjaastad, Pettersen, & Bakketeig, 2003).

Contrary to the experience in adults, the literature suggests PSH in children is not usually accompanied by other forms of headache (Soriani et al., 1996). Our clinical experience is that careful inquiry in children will often result in reports of PSH in association with other primary headaches.

Jabs and Jolts Syndrome

Sjaastad (1992) first referred to sharp pains associated with chronic paroxysmal hemicrania (CPH) in 1979. He describes jabs and jolts as sharp, knifelike pains less than 1 minute in duration, occurring in patients with tension headache, migraine, or cluster headache as well as in headache-free individuals. These sensations are probably a variation on ice-pick pains but last longer and must be distinguished from episodes of CPH, which last a minimum of 3 minutes. Medina and Diamond (1981) reported multiple jabbing pains with episodic headaches, which they regarded as a cluster variant.

Ophthalmodynia

Researchers have described sudden stabbing pain in the eye as ophthalmodynia periodica. Lansche (1964) reported that more than 60% of patients with this syndrome suffered from migraine.

Pathophysiology and Treatment

Although researchers have not learned the mechanism of these transient pains, the lancinating quality of the pain resembles that of trigeminal neuralgia and suggests a paroxysmal neuronal discharge. The localization of stabbing pains to the habitual site of migraine or cluster headache may point to the pathophysiology of these conditions. Although a source of irritation may lie in the peripheral branches of the trigeminal nerve, more likely an intermittent deficit in central pain control mechanisms permits the spontaneous synchronous discharge of neurons receiving impulses from the area to which headache is referred.

Mathew (1981) reported that five patients with this syndrome improved substantially while treated with indomethacin 50 mg 3 times daily and did not respond to aspirin or placebo. Medina and Diamond (1981) found that 20 patients who were subject to frequent jabbing pains (unilateral in 13 cases) in association with atypical vascular headaches responded well to indomethacin, whereas Sjaastad (1992) stated that the response of jabs and jolts to indomethacin was partial or lacking.

Piovesan et al. (2002) reported that ice-pick pains secondary to a stroke responded to the cyclooxygenase 2 (COX-2) inhibitor celecoxib.

COUGH HEADACHE

Clinicians have long regarded sharp pain in the head on coughing, sneezing, straining, laughing, or stooping as a symptom of organic intracranial disease, commonly associated with obstruction of the cerebrospinal fluid (CSF) pathways. Symonds (1956) presented the case histories of six patients in whom cough headache was a symptom of a space-occupying lesion in the posterior fossa or of basilar impression from Paget's disease. He then described 21 patients with the same symptom in whom no intracranial disease became apparent. Cough headache disappeared in nine patients and improved spontaneously in another six patients. Two patients died of heart disease, and four were lost to follow-up. Symonds concluded that there was a syndrome of benign cough headache, now known as primary cough headache, which he attributed to the stretching of a pain-sensitive structure in the posterior fossa, possibly the result of an adhesive arachnoiditis. Of Symonds's 21 patients, 18 were males, and ages ranged from 37 to 77 years, with an average age of 55.

Ekbom (1986) cites an earlier description in the French literature by Tinel in 1932 concerning four patients whose headaches were brought on by coughing, nose blowing, breath holding, and bending the head forward. He also quotes observations by Nick on 15 patients, 12 of whom were men, ranging in age from 19 to 73 years.

Rooke (1968) considered cough headache a variety of exertional headache and recorded his experience with 103 patients who developed transient headaches on running, bending, coughing, sneezing, lifting, or straining at stool, in whom no intracranial disease could be detected and who were followed for 3 years or more. During the follow-up period, reinvestigation discovered structural lesions such as Chiari type 1 malformation, platybasia, subdural hematoma, and cerebral or cerebellar tumor in 10 patients. Of the remaining 93, within 5 years 30 were free of headache, and after 10 years 73 were improved or free of headache. This type of headache appeared in men more often than women, in the ratio 4:1. Rooke noted that this form of headache may appear for the first time after a respiratory infection with cough and that some patients reported an abrupt recovery after having abscessed teeth extracted, which Symonds had also noted.

We prefer to maintain the separation between primary cough headache and primary exertional headache (which is more common at a younger age), although the two obviously overlap.

Pascual et al. (1996) reported that on average their patients with cough headache were 43 years older than their patients with exertional headache. They analyzed their experience with 72 patients whose headaches were precipitated by coughing (30), physical exercise (28), or sexual activity (14). Of the patients with cough headache, 17 cases were secondary to Chiari type 1 malformations (see Figure 19.2). The remaining 13 patients, 10 men and 3 women, were diagnosed as having "benign cough headaches." Their ages range from 44 to 81 years (mean 67 ±11 years). Headache was also brought on by a sudden Valsalva maneuver in four subjects but never by physical exertion. Headache was bilateral in 12 cases and unilateral in 1. Doppler ultrasound showed no evidence of carotid disease in this last case. Indomethacin 75 mg daily was effective in the six patients for whom the physician prescribed it but not for patients with Chiari type 1 malformation. The tendency to primary cough headache persisted for 2 months to 2 years.

An atypical cough headache in a 57-year-old man was unilateral and recurred in bouts of 30 to 60 days reminiscent of episodic cluster headache (Perini & Toso, 1998). The headaches involved one supraorbital region, were very severe, and lasted for 1 to 10 minutes without any autonomic features. The pain was eased by a nonsteroid anti-inflammatory agent, nimesulide.

Pathophysiology

Williams (1976) recorded CSF pressure from the cisterna magna and lumbar region during coughing. He found a phase in which lumbar pressure exceeded cisternal pressure, followed by a phase in which the pressure gradient was reversed. He postulated that cough headache may be caused by a valvelike blockage at the foramen magnum that interferes with the downward or rebound pulsation. Williams (1980) later studied two patients with cough headache whose cerebellar tonsils descended below the foramen magnum without any obvious obstruction and confirmed a severe craniospinal pressure dissociation during the rebound after a Valsalva maneuver. Decompressing the cerebellar tonsils relieved the headache and eliminated the steep pressure gradient on coughing. He commented that coughing increased intrathoracic and intra-abdominal pressure, which transmitted to the epidural veins, creating a pressure wave and moving CSF rostrally. Presumably when the subject relaxed and the pressure gradient then reversed, temporary impaction of the cerebellar tonsils caused the headache. Whether this explanation applies to those patients without a Chiari type 1 malformation remains uncertain. The possibility of a sudden increase in venous pressure being sufficient by itself to cause headache must be considered. Lance (1991) reported the case of a man with a goiter large enough to cause sudden headache when his arms were elevated and the jugular veins distended (see Figure 15.7).

Symptomatic Cases

The most common secondary cough headaches are those caused by Chiari type 1 malformation in which a tongue of cerebellum projects through the foramen magnum and provides a valvelike obstruction to the flow of CSF on coughing. Patients with this Chiari type 1 malformation are significantly younger than patients with primary cough headache. Pascual et al. (1996) found that the age of onset in the secondary cases varied from 15 to 64 years (mean 39 ± 14 years). His patients complained of occipital and suboccipital pain precipitated by laughing, weight lifting, or sudden changes in posture, as well as by coughing. All patients later developed posterior fossa symptoms or signs. Eight patients underwent operation, which improved headache in seven.

Smith and Messing (1993) reported cough headache as the presenting feature of a cerebral aneurysm. Their patient described a severe right temporal ache on coughing or bending lasting 1 to 5 minutes, not relieved by indomethacin. After 24 days the pain became continuous, and a right third cranial nerve palsy developed. The clinicians found she had a posterior communicating artery aneurysm. After the operation, her headache disappeared.

Britton and Guiloff (1988) also reported cough headache as the presenting symptom of carotid stenosis persisting for a year before other neurologic symptoms appeared. After the artery occluded, causing a hemiparetic stroke, the headache disappeared.

Before cough headache is considered primary, these conditions must be excluded.

Treatment

Boes, Mathuru, and Goadsby (2002) in a comprehensive review of the subject reported that indomethacin 25 to 150 mg/day, combined with a protein-pump inhibitor for long-term use, was usually effective, but that 250 mg daily may be necessary in some cases. Indomethacin probably works by decreasing intracranial pressure. Acetazolamide and methysergide have also been effective (Boes, Mathuru, & Goadsby, 2002).

Raskin (1995) found that lumbar puncture relieved 6 out of 14 patients with cough headaches. Another 6 of these patients and 14 of 16 patients in a comparison group responded to indomethacin.

EXERTIONAL HEADACHE

Headache may be precipitated by any form of exercise and often has the pulsatile quality of migraine. Credit must be given to Hippocrates for first recognizing this syndrome, as he wrote, "One should be able to recognize those who have headaches from gymnastic exercises, or running, or walking, or hunting, or any other unseasonable labor, or from immoderate venery" (Adams, 1848).

Dalessio (1974) drew attention to this form of headache in an editorial in which he cited running, rowing, tennis, and wrestling as possible causes, and mentioned that heat, high humidity, lack of training, and performance at high altitudes (such as the Olympic games in Mexico City) were contributing factors. Massey (1982) presented three cases of headaches resembling migraine, one with visual disturbance and mild hemiparesis, precipitated by running short or long distances. Sudden, severe headache can also be precipitated by swimming (Indo & Takahashi, 1990) and weight lifting (Paulson, 1983). Paulson considered strain or stretch of cervical ligaments as a possible cause of weight-lifter's headaches, but the sudden onset and persisting sensitivity to coughing, sneezing, and straining suggests acute venous distension as a possible mechanism for these. Headache after sustained exertion, particularly in hot conditions, is more likely to develop from arterial dilation, but objective evidence is lacking.

Symptomatic Cases

Cardiac ischemia may present as unilateral or bilateral exertional headache, relieved promptly by rest, as an unusual referral pattern of angina that may precede chest pain (Grace et al., 1997; Lance & Lambros, 1997) (see Figure 13.1). Stress testing (exercise on a treadmill) will confirm the diagnosis as ST changes develop in the electrocardiogram (ECG) at the onset of headache. Coronary angiography followed by angioplasty or bypass surgery relieves the symptom.

Clinicians have reported exertional headache with pheochromocytoma (Paulson, Zipf, & Beckman, 1979), spontaneous CSF leaks (Mokri, 2002), and Paget's disease (Queiroz, Dach, & Silva, 2003). Gadolinium enhancement of the meninges on magnetic resonance imaging (MRI) may detect low CSF pressure syndromes (see Chapter 16). The clinician may have to exclude intracranial

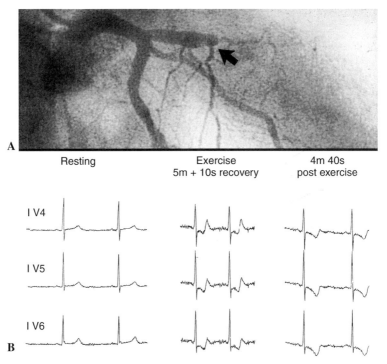

FIGURE 13.1   *A,* Anginal headache, appearing at the same time as ST changes in the ECG during stress testing. *B,* Occlusion of the left anterior descending branch of the coronary artery. Anginal headache was cured by coronary artery bypass grafting. (From Lance and Lambros, 1997. Reproduced by permission from the editor of *Headache.*)

lesions or stenosis of the carotid arteries, as discussed for benign cough headache.

Treatment

The most logical form of treatment is to take exercise gradually and progressively whenever possible. Lambert and Burnet (1985) described how a prescribed warm-up period prevented "swimmer's headache." Diamond and Medina (1979) reported that taking indomethacin over a follow-up period of 3 to 18 months relieved exertional headache in 9 out of 11 patients. Mathew (1981) recorded similar success with indomethacin 50 mg three times daily (with an antacid). Diamond (1982) described 15 patients, aged 8 to 54 years, with exertional headaches lasting for an average of 4 hours. Indomethacin in daily doses varying from 25 to 150 mg controlled the headaches almost completely in 13 patients. Ergotamine tartrate 1 to 2 mg orally or methysergide 1 to 2 mg orally given 30 minutes before exercise begins is also a useful prophylactic measure.

HEADACHE ASSOCIATED WITH SEXUAL ACTIVITY

Hippocrates included immoderate venery (defined as "the practice or pursuit of sexual pleasure" or "indulgence of sexual desire" by the Oxford English Dictionary) as a cause of exertional headache (Adams, 1848). However, "sex headaches" can arise with little or no physical exertion by the participant.

Headaches developing at the time of orgasm are not always benign. Sexual intercourse precipitated subarachnoid hemorrhage in 3 of 66 cases (4.5%) that Fisher (1968) reported and 6 (12%) of 50 cases Lundberg and Osterman (1974) studied. Cerebral or brainstem infarction has also been reported. One young man developed a brainstem thrombosis (Lance, 1976), and another, a left hemisphere infarction (Levy, 1981). Martinez, Roig, and Arboix (1988) described three patients whose neurologic deficits began at the moment of orgasm. A 50-year-old woman developed confusion and amnesia lasting 3 days, with a right Babinski sign for 20 days; a man aged 40 years had a right hemisensory defect for 24 hours; and a 36-year-old man had a left homonymous hemianopia, which cleared over 2 weeks. Cerebral angiography was normal in the first two patients but showed poor filling of the right posterior cerebral artery in the third. These authors cite another three cases that Nick and Bakouche described in 1980.

Wolff (1963) probably first recognized that most headaches occurring during sexual activity are not associated with an underlying vascular malformation and have a benign prognosis, but Kriz later reported 25 cases from Czechoslovakia in 1970, which Martin (1973) cited. Martin related the histories of five male patients subject to severe headache toward the end of intercourse, three of whom had a past history of migraine. Paulson and Klawans (1974) reported 14 patients with this condition as having "benign orgasmic cephalgia," but this term does not cover those patients whose headache begins before orgasm.

Sex headache affects men more than women and may occur at any time during the years of sexual activity. Capriciously, it may develop on several occasions in succession and then not trouble the patient again, although there is no obvious change in sexual technique. In a description of 21 patients (Lance, 1976), 16 were male and 5 female, aged from 18 to 58 years. Three patients experienced headache with masturbation, two of whom also complained of similar headaches during sexual intercourse. The headaches of the remaining patients were confined to sexual intercourse. Those patients who stopped sexual activity when they first noticed headache found it subsided within a period of 5 minutes to 2 hours. Those who proceeded to orgasm reported that a severe headache persisted for 3 minutes to 4 hours, and a milder headache lingered for 1 to 48 hours afterward. Only four patients had previously suffered from migraine, and two had experienced exertional headaches. Seven were hypertensive.

The headaches were more likely to occur when the patient attempted intercourse for a second time after a brief interval. One young man complained of headaches at orgasm while he was on vacation for a month, engaging in sexual intercourse two or three times daily. When the vacation was over and intercourse frequency declined to once daily, he remained free of headache. Carotid or vertebral angiography, performed in nine of the patients with this syndrome, was completely normal. As familiarity with the syndrome increases, investigation can be reserved for patients who may have an underlying lesion.

Three kinds of headache are associated with sexual activity. The first is a dull headache, commonly bilateral and occipital in site, that comes on as sexual excitement mounts. It is probably related to excessive contraction of head and neck muscles, because it can be prevented or relieved by deliberately relaxing these muscle groups. The second type of headache, more severe and explosive in onset, appears immediately before or at the moment of orgasm, presumably caused by the increase in blood pressure at this time. A third type, was described by Paulson and Klawans (1974) in 3 of their 14 patients with headaches arising during coitus. This form of headache was worse on standing up and thus resembles the low-pressure headache following lumbar puncture. We have now seen patients with diffuse meningeal enhancement on MRI after vigorous or repeated sexual activity and subsequent postural headache. The MRI changes and clinical picture are typical of low CSF volume headache and often respond to intravenous caffeine.

What is the relationship between sex headaches and physical exertion? Silbert et al. (1991) found that 18 of their 45 patients subject to acute vascular headaches during sexual intercourse had also experienced headaches on exertion. Nine patients described a close link between the two sorts of headache, with one following the other within a few days and a dull, generalized headache persisting between the two acute events. During follow-up for an average of 6 years, two fifths of these patients had recurrences of their sex headaches, usually at times of fatigue or stress. Selwyn (1985) reported that, of 32 patients with headaches related to coitus who replied to a questionnaire, 11 had experienced similar headaches after both exercise and sexual intercourse. Of the 32, 9 had a history of hypertension and 15 a background of migraine. Of 10 patients whose headaches developed at the time of orgasm, 5 had previously suffered from migraine. Taking all 32 patients, 21 had a history of migraine and 11 of hypertension. Two patients had experienced such headaches with masturbation and one after a nocturnal emission following dreaming during sleep. Pascual et al. (1996) found a relationship between sex headaches and exertional headaches, but not with cough headaches.

Johns (1986) summarized 110 cases in the literature at that time, 86 male and 24 female. Of these, 5 had a low CSF pressure syndrome after intercourse, 17 had a diffuse dull type of headache, and the remaining headaches had migrainous features, with 40 occurring at orgasm. He also described four sisters with this syndrome. Ostergaard and Kraft (1992) followed 26 patients for up to 14 years. Half the patients lost their headaches after periods of 6 weeks to 6 months, but half had recurrences after freedom for up to 6 years.

Frese et al. (2003) interviewed 51 patients with headaches associated with sexual activity (HSA) and found that the mean age of onset was 39.2 (± 11.1) years, and the male-to-female ratio was 2.9:1. Eleven patients had the dull type of headache (HAS type 1), and forty had an explosive onset (HSA type 2). These authors found a strong association with migraine (25%), exertional headache (29%), and tension-type headache (45%).

Pathophysiology

The possible relationship of sex headaches with migraine, hypertension, and exertional headaches has been discussed previously.

Muscle contraction, or at least the sensation of diffuse constriction, appears to be a major feature in the milder headache that becomes more severe as sexual excitement increases. Of 21 patients (Lance, 1976), 10 stated they were subject to headaches at times of emotional tension unrelated to sexual activity. In seven patients the tension headache was similar but milder than the headache experienced with intercourse. Five patients stated they were aware of excessive muscle contraction, particularly involving the jaw and neck muscles, and found they could reduce the intensity of the headache by deliberately relaxing those muscles while continuing with intercourse or masturbation. The headache seemed related to the degree of sexual excitement and not to physical exertion. If patients with such "muscle contraction headaches" continued to orgasm, the headache usually became very intense and persisted for up to 48 hours afterward. Masters and Johnson (1966) have commented on the excessive contraction of facial, jaw, and neck muscles as sexual excitement mounts.

The vascular aspect of sex headaches may be superimposed on the tension-type headache or may occur without warning at orgasm. It is abrupt in onset, occipital or generalized, frequently throbbing, and sometimes associated with palpitations, resembling the headache of pheochromocytoma (Lance & Hinterberger, 1976). Masters and Johnson observed that blood pressure rose by 40 to 100 mm Hg systolic and 20 to 50 mm Hg diastolic during orgasm, figures quite comparable with the paroxysms caused by pheochromocytoma. Littler, Honour, and Sleight (1974) recorded similar increases of up to 214/135 mm Hg. One of our patients experienced a headache comparable in severity with her sex headache after taking a tablet of the sympathomimetic drug pseudoephedrine, supporting the concept that a sudden increase in blood pressure at orgasm may cause the explosive nature of these headaches. Staunton and Moore (1978) provided an interesting example of a pressor response causing coital cephalgia. A patient with obstruction of the lower aorta reported this problem, developing a blood pressure of 250/130 mm Hg after 3 minutes exercise on a bicycle ergometer. After a successful aortic-iliac bypass, his coital headaches disappeared.

Clinicians found multiple areas of cerebral arterial spasm in a 30-year-old man after a coital headache exacerbated by exertion (Silbert et al., 1989). If cerebral arterial spasm is a feature of the explosive orgasmic headache, it is not surprising that strokes have resulted on some occasions.

We can thus conclude that an acute pressor response with or without pre-existing hypertension and arterial disease causes the "thunderclap headache" that may occur at orgasm.

Management

Primary (benign) sex headaches are usually irregular and recur infrequently, so management can often be limited to reassurance and advice about ceasing sexual activity if a milder warning headache develops. When the condition recurs regularly or frequently, the patient can prevent it by taking propranolol, but the dosage required varies from 40 to 200 mg daily (Porter & Jankovic, 1981). Beta-blockers presumably act by limiting the surge of blood pressure at orgasm. One patient was successfully treated by the calcium-channel blocking agent diltiazem 60 mg three times daily (Akpunonu & Ahrens, 1991), and we have used this medicine with good effect. Ergotamine tartrate, indomethacin, or methysergide taken before sexual activity may also prevent such headache. An explanation of the natural history to settle and some sympathy, understanding, and patience by the sufferer's partner fixes much of this problem.

PRIMARY HYPNIC HEADACHE

Raskin (1988) first drew attention to the uncommon syndrome of primary hypnic headache. He reported six patients, five of whom were male, all aged 60 years or older, who were waking up consistently with generalized headaches that persisted for 30 to 60 minutes. Two volunteered that these headaches always woke them from a dream. Three patients reported accompanying nausea. The headaches were not alleviated by amitriptyline but responded to lithium 300 mg or propranolol 600 mg at night. Raskin attributed the condition to a disorder of the brain's "biological clock" in the hypothalamus, pointing out that cluster headache, cyclic migraine, and manic-depressive disorder are also tied to bodily rhythms and responded to lithium.

Evers and Goadsby (2003) have reviewed the 71 cases of hypnic headache reported in the literature to date. Of the 65 patients whose sex was mentioned, 24 were men and 41 were women ranging in age from 26 to 83 years. The headache was bilateral in 61% and unilateral in 39%. It varied in frequency from one each week to six per night. Headache usually started 2 to 4 hours after falling asleep, was moderate in intensity, and persisted for 15 minutes to 3 hours.

Nausea affected 19.4%, and 6.8% experienced mild photophobia, phonophobia, or both. Some autonomic features such as lacrimation arose in six patients, two of whom developed ptosis. No relevant abnormality appeared on computed tomography (CT), MRI, electroencephalogram (EEG), or carotid Doppler ultrasound studies.

Pathophysiology

Most episodes start during rapid eye movement (REM) sleep with or without oxygen desaturation at that time.

Cells that switch REM sleep cells off lie in the locus ceruleus and dorsal raphe nucleus and discharge regularly during waking hours, ceasing during REM sleep. Their action depends on noradrenergic and serotonergic transmission, respectively. Because pathways from these areas form part of the body's endogenous pain-control system, their switching off could account for the onset of pain with REM sleep (Dodick, Eross, & Parish, 2003; Pinessi et al., 2003).

The suprachiasmatic nucleus of the hypothalamus controls the sleep-wake cycle, and researchers believe that reduced melatonin secretion plays a part in initiating hypnic headache.

Treatment

Evers and Goadsby (2003) summarized the response to treatment in reported cases. Lithium achieved good results in 26 of 35 patients, caffeine in 6 of 16, indomethacin in 7 of 18, flunarizine in 4 of 5, melatonin in 3 of 7, and prednisone in the only 2 patients in whom it had been tried. On going to bed at night, the patient usually takes caffeine 100 mg or lithium 300 to 600 mg.

PRIMARY AND SECONDARY THUNDERCLAP HEADACHE

Day and Raskin (1986) called headaches of explosive onset described as a sudden blow to the head "thunderclap headache." They reported a woman with three such episodes who was found to have an unruptured aneurysm of the internal carotid artery with adjacent areas of segmental vasospasm. Abbott and van Hille (1986) questioned the relationship between thunderclap headache and aneurysm in the absence of CT scan or CSF evidence of subarachnoid hemorrhage, describing 14 patients, 6 of whom had normal four-vessel cerebral angiography. Wijdicks, Kerkhoff, and van Gijn (1988) followed 71 patients, whose CT scan and CSF findings were negative, for an average of 3.3 years. Of these, 12 patients had further such headaches, and 31 (44%) later had regular episodes of migraine or tension headache. Factors identified as precipitating the headaches were sexual intercourse in 3 cases, coughing in 4, and exertion in 12, whereas the remainder had no obvious cause. A history of hypertension marked 11 and previous headache was reported in 22.

Markus (1991) compared the presentation of 37 patients with subarachnoid hemorrhage and 18 with a similar thunderclap headache but normal CSF examination (primary thunderclap headache) and could not discern any characteristic to distinguish the two conditions on clinical grounds. Landtblom et al. (2002), who undertook a prospective study of 137 consecutive patients with thunderclap headache, reached the same conclusion. They found the cause to be subarachnoid hemorrhage in 23, cerebral infarction in 5, intracerebral hematoma in 3, aseptic meningitis in 4, cerebral edema in 1, and venous sinus thrombosis in 1. They could not identify a cause in the remainder. The attacks occurred in 11 cases during sexual activity, and 2 of these had a subarachnoid hemorrhage.

Other causes of thunderclap headache to consider are pressor responses, as in patients with pheochromocytoma or who ingest tyramine-containing substances while on monoamine oxidase inhibitors. Obstructive hydrocephalus (e.g., a colloid cyst of the third ventricle) and carotid or vertebral artery dissection also must be considered. Chapter 19 summarizes the differential diagnosis.

We can conclude that the investigations of thunderclap headache unrelated to coitus should include a CT or MRI scan and CSF examination, but that cerebral angiography is usually unnecessary. When a typical explosive headache occurs at orgasm, particularly if after an escalating tension-type headache, investigation could consist of CT or MRI scanning unless other features, such as neck stiffness, mandate a CSF examination.

Call-Fleming Syndrome

Arterial spasm has been demonstrated angiographically in some cases of thunderclap headache (Silbert et al., 1989; Slivka & Philbrook, 1995). Call et al. (1988) described a more malignant disorder of segmental cerebral vasospasm in which nausea, vomiting, and photophobia accompanied recurrent thunder-clap headaches. Generalized epileptic seizures occurred in 7 of 19 patients, neurologic symptoms also in 7 of 19 patients, and a permanent neurologic deficit in 4. Infarction in reported cases often involves the parieto-occipital area.

In an editorial commentary, Dodick (2003) wrote that the syndrome of thunderclap headache, diffuse reversible vasospasm, and delayed ischemic deficits may occur spontaneously or secondary to an underlying metabolic, hemodynamic, or biochemical insult. Intravenous nimodipine or oral calcium-channel antagonists appear useful in treatment, but take care not to cause hypotension sufficient to further impair cerebral perfusion.

Reversible Posterior Leukoencephalopathy

Hinchey et al. (1996) reported a similar clinical picture associated with a sudden increase in blood pressure in renal disease or postpartum eclampsia, as affecting the parieto-occipital area, and termed it a "reversible posterior leukoen-cephalopathy syndrome." It can also develop during treatment with immunosup-pressant drugs. Usually such patients urgently require antihypertensive therapy (Dodick, 2003).

HEADACHE AS A SYMPTOM OF EPILEPSY

Young and Blume (1983) examined the seizure pattern of 358 patients with epilepsy and found 24 who experienced pain during their attacks, including 11 with headache as a symptom. Unilateral or bilateral headache was the first indi-cation of a seizure in seven and followed other ictal symptoms in four patients. The epilepsy for 8 out of 11 had a temporal lobe origin, but the area affected by their headache bore no relation to the epileptogenic focus. In some of these patients, headaches were migrainous, in which case diminished cerebral blood flow during an aura may have precipitated the epileptic manifestations, but in others the headache was clearly a part of the ictal discharge. Laplante, Saint-Hilaire, and Bouvier (1983) discovered two patients with ictal headaches who had a right temporal origin for their attacks, which vanished after right temporal lobectomy. The headaches were paroxysmal, lasting for less than a minute, and were described as "not like any headache before."

HEADACHES CAUSED BY VASOACTIVE SUBSTANCES

Headaches resulting from dilation of intracranial vessels are characteristi-cally throbbing in nature and made worse by jarring of the head or any sudden movement. Vasodilator medications—for example, phosphodiesterase (PDE) inhibitors such as sildenafil (Viagra)—may cause headaches and induce migraine attacks.

Alcohol

Ethyl alcohol is a vasodilator agent and may trigger migraine or cluster headache in this way although the issue has never been adequately studied. The cause of "hangover headache," which happens the day after excessive alcohol intake, is still uncertain. The average rate at which a normal-sized adult metabolizes alcohol is about 10 mL/hour (Ritchie, 1970). It is first oxidated to acetaldehyde by alcohol dehydrogenase, and acetaldehyde is then converted to acetyl-coenzyme A, which is oxidated or used in the synthesis of cholesterol and fatty acids. Disulfiram, administered to discourage the intake of alcohol, increases the blood acetaldehyde concentration 5 to 10 times and produces the "aldehyde syndrome." The face becomes flushed and a throbbing headache may develop, which is associated with nausea, vomiting, and giddiness followed by hypotension and pallor. Whether the headache of a hangover can be attributed solely to acetaldehyde or other break-down products of alcohol remains unknown. Raskin and Appenzeller (1980) reviewed the subject and concluded by stating that "the performance of experi-ments that very often must take place on Sunday mornings may be an important factor in perpetuating our ignorance."

Marijuana

Dry mouth, paresthesias, a sensation of warmth, and suffusion of the conjuncti-vae are common after ingestion of 60 mg of *Cannabis sativa.* Of 10 subjects studied by Ames (1958), 5 complained of mild frontal headache, presumably related to vasodilation. Some tension-type headaches are relieved by smoking marijuana, so its relaxing and vasodilator properties may combine to help this form of headache, just as alcohol does.

Cocaine

Clinicians should take seriously the complaint of headache in cocaine abusers, because some researchers have reported intracranial hemorrhage, ischemic stroke, endocarditis, and brain abscess (Dhuna, Pascual-Leone, & Belgrade, 1991). Dhuna et al. described headaches with migrainous features during cocaine intoxication. Some developed acutely, some during the course of a cocaine binge, and others on withdrawal. Associated neurologic symptoms and signs were attributed to the sympathomimetic effect of cocaine causing cerebral vasoconstriction.

Monosodium Glutamate: "Chinese Restaurant Syndrome"

Headache has been reported as part of the Chinese restaurant syndrome (Schaumburg et al., 1969)—a symptom complex of pressure and tightness in the face; burning over the trunk, neck, and shoulders; and a pressing pain in the chest, which may arise 25 minutes after the patient eats a Chinese meal. The headache, a pressure or throbbing over the temples, and a bandlike sensation around the forehead, has been attributed to monosodium glutamate (MSG), which is used abundantly in Chinese cooking. About 3 g of MSG, contained in 200 mL of wonton ("short") soup, may provoke headache in people sensitive to it.

Nitrites and Nitrates: "Hot Dog Headache" (Nitric Oxide Donor–Induced Headaches)

When clinicians used inhalation of amyl nitrite to treat angina pectoris, it often caused a sudden bilateral throbbing headache as a complication of its vasodilator action. Glyceryl trinitrate may have the same effect in patients who are not usually subject to headache, and it reliably precipitates cluster headache during a bout after a latent period of 1 to 2 hours. Normal subjects rarely get delayed headaches, but people with migraine or tension-type headache may. Glyceryl trinitrate is a donor of nitric oxide, which plays an intermediary role in vasodilation.

An uncommon but interesting variation on this theme is a headache that afflicts some people after eating cured meat. Meat processors add nitrites or nitrates to salt to give a uniform red appearance to cured meat. The concentration of nitrite in the cooked meat is only 50 to 130 parts per million, but this is enough to cause headache in some susceptible individuals after eating hot dogs, bacon, ham, salami, and other such products. Henderson and Raskin (1972) described such a patient who developed headache on most occasions after ingesting 10 mg of sodium nitrite but not after a placebo of sodium bicarbonate.

Histamine Headache

Pickering and Hess (1933) found that the intravenous infusion of histamine caused flushing of the face followed by a generalized throbbing headache. Wolff (1963) and his colleagues showed that headache came on after the scalp arteries had returned to their normal caliber, whereas CSF pulsation was still increased by 250% while histamine headache was in progress. Increasing intracranial pressure to 1000 mm CSF relieved histamine headache immediately, confirming the idea that it was caused by dilation of intracranial vessels rather than of scalp arteries. The intravenous infusion of histamine, in doses that did not cause headache in normal subjects, evoked headache in 24 of 25 migraine patients and in 5 out of 10 patients susceptible to tension headache (Krabbe & Olesen, 1980).

Rebound Headache—Nicotine and Caffeine

Unlike vasodilators, vasoconstrictor agents do not in themselves induce headache, but a rebound dilation may follow the constriction nicotine induces as the result of excessive tobacco smoking or the vasoconstrictor effect of caffeine contained in tea, coffee, cola drinks, or commercial analgesic preparations. Children and adolescents may suffer caffeine headaches from a heavy consumption of cola drinks. Hering-Hanit and Gadoth (2003) reported 36 youngsters with near-daily headaches from drinking at least 1.5 liters (containing almost 200 mg of caffeine) each day. As the effect of the last dose wears off, a dull headache may become apparent, which is relieved by repeating the dose, one of the factors in habituation (Greden et al., 1980). Whether this is a vascular rebound or second messages, rebound is undertermined.

Regional cerebral blood flow decreased after the ingestion of 250 mg of caffeine and increased in the frontal areas during abstinence in a group with high habitual caffeine consumption, involving more than six cups of coffee daily for at least 3 years (Mathew & Wilson, 1985).

Peptide-Secreting Tumors

Lance (1991) reported the rare association of episodic flushing and headache with an abdominal tumor (renal oncocytoma). The vacuoles of some cells stained for calcitonin gene–related peptide (CGRP). Headaches and flushing ceased after the tumor was removed. CGRP causes an immediate headache when infused by dilating extracranial rather than intracranial arteries (Petersen et al., 2003).

Drug-Induced Headaches

Headache may be a side effect of some drugs other than vasodilators, possibly by interference with 5-HT mechanisms. Zemelidine, indomethacin, cimetidine, and ranitidine were commonly reported by clinicians to the World Health Organization (WHO) as being responsible for headaches (Askmark, Lundberg, & Olsson, 1989). Agents that lower serum cholesterol, such as gemfibrozil and bezafibrate, may cause generalized pulsatile headaches (Hodgetts & Tunnicliffe. 1989). Simvastatin has also been reported as being a cause of headache and muscle pains. The frequent consumption of opioids, analgesics, ergotamine tartrate, or triptans is now considered a cause of chronic daily headache. The Headache Classification Subcommittee of the IHS (2004) lists a large number of drugs that have been reputed to induce headaches. Headache, often of the "thunderclap" variety, has followed the use of cyclosporin (Steiger et al., 1994), tacrolimus (Kiemeneij et al., 2003), and other immunosuppressant agents.

HEADACHE ASSOCIATED WITH SYSTEMIC INFECTIONS

Most febrile illnesses entail headache, presumably because bacterial or viral toxins effect trigemine vascular afferents. Neck stiffness (meningismus) may be present even in the absence of aseptic or bacterial meningitis but warrants immediate investigation—and urgent treatment if bacterial meningitis is suspected. Injections of typhoid and other vaccines may induce a febrile reaction with headache.

METABOLIC CAUSES OF HEADACHE

Hypoxia and Hypercapnia

Carbon dioxide is the most efficient cerebral vasodilator, and the headache caused by prolonged exposure to an overcrowded, underventilated room presumably owes its origin to this effect. Gilbert (1972) coined the term *turtle headache* for patients who pulled the bedcovers over their head on settling down to sleep. Ceasing the habit cured the headache. Conversely, oxygen constricts cerebral vessels that dilate under conditions of hypoxia. Headache may be a symptom of sleep apnea, mountain sickness, or chronic pulmonary insufficiency.

Carbon monoxide poisoning may induce headache by hypoxia. In 1931, Charles Kingsford Smith set out to fly from Australia to England in an Avro Avian named Southern Cross Minor in an attempt to break the record. The plane developed a leak in the exhaust pipe, allowing carbon monoxide to leak into the cockpit. Before the defect was remedied, he wrote in his diary that he felt awful: "a rotten night . . . my head bashed away like a bloody drum" (McNally, 1966).

Sleep Apnea

Sleep apnea commonly affects overweight men and is characterized by snoring during sleep and long pauses without respiration followed by a loud inspiratory gasp, producing a restless night followed by daytime drowsiness. Pocera and Dalessio (1995) found that morning headache was not more frequent after sleep apnea than in other sleep disorders, but 30% of patients did improve with the use of intranasal continuous positive airway pressure (CPAP) treatment. Although headache is a common complaint in patients referred for sleep studies, researchers found no correlation between headache and snoring (Neau et al., 2002), the severity of sleep apnea, or oxygen desaturation (Sand, Hagen, & Schroder, 2003).

Mountain Sickness

Headache is the most frequent and severe symptom of acute mountain sickness (Appenzeller, 1972; King & Robinson, 1972). Of 30 young men subjected for 30 hours to simulated altitudes of 14,000 to 15,000 feet in a hypobaric chamber, 28 developed headache. This was usually bilateral but was localized to one side in 25%. The headache was more completely relieved by compressing the superficial temporal arteries than by the Valsalva maneuver, suggesting that the extracranial arteries were more important in producing headache than was intracranial vasodilation.

Silber et al. (2003) studied the nature of high-altitude headaches in 60 members of an expedition to Nepal. Fifty experienced from 1 to 10 headaches at altitudes above 3000 m (mean 4723 m). Headaches occurred more often in those who had been prone to headache at other times. About half of those with headache had other symptoms of acute mountain sickness such as loss of appetite, nausea, fatigue, dizziness, and sleep disorders. Most of the headaches were bilateral and lasted between 4 and 8 hours. They were aggravated by bending, coughing, or sneezing, suggesting the possibility of intracranial hypertension.

The cause of the headache is not necessarily hypoxia, because inhaling oxygen does not provide relief, and similar headaches resembling migraine have been reported after exposure to a hyperbaric chamber. Other factors such as fluid and electrolyte changes may play a part. Spironolactone, an aldosterone antagonist, prevents the headache of mountain sickness if taken prophylactically. Acetazolamide 500 mg daily proved an effective preventive agent in a double-blind crossover trial, the crossing over taking place between Mount Kenya and Mount Kilimanjaro (Greene et al., 1981). Diuretics such as frusemide can also be used to treat altitude headache.

Hypoglycemia

Hypoglycemia may produce a migrainous headache in some people who miss a regular meal or in those with carbohydrate intolerance, in which case headache appears several hours after meals. Amery (1987) discusses the relationship of hypoglycemia to migraine. Fasting enforced by religious practices may be responsible, exemplified by "Yom Kippur headache" (Mosek & Korczyn, 1995), although dehydration may also play a part, because these headaches may be eased by lying down.

Headache During Hemodialysis

Bana, Yap, and Graham (1972) reported that 70% of 44 patients had experienced headache during hemodialysis. Six patients described generalized constricting headaches, and eleven of twelve migraine patients had their usual headache precipitated by dialysis. The authors described a new entity of "dialysis headache," which started a few hours after the procedure as a mild bifrontal ache and later became throbbing, sometimes accompanied by nausea and vomiting. The severity of the headache correlated with hypertension, longer intervals between each dialysis, fall in blood pressure during dialysis, decrease in serum sodium, and decrease in osmolality. Bilateral nephrectomy and successful renal transplant relieved headaches. Dialysis headache appears to be of vascular origin, is associated with the release of vasodilator peptides, and responds to small doses of ergotamine. The IHS diagnostic criteria state that the headaches should develop during at least half of the dialysis sessions, resolve within 72 hours, and cease after successful kidney transplant.

Headache Following Epileptic Seizures

Cerebral vasodilation is probably responsible for the headache that follows a major (tonic-clonic) epileptic seizure. Plum, Posner, and Troy (1968) have analyzed the effects on the monkey's cerebral circulation of the direct metabolic changes resulting from the seizure discharge itself and of indirect effects from alterations in respiration and muscle metabolism. Although the animals were anesthetized, paralyzed, and adequately ventilated with oxygen, during an induced seizure cerebral blood flow increased to a mean of 264% over the resting level. This was caused by increased carbon dioxide production and loss of autoregulation of the cerebral blood vessels, so that flow increased passively with the neurogenic elevation of blood pressure accompanying a seizure. Despite an increase in cerebral metabolism of 60%, venous oxygen tension actually rose and there was no demonstrable cerebral acidosis. The same group of researchers has reported similar findings in humans. In a spontaneous epileptic seizure, hypoxia from respiratory arrest is an added factor.

Of 100 patients with epilepsy studied by Schon and Blau (1987), 51 suffered postictal headaches. In eight out of nine patients who had had migraine, the postictal headache resembled a mild attack of their usual migraine, and half of the remainder had migrainous symptoms such as nausea and photophobia associated with their headaches. Of the 51 patients, 13 were subject only to "minor seizures," which throws doubt on the idea that metabolically induced changes in cerebral blood are the sole causative factor. Following this line of thought, D'Alessandro et al. (1987) examined 174 patients with nonconvulsive epileptic attacks and found that the 23 patients prone to postictal headache all suffered from complex partial seizures. These patients showed no greater tendency to suffer interictal headaches than those who had simple partial seizures or generalized nonconvulsive attacks (absences with or without myoclonic jerks). The authors postulated that neuronal discharges originating in the locus ceruleus and brainstem raphe nuclei might trigger the vascular changes responsible for postictal headaches.

CONCLUSION

The primary syndromes described in this chapter are "benign" in the sense that no structural lesion can be held responsible and the prognosis is favorable. Because of the association of similar symptoms with the presence of space-occupying intracranial lesions, aneurysms, cerebral atherosclerosis, or cardiac ischemia in some instances, the physician must use clinical judgment to determine the extent of investigation required in each individual.

References

Abbott, R. J., & van Hille, P. (1986). Thunderclap headache and unruptured cerebral aneurysm. *Lancet, ii,* 1459.

Adams, F. (1848). *The genuine works of Hippocrates* (p. 94). London: Sydenham Society. (Reprinted 1939, Baltimore: Williams and Wilkins)

Akpunonu, S. E., & Ahrens, J. (1991). Sexual headaches: Case report, review, and treatment with calcium blocker. *Headache, 31,* 141–145.

Amery, W. K. (1987) The oxygen theory of migraine. In J. N. Blau (Ed.), *Migraine, clinical and research aspects* (pp. 411–412). Baltimore: Johns Hopkins University Press.

Ames, F. (1958). A clinical and metabolic study of acute intoxication with *Cannabis sativa* and its role in the model psychoses. *J Ment Sci, 104,* 977–999.

Appenzeller, O. (1972). Altitude headache. *Headache, 12,* 126–179.

Askmark, H., Lundberg, P. O., & Olsson, S. (1989). Drug-related headache. *Headache, 29,* 441–444.

Bana, D. S., Yap, A. U., & Graham, J. R. (1972). Headache during hemodialysis. *Headache, 2,* 1–14.

Boes, C. J., Mathuru, M. S., & Goadsby, P. J. (2002). Benign cough headache. *Cephalalgia, 22,* 772–779.

Britton, T. C., & Guiloff, R. J. (1988). Carotid artery disease presenting as cough headache. *Lancet, i,* 1406–1407.

Call, G. K., Fleming, M. C., Sealfen, S., et al. (1988). Reversible segmental vasoconstriction. *Stroke, 19,* 1159–1170.

D'Alessandro, R., Sacquegna, T., Pazzaglia, P., & Lugaresi, E. (1987). Headache after partial complex seizures. In F. Andermann & E. Lugaresi (Eds.), *Migraine and epilepsy* (pp. 273–278). Boston: Butterworths.

Dalessio, D. J. (1974). Editorial. Effort migraine. *Headache, 14,* 53.

Day, J. W., & Raskin, N. H. (1986). Thunderclap headache: Symptom of unruptured cerebral aneurysm. *Lancet, ii,* 1247–1248.

Dhuna, A., Pascual-Leone, A., & Belgrade, M. (1991). Cocaine-related vascular headaches. *J Neurol Neurosurg Psychiatry, 54,* 803–806.

Diamond, S. (1982). Prolonged benign exertional headache: Its clinical characteristics and response to indomethacin. *Headache, 22,* 96–98.

Diamond, S., & Medina, J. L. (1979). Benign exertional headache: Successful treatment with indomethacin. *Headache, 19,* 249.

Dodick, D. W. (2003). Reversible segmental cerebral vasoconstriction (Call-Fleming syndrome): The role of calcium antagonists. *Cephalalgia, 23,* 163–165.

Dodick, D. W., Eross, E. J., & Parish, J. M. (2003). Clinical, anatomical and physiologic relationship between sleep and headache. *Headache, 43,* 282–292.

Drummond. P. D., & Lance, J. W. (1984). Neurovascular disturbances in headache patients. *Clin Exp Neurol, 20,* 93–99.

Ekbom, K. (1975). Some observations on pain in cluster headache. *Headache, 14,* 219–225.

Ekbom, K. (1986). Cough headache. In F. Clifford Rose (Ed.), *Handbook of clinical neurology.* Vol. 4(48). *Headache* (pp. 367–371). Amsterdam: Elsevier.

Evers, S., & Goadsby P. J. (2003). Hypnic headache. Clinical features, pathophysiology and treatment. *Neurology, 60,* 905–909.

Fisher, C. M. (1968). Headache in cerebrovascular disease. In P. J. Vinken & G. W. Bruyn (Eds.), *Handbook of clinical neurology.* Vol. 5. *Headaches and cranial neuralgias* (pp. 124–156). Amsterdam: Elsevier.

Frese, A., Eikermann, A., Frese, K., Schwaag, S., Hussedt, I.-W., & Evers, S. (2003). Headache associated with sexual activity: Demography, clinical features and comorbidity. *Neurology, 61,* 796–800.

Gilbert, G. J. (1972). Hypoxia and bedcovers. *JAMA, 221,* 1165–1166.

Grace, A., Horgan, J., Breathnach, K., & Staunton, H. (1997). Anginal headache and its basis. *Cephalalgia, 17,* 195–196.

Greden, J. F., Victor, B. S., Fontaine, P., & Lubelsky, M. (1980). Caffeine-withdrawal headache: A clinical profile. *Psychosomatics, 21,* 411–418.

Greene, M. K., Kerr, A. M., McIntosh, I. B., & Prescott, R. J. (1981). Acetazolamide in prevention of acute mountain sickness: A double-blind controlled cross-over study. *BMJ, 283,* 811–813.

Headache Classification Subcommittee of the International Headache Society. The International Classification of Headache Disorders, 2nd edition (2004). *Cephalalgia, 24*(Suppl. 1), 88–101.

Henderson, W. R., & Raskin, N. H. (1972). Hot-dog headache: Individual susceptibility to nitrite. *Lancet, ii,* 1162–1163.

Hering-Hanit, R., & Gadoth, N. (2003). Caffeine-induced headache in children and adolescents. *Cephalalgia, 23,* 332–335.

Hinchey, J., Chaves, C., Appignani, B., Breen, J., Pao, L., Wang, A., et al. (1996). A reversible posterior leukoencephalopathy syndrome. *N Engl J Med, 334,* 494–500.

Hodgetts, T. J., & Tunnicliffe, C. (1989). Bezafibrate-induced headache. *Lancet, i,* 163.

Indo, T., & Takahashi, A. (1990). Swimmer's migraine. *Headache, 30,* 485–487.

Johns, D. R. (1986). Benign sexual headache within a family. *Arch Neurol, 43,* 1158–1160.

Kiemeneij, I. M., de Leeww, F-E., Ramos, L. M. P., & van Gijn, J. (2003). Acute headache as a presenting symptom of tacrolimus encephalopathy. *J Neurol Neurosurg Psychiatry, 74,* 1126–1127.

King, A. B., & Robinson, S. M. (1972, August). Vascular headaches of acute mountain sickness. *Aerospace Med,* pp. 849–851.

Krabbe, A. A., & Olesen, J. (1980). Headache provocation by continuous intravenous infusion of histamine. Clinical results and receptor mechanisms. *Pain, 8,* 253–259.

Lambert, R. W., & Burnet, D. L. (1985). Prevention of exercise-induced migraine by quantitative warm-up. *Headache, 25,* 317–319.

Lance, J. W. (1976). Headaches related to sexual activity. *J Neurol Neurosurg Psychiatry, 39,* 1226–1230.

Lance, J. W. (1991). Solved and unsolved headache problems. *Headache, 31,* 439–445.

Lance, J. W., & Anthony, M. (1971). Migrainous neuralgia or cluster headache? *J Neurol Sci, 13,* 401–411.

Lance, J. W., & Hinterberger, H. (1976). Symptoms of phaeochromocytoma with particular reference to headache, correlated with catecholamine production. *Arch Neurol, 33,* 281–288.

Lance, J.W., & Lambros, J. (1997). Headache associated with cardiac ischaemia. *Headache, 38,* 315–316.

Landtblom, A.-M., Fridriksson, S., Boivie, J., et al. (2002). Sudden onset headache: A prospective study of features, incidence and causes. *Cephalalgia, 22,* 354–360.

Lane, J. M. R., & Routledge, P. A. (1983). Drug-induced neurological disorders. *Drugs, 26,* 124–147.

Lansche, R. K. (1964). Ophthalmodynia periodica. *Headache, 4,* 247–249.

Laplante. P., Saint-Hilaire, J. M., & Bouvier, G. (1983). Headache as an epileptic manifestation. *Neurology, 33,* 1493–1495.

Levy, R. L. (1981). Stroke and orgasmic cephalalgia. *Headache, 21,* 12–13.

Littler, W. A., Honour, A. J., & Sleight, P. (1974). Direct arterial pressure, heart rate and electrocardiogram during human coitus. *J Reprod Fertil 40,* 321–331.

Lundberg, P. O., & Osterman, P. O. (1974). The benign and malignant forms of orgasmic cephalgia. *Headache, 14,* 164–165.

Markus, H. S. (1991). A prospective follow-up of thunderclap headache mimicking subarachnoid haemorrhage. *J Neurol Neurosurg Psychiatry, 54,* 1117–1125.

Martin, E. A. (1973). Severe headache accompanying orgasm. *BMJ, 4,* 44.

Martinez, J. M., Roig, C., & Arboix, A. (1988). Complicated coital cephalalgia. Three cases with benign evolution. *Cephalalgia, 8,* 265–268.

Massey, E. W. (1982). Effort headache in runners. *Headache, 22,* 99–100.

Masters, W. H., & Johnson, V. E. (1966). *Human sexual response* (pp. 278–294). Boston: Little, Brown.

Mathew, N. T. (1981). Indomethacin-responsive headache syndromes. *Headache, 21,* 147–150.

Mathew, R. J., & Wilson, W. H. (1985). Caffeine consumption, withdrawal and cerebral blood flow. *Headache, 25,* 305–309.

McNally, W. (1966). *Smithy: The Kingsford Smith story.* London: Robert Hale.

Medina, J. L., & Diamond, S. (1981). Cluster headache variant: Spectrum of a new headache syndrome. *Arch Neurol, 38,* 705–709.

Mokri, B. (2002). Spontaneous CSF leaks mimicking benign exertional headaches. *Cephalalgia, 22,* 780–783.

Mosek, A., & Korczyn, A. D. (1995). Yom Kippur headache. *Neurology, 45,* 1953–1955.

Neau, J.-P., Paqueseau, J., Bailbe, M., Ingrand, P., & Gil, R. (2002). Relationship between sleep apnoea syndrome, snoring and headaches. *Cephalalgia, 22,* 333–339.

Odell-Smith, R. (1968). Ice-cream headache. In P. J. Vinken & G. W. Bruyn (Eds.), *Handbook of clinical neurology.* Vol. 5. *Headaches and cranial neuralgias* (pp. 188–191). Amsterdam: Elsevier.

Ostergaard, J. R., & Kraft, M. (1992). Natural history of benign coital headache. *BMJ, 305,* 1129.

Pareja, J. A., Kruszewski, P., & Caminero, A. B. (1999). SUNCT syndrome versus idiopathic stabbing headache (jabs and jolts syndrome). *Cephalalgia, 19*(Suppl. 25), 46–48.

Pareja, J. A., Ruiz, J., de Isla, C., al-Sabbah, H., & Espejo, J. (1996). Idiopathic stabbing headache (jabs and jolts syndrome). *Cephalalgia, 16,* 93–96.

Pascual, J., Iglesias, F., Oterino, A., Vasquez-Barquero, A., & Berciano, J. (1996). Cough, exertional and sexual headaches. *Neurology, 46,* 1520–1524.

Paulson, G. W. (1983). Weightlifter's headache. *Headache, 23,* 193–194.

Paulson, G. W., & Klawans, H. L. (1974). Benign orgasmic cephalalgia. *Headache, 13,* 181–187.

Paulson, G. W., Zipf, R. E., & Beekman, J. F. (1979). Phaeochromocytoma causing exercise-related headache and pulmonary edema. *Ann Neurol, 5,* 96–99.

Pearce, J. M. S. (1988). Exploding head syndrome. *Lancet, ii,* 270–271.

Perini, F., & Toso, V. (1998). Benign cough "cluster" headache. *Cephalalgia, 18,* 493–494.

Pestronk, A., & Pestronk, S. (1983). Goggle migraine. *N Engl J Med, 308,* 226.

Petersen, K. A., Lassen, L. H., Birk, S., & Olesen, J. (2003). The effect of the nonpeptide CGRP-antagonist, BIBN4096 BS on human-alpha CGRP induced headache and hemodynamics in healthy volunteers. *Cephalalgia, 23,* 725.

Pickering, G. W., & Hess, W. (1933). Observations on the mechanism of headache produced by histamine. *Clin Sci (Colch), 1,* 77–101.

Pinessi, L., Rainero, I., Cicolin, A., Zibetti, M., Gentile, S., & Mutani, R., (2003). Hypnic headache syndrome: Association of the attacks with REM sleep. *Cephalalgia, 23,* 150–154.

Piovesan, E. J., Zukerman, E., Kowacs, P. A., & Werneck, L. C. (2002). COX-2 inhibitor for the treatment of idiopathic stabbing headache secondary to cerebrovascular disease. *Cephalalgia, 22,* 197–200.

Plum, F., Posner, J. B., & Troy, B. (1968). Cerebral metabolic and circulatory responses to induced convulsions in animals. *Arch Neurol, 18,* 1–13.

Pocera, J. S., & Dalessio, D. J. (1995). Identification and treatment of sleep apnea in patients with chronic headache. *Headache, 35,* 586–589.

Porter, M., & Jankovic, J. (1981). Benign coital cephalalgia. Differential diagnosis and treatment. *Arch Neurol, 38,* 710–712.

Queiroz, L. P., Dach, F., & Silva, F. M. (2003). Exertional headache associated with Paget's disease: Two cases. *Cephalalgia, 23,* 670.

Raskin, N. H. (1988). The hypnic headache syndrome. *Headache, 28,* 534–536.

Raskin, N. H. (1995). The cough headache syndrome: Treatment. *Neurology, 46,* 1784.

Raskin, N. H., & Appenzeller, O. (1980). In J. H. Smith, Jr. (Ed.), *Headache. Major problems in internal medicine* (Vol. 19, p. 16). Philadelphia: Saunders.

Raskin, N. H., & Schwartz. R. K. (1980). Icepick-like pain. *Neurology, 30,* 203–205.

Rasmussen, B. K., & Olesen, J. (1992). Symptomatic and non-symptomatic headaches in a general population. *Neurology, 42,* 1225–1231.

Ritchie, J. M. (1970). The aliphatic alcohols. In L. S. Goodman & A. Gilman (Eds.), *The pharmacological basis of therapeutics* (4th ed., p. 135). London: Collier-Macmillan.

Rooke, E. D. (1968). Benign exertional headache. *Med Clin North Am, 52,* 801–808.

Sand, T., Hagen, K., & Schrader, H. (2003). Sleep apnoea and chronic headache. *Cephalalgia, 23,* 90–95.

Schaumburg, H. H., Byck, R., Gerstl, R., & Mashman, J. H. (1969). Monosodium l-glutamate. Its pharmacology and role in the Chinese restaurant syndrome. *Science NY, 163,* 826–828.

Schon, F., & Blau, J. N. (1987). Post-epileptic headache and migraine. *J Neurol Neurosurg Psychiatry, 50,* 1148–1152.

Selwyn, D. L. (1985). A study of coital related headaches in 32 patients. *Cephalalgia, 5*(Suppl. 3), 300–301.

Silber, E., Sonnenberg, P., Colier, D. J., Pollard, A. J., Murdoch, D. R., & Goadsby, P. J. (2003). Clinical features of headache at altitude. A prospective study. *Neurology, 60,* 1167–1171.

Silbert, P. L.. Edis, R. H., Stewart-Wynne, E. G., & Gubbay, S. S. (1991). Benign vascular sexual headache and exertional headache: Interrelationships and long term prognosis. *J Neurol Neurosurg Psychiatry, 54,* 417–421.

Silbert, P. L., Hankey, G. J., Prentice, D. A., & Apsimon, H. T. (1989). Angiographically demonstrated arterial spasm in a case of benign sexual headache and benign exertional headache. *Aust N Z J Med, 19,* 466–468.

Sjaastad, O. (1992). *Cluster headache syndrome* (pp. 310–312). London: Saunders.

Sjaastad, O., Pettersen, H., & Bakketeig, L. S. (2001). The Vaga study; epidemiology of headache. *Cephalalgia, 21,* 207–215.

Sjaastad, O., Pettersen, H., & Bakketeig, L. S. (2003). Extracephalic jabs/idiopathic stabs. Vaga study of headache epidemiology. *Cephalalgia, 23,* 50–54.

Slivka, A., & Philbrook, B. (1995). Clinical and angiographic features of thunderclap headache. *Headache, 35,* 1–6.

Smith, W. S., & Messing, R. O. (1993). Cerebral aneurysm presenting as cough headache. *Headache, 33,* 203–204.

Soriani, G., Battistella, P. A., Arnaldi, C., De Carlo, L., Cernetti, R., Corra, S., & Tosato, G. (1996). Juvenile idiopathic stabbing headache. *Headache, 36,* 565–567.

Staunton, H. P., & Moore, J. (1978). Coital cephalgia and ischaemic muscle work of the lower limbs. *J Neurol Neurosurg Psychiatry, 41,* 930–933.

Steiger, M. J., Farrah, T., Rolles, K., Harvey, P., & Burrows, A. K. (1994). Cyclosporin associated with headache. *J Neurol Neurosurg Psychiatry, 57,* 1258–1259.

Symonds, C. (1956). Cough headache. *Brain, 79,* 557–568.

Wijdicks, E. F. M., Kerkhoff, H., & van Gijn, J. (1988). Long-term follow-up of 71 patients with thunderclap headache, mimicking subarachnoid haemorrhage. *Lancet, ii,* 68–70,

Williams, B. (1976). Cerebrospinal fluid changes in response to coughing. *Brain, 99,* 331–346,

Williams, B. (1980). Cough headache due to craniospinal pressure dissociation. *Arch Neurol, 37,* 226–230.

Wolff, H. G. (1963). *Headache and other head pain.* New York: Oxford University Press.

Young, G. B., & Blume, W. T. (1983). Painful epileptic seizures. *Brain, 106,* 537–554.

Chapter 14
Post-Traumatic Headache and Whiplash Injury

The Headache Classification Committee of the International Headache Society (2004) considered post-traumatic headache in two categories, acute and chronic, subdivided into those whose head injury was moderate or severe and those whose headaches followed a minor injury.

The IHS defined acute headache as developing within 7 days of head trauma, or after regaining consciousness, and resolving within 3 months. If headaches persist for more than 3 months, they are classified as chronic.

A moderate or severe head injury was characterized by the following:

1. Loss of consciousness for more than 30 minutes
2. A Glasgow Coma Scale (GCS) score of less than 13 (Table 14.1)
3. Post-traumatic amnesia for more than 48 hours
4. Imaging demonstration of a traumatic brain lesion

For the designation of "moderate to severe," the IHS required that at least one of these criteria be fulfilled. A minor head injury involved loss of consciousness for less than 30 minutes or not at all and involved a GCS score of 13 or more with symptoms or signs of concussion.

Headaches attributed to sudden and significant acceleration/deceleration movement of the neck (whiplash injury) are regarded as acute if they start within 7 days after an injury associated with neck pain and resolve within 3 months and as chronic if they persist beyond that time. Headaches associated with extradural and subdural hematomas are described in Chapter 15 of this book, but we have included a discussion of postcraniotomy headaches in this chapter, with apologies to our neurosurgical colleagues for considering operations as trauma.

INCIDENCE

Head injury has an annual incidence of 180 to 220 per 100,000 in North America and about 350 per 100,000 in Europe, with frequency of acute post-traumatic

TABLE 14.1   Glasgow Coma Scale (GCS)

Eye Opening

1. Nil

2. To pain

3. To speech

4. Spontaneously

Motor Response

1. Nil

2. Extensor

3. Flexor

4. Withdrawal

5. Localizing

6. Voluntary

Verbal Response

1. Nil

2. Groans

3. Inappropriate

4. Confused

5. Oriented

FULL SCORE 15

headaches cited in various series as 31% to 90% (Keidel & Ramadan, 2000). The characteristics of post-traumatic headache resemble tension-type headache in 85% of cases, cervicogenic headache in 8%, migraine in 2.5%, and other forms including cluster headache in the remainder.

Head injuries are considered mild in 75% of cases, but up to 32% of patients report persistent headaches 6 months after injury, and some 25% still complain of headaches after 4 years (Ramadan & Keidel, 2000). In fact, as some research shows, "It may not be so much what happens to the head but to whose head it happens" (Saper, 2000).

PATHOPHYSIOLOGY

People may become subject to headaches after what seems a relatively minor head injury, with or without loss of consciousness. Povlishock et al. (1983) studied the effect of head injury in anesthetized cats, administered by the impact of a 4.8-kg pendulum swinging through 12 degrees. Researchers studied axonal function by applying horseradish peroxidase to the motor cortex and cerebellar nuclei 24 hours before the injury. They found axonal swelling and, eventually, disruption without parenchymal or vascular damage, indicating that axonal changes could result from minor head injury.

Taylor and Kakulas (1991) examined the cervical spine in 43 patients who died after trauma. Only 28% had fractures, whereas disc injuries were found in 96%, and soft tissue injuries of the facet joints were found in 72%. They reported two cases of extension neck injury, with persisting pain in the neck, shoulder, or arm in individuals who had no convincing radiographic abnormality but at autopsy showed disc pathology. These researchers observed that clefts in the cervical discs of trauma patients persist for a year or more in the innervated parts of the anterior annulus and commented that "it is unreasonable to assume that chronic pain in such cases has a psychosomatic basis."

These histologic studies make clear that injury to the head and neck can produce changes our present methods of investigation cannot detect, which should caution clinicians against leaping to the conclusion that symptoms without signs indicate a psychosomatic origin. This finding is not surprising, because research has as yet demonstrated no structural basis for migraine and cluster headache.

Simons and Wolff (1946) found that the intravenous injection of 0.1 to 0.2 mg histamine in 16 patients with post-traumatic headache gave rise to a deep ache, sometimes throbbing, that was most intense in the occipital and frontal regions. The sensitivity of the patients to histamine was no greater than that of normal subjects, but in three cases the headache was most severe at the site of head injury.

Ramadan, Norris, and Shultz (1995) demonstrated abnormal asymmetry of cerebral blood flow in patients with chronic post-traumatic headache by xenon-inhalation single-photon emission computed tomography (SPECT). Changes correlated with the severity of headache and could provide an objective assessment of abnormality in patients who usually lack computed tomography (CT) or magnetic resonance imaging (MRI) support for their complaint of continuing headache. Expanding these findings, Gilkey et al. (1997) examined regional cerebral blood flow in 35 patients with chronic post-traumatic headache in comparison with 49 headache-free patients and 92 patients with migraine. Patients with chronic post-traumatic headache had less regional cerebral blood flow and greater regional and hemispheric asymmetry than did the other two groups.

Abdel-Dayem et al. (1998) reviewed the SPECT images of 228 patients, ranging in age from 11 to 88 years, who had experienced mild to moderate traumatic brain injury. The review excluded patients with abnormalities on CT or MRI scans. The common symptoms were headache (60.9%), memory problems (27.6%), and dizziness (26.7%). Of 41 patients who had had a mild head injury without loss of consciousness and with a normal CT scan of the brain, 28 studies were abnormal. In the total of 228 patients, focal areas of hypoperfusion appeared in 77%. The evaluators noted abnormalities in basal ganglia and thalami (55.2%), frontal lobes (23.8%), temporal lobes (13%), parietal lobes (3.7%), and insular and occipital lobes (4.6%). All studies were randomized with controls and read twice by a nuclear medicine physician in the field of traumatic brain injury. Saper (2000) marshaled the facts in support of an organic explanation for chronic headache after head injury. Warner (2000) took the other side in this controversy, claiming that such patients lost their headaches if weaned from analgesics. We discuss the role of psychologic factors and the influence of litigation later.

CLASSIFICATION

Simons and Wolff (1946) divided post-traumatic headache into three groups. The first was a dull pressure sensation associated with nervous tension and depression, in which electromyogram (EMG) recordings from the scalp muscles correlated with headache severity. Injecting local anesthetic into areas of deep tenderness reduced or abolished the headache. They concluded this form resulted from sustained contraction of skeletal muscle. The second variety of headache was local pain and tenderness in an area of scarring and was superimposed on a generalized dull headache of the first type. The third variety was a unilateral throbbing headache with nausea, accompanied by dilation of arteries and veins and relieved by ergotamine. We refer to this third type as extracranial vascular headache or post-traumatic migraine. With the present state of knowledge, clinicians cannot with certainty classify headache following injury. Probably at least six distinct types of post-traumatic headache exist, with overlap among the groups.

Intracranial Vascular Headache

Concussion is followed by dilation of intracranial vessels, giving rise to a pulsating headache made worse by head movement, jolting, coughing, sneezing, and straining. Tubbs and Potter (1970) found that 83 of 200 patients admitted to a hospital had a headache in the day or so after head injury. Headache was complained of spontaneously by 22 patients (11%), of whom 3 required an analgesic. The remainder admitted to headache only on questioning. Sensitivity to jolting, coughing, or straining may persist in some patients without any obvious neurologic signs being present. It may accompany other symptoms of organic origin, such as giddiness on looking upward or on lying down with the head on one side or the other (benign positional vertigo). The same type of headache may develop, or intensify, if extradural or subdural hematoma complicates head injury.

Extracranial Vascular Headache

Patients who have experienced local damage to the scalp overlying a main extracranial vessel not uncommonly become subject to periodic headache in the distribution of that vessel. Such headaches may recur with the periodicity of migraine and may accompany nausea and photophobia. Jabbing pains may also arise from any scalp nerve damaged by the blow or from subsequent development of scar tissue. Ligation and section of the affected nerve and vessel may help abolish this syndrome. Apart from surgical measures, the management is the same as for migraine.

Post-Traumatic Migraine

A sharp blow to the head may precipitate migraine with aura in children or adults ("footballer's migraine"; see Chapter 7). Migrainous headaches not uncommonly begin after open or closed head injury, which poses the medicolegal question, Was the migraine caused by the injury, or would it have started spontaneously? To examine this problem, Russell and Olesen (1996) looked at the family histories of 29 patients with no past history of migraine who developed migrainous headaches after head injury, fulfilling IHS criteria for significant trauma in 11 cases and minor trauma in 18 cases. Three patients had migraine with aura, and twenty-six had migraine-type headaches without aura. The first-degree relatives of patients with post-traumatic migraine had a significantly lower prevalence of migraine than patients who had migraine without any history of head trauma. The authors concluded that head trauma, even a minor one, can very likely cause migraine without aura. The number of patients with aura was too small for conclusions to be drawn. Haas (1996) examined 48 patients with chronic post-traumatic headache, concluding that, in 21%, the headaches had the characteristics of migraine without aura, indistinguishable from the histories of patients with migraine and without any previous head injury. Weiss, Stern, and Goldberg (1992) pointed out that the response of post-traumatic migraine to propranolol, amitriptyline, or both in combination was often gratifying.

Post-Traumatic Dysautonomic Cephalalgia

Vijayan and Dreyfus (1975) described five patients with a distinctive syndrome that followed injury to the anterior triangle of the neck, presumably involving the carotid artery sheath. All patients complained of pain and tenderness in this area for some weeks after the injury. Some weeks or months after the injury the patients began to suffer from severe unilateral episodic headaches on the side previously injured. The headaches were frontotemporal in site and associated with severe sweating over the same side of the face, dilation of the pupil on that side, blurring of vision and photophobia in the ipsilateral eye, and nausea. The headaches recurred several times each month and lasted from 8 hours to 3 days. After the headache subsided, three patients had ptosis and miosis on the affected side. They attributed the attacks to a paroxysmal excess of sympathetic activity followed by a period of diminished activity, as a result of trauma to the pericarotid sympathetic plexus. Partial sympathetic denervation was confirmed by the fact that the pupil on the affected side dilated in response to a 1:1000 solution of adrenaline. The headaches did not improve with ergotamine but responded promptly to propranolol, 40 mg daily. We have never encountered this syndrome.

Pain in the Neck and Occipital Region from Injury to the Upper Cervical Spine ("Whiplash" Injury)

The part played by whiplash injury of the cervical spine is difficult to assess in the absence of definite radiologic changes. Positron-emission tomography (PET) and SPECT scanning have demonstrated hypoperfusion and hypometabolism in both parieto-occipital regions in patients with neck pain and headache after whiplash injury in comparison with normal controls (Otte et al., 1997). Keidel et al. (2001) investigated brainstem-mediated inhibitory reflexes of the temporalis muscle in 82 patients on average 5 days after a whiplash injury. After stimulation of the second or third branches of the trigeminal nerve, temporalis contraction is suppressed, as a protective bite-regulating reflex. In patients with acute post-traumatic headache, they found significantly altered silent periods evoked in the temporalis muscle, which they attributed to alteration of the pain control pathway after whiplash. These studies give objective support to the existence of an organic syndrome in patients with no obvious structural basis for continuing headache.

Balla (1980) analyzed the symptoms attributed to whiplash injury in 300 patients, two thirds of whom were female, examined 6 months or more after the accident that was considered responsible. Of these, 219 patients complained of daily aching in the neck, and 58 had aching in the arms. Headache recurred daily in 176 patients (59%), every week or so in 42 patients (14%), and occasionally or not at all in 82 patients (27%). The patients with daily headaches described them as a generalized ache, worse toward the back of the head. Occasional or weekly headaches resembled migraine without aura.

When a vehicle traveling at about 15 miles (24 km) per hour hits a stationary car in the rear, the neck of any person sitting in the stationary car is hyperextended well beyond the normal range of movement. Anatomic studies after such acceleration injuries in monkeys show apophyseal joint damage that was not visible on radiologic examination (La Rocca, 1978). Taylor and Kakulas (1991) produced similar evidence for human whiplash injuries. In reviewing the problems of whiplash injury, La Rocca pointed out that degenerative changes in the cervical spine in patients who have experienced whiplash injury are six times as common as would be expected for that age group.

After cervical disc injury, the person may hold the neck at a slightly tilted or rigidly fixed position. Points of referred tenderness often appear, not only in the suboccipital and cervical regions, but over the upper part of the medial edge of the scapula, the deltoid muscle, and around the elbow on the affected side. Ryan et al. (1993) analyzed the symptoms of 32 individuals with neck strain after a car accident in relation to the dynamics of the impact. Approximately 80% complained of pain in the back of the neck, head, and shoulders, whereas others experienced pain in the upper back or arms. The initial severity of neck symptoms correlated with the severity of the crash. Examination evoked tenderness, spasm, or pain more often over the middle segments of the cervical spine than at the upper and lower ends. Those people who had been aware of the impending crash had a greater range of neck movement and fewer adverse responses to palpation than those who were taken unaware.

Neck injury can cause dissection of a vertebral artery with resulting infarction of the brainstem and occipital cortex at the time of the accident or even 2 or 3 months later (Tulyapronchote et al., 1994). Jacome (1986) has also reported basilar artery migraine after whiplash injury.

Cervicogenic Headache

Lord et al. (1994) studied 100 patients with neck pain persisting more than 3 months after whiplash injury. Headache was the main complaint in 40% and a secondary problem in 31%. By blocking the third occipital nerve, they assessed the part played by trauma to the upper cervical facet joints. This technique provided temporary relief to 27% of patients, increasing to 53% of those patients with associated headache. Tenderness over the C2–3 facet joint was more common in those who responded. The same group (Lord et al., 1996) completed a double-blind controlled study of radiofrequency neurotomy in 24 patients. Of 12 submitted to the genuine procedure, the mean duration of pain relief before returning to 50% of baseline level was 263 days, compared with 8 days for those who had a placebo procedure.

Drottning, Staff, and Sjaastad (2002) examined 222 patients who still had a headache 1 month after injury (out of 587 who had sustained whiplash injury) and followed them for a year. Unilateral headache, aggravated by neck movement and usually relieved by local anesthetic block of occipital nerves, was present in 8.2% at 6 weeks, 4.4% at 6 months, and 3.4% at 1 year.

Clinicians usually place much store on limited range of neck movement in assessing patients with whiplash injury. In our experience of chronic post-whiplash headache, the more rigidly the patient holds the neck, the less the underlying organic lesion and the greater the functional overlay. Ferrari and Schrader (2001) comment that "less research is needed in trying to pinpoint an anatomical source for pain, and more research in trying to find the cultural source for behaviour in response to an acute pain—a simple neck sprain."

Treatment

Some patients respond to application of heat, cervical traction, mobilization of the neck, or to injection of a local anesthetic agent and long-acting corticosteroids, such as Depo-Medrol (methylprednisolone acetate), into tender areas of the suboccipital region. Transcutaneous electrical nerve stimulation (TENS) may relieve pain and thus restore mobility more rapidly (Nordemar & Thorner, 1981). Relaxation training is a useful adjunct to other forms of treatment, because the muscles are commonly overcontracted. Psychologic management and the use of antidepressants may be equally important (Tyler, McNeely, & Dick, 1980). Releasing the occipital nerve in 13 patients with occipital neuralgia after a whiplash injury caused improvement but not complete pain relief in most (Magnusson, Ragnarsson, & Bjornsson, 1966). In a few patients resistant to other forms of therapy, a physician may consider division of the posterior rami or radiofrequency lesions of the facet joints or dorsal root ganglia (Sluijter & Koetsveld-Baart, 1980).

More research is needed to establish which components of the whiplash syndrome stem from damage to cervical discs, ligaments, or soft tissues, and which stem from excessive muscle contraction associated with anxiety and depression, daily intake of analgesics, or simply the expectation of continuous symptoms after neck injury.

Muscle Contraction (Tension) Headache

Authors have amply pointed out in the medical literature that multiple symptoms may follow minor head injuries where compensation or litigation is involved, that after head injury self-employed or professional workers return to work more rapidly than employees, and that disability does not usually follow sports injuries. Head injury seems to accentuate any tendency to anxiety or depression, and the personality of the patient before the accident plays a large part in how he or she reacts to injury. Some post-traumatic headaches have all the qualities of tension-type headache and respond, at least in part, to tricyclic antidepressant drugs. This form of headache often arises from that natural worry resulting from the possibility of brain damage and is reinforced by some legal advisers who instruct their clients not to resume work or normal activities until the case is settled.

Other Post-Traumatic Headaches

Cluster-like headache has arisen after head injury and is more common after injury near the eye or forehead. Newman et al. (1997) reported three patients with hemicrania continua after head injury.

PSYCHOLOGIC ASPECT

Miller (1961) made a strong case for the concept of accident neurosis being the most important factor in post-traumatic symptoms. Certainly clinicians encounter cases of "functional overlay" and even frank malingering. Ellard (1970) has summarized the psychologic reactions he has met in patients with a compensatable injury:

Attitudinal pathosis. This label characterizes patients who do not seek to be healed but to be justified. They are not incapacitated by symptoms but have a grievance and believe they cannot work because they have been handled unjustly.

Schizophrenic reaction. This type of reaction is commonly paranoid, with feelings of persecution by doctors, solicitors, and even the law courts.

Bizarre hypochondriasis. This syndrome marks a group of patients who before injury were fitness fanatics, narcissistic, and preoccupied with health foods and sporting activities. They commonly describe their headache in an exaggerated manner and are often diagnosed as hysterical.

Traumatic neurosis. Here the accident may have symbolic significance, but more commonly the patient's anxiety is conditioned by the accident. Such patients may respond to behavior therapy.

Depression. Many patients who become depressed have a compulsive personality, for whom work has become an important defense mechanism. Losing their normal work pattern brings on typical depressive symptoms.

Compensation neurosis. Here, symptoms of anxiety usually overshadow those of depression. The patient often becomes aggressive at work as well as at home. Hysterical manifestations may become superimposed. The total amount of disability is usually greater than the sum of its parts.

Malingering. Malingerers exhibit the paradox of the person who remains sick because of the hope of financial reward.

Ellard stresses the need to assess each patient in light of the specific racial, cultural, and educational background as well as the premorbid personality. Patients with an excessive psychologic reaction to injury look well despite their description of suffering. They lack motivation to get well, and their attitude to treatment is unusual and may be resentful.

Ham et al. (1994) examined 31 patients with post-traumatic headache in comparison with 28 patients who had combined migraine and tension-type headache as well as 18 subjects with low back pain and 28 normal controls. The post-traumatic headache group showed the highest level of psychopathology over a range of tests for anxiety, depression, and anger expression. A somewhat similar study by Tatrow et al. (2003) involved subjects with post-traumatic headache (14), nontraumatic headache (16), healthy controls (16), and people who had been involved in a motor vehicle accident without developing headache (16) evaluated over a range of psychologic tests. The post-traumatic group had more functional symptoms (such as dizziness, fatigue, nausea, and weakness), as well as anxiety and depression, than did the other groups.

The field would benefit from studies with larger sample sizes and more explanation about the meaning of many psychologic tests employed and their interpretation.

LITIGATION

The frequency of post-traumatic headache varies greatly from country to country, bearing some relation to the nature of each legal system and the culture of each community. The most striking example is Lithuania, where citizens hold no expectation of chronic disability resulting from whiplash injury and no insurance or other source of financial compensation for such injuries. Obelieniene et al. (1998) compared a questionnaire survey of 202 patients 1 to 3 years after a rear-end car collision with that of 202 matched control subjects and sent those reporting headaches a second questionnaire. Headache on more than 7 days a month was reported by 9.4% in the whiplash group and 5.9% of the controls ($p = .26$). Possible cervicogenic headaches were reported by 10 of the whiplash patients and 5 of the controls, not a statistically significant difference. Surprisingly, 10 out of 98 "normal" controls who reported headaches suffered from chronic tension-type headaches. The same group later undertook another study using a questionnaire applied between 2 and 7 days after a rear-end collision and repeated after 2 months and after 1 year. Initially neck pain alone was felt by 10%, headache alone by 19%, and both by 18%. Neck pain resolved within 17 days and headache within 20 days. After 1 year no difference distinguished the accident victims from a control group. Frequent neck pain (more than 7 days a month) was reported by 4.0% of whiplash patients and, remarkably, by 6.2% of controls. Headaches occurring more than 7 days each month were reported by 5.1% of the accident group and 6.7% of controls. This community thus showed no evidence of late headaches after whiplash.

It is therefore interesting to hear of any change in incidence of neck pain and headache when laws are changed to reduce or abolish compensation for pain and suffering after motor vehicle injuries. Such a change took place in Saskatchewan, Canada, on January 1, 1995. The number of claims dropped from 417 per 100,000 population in the 6 months before the change in legislation to 302 and 296 per 100,000 in the next two 6-month periods. The median time from the date of injury to closure of a claim decreased from 433 days to less than half that. Eliminating compensation thus correlated with a decreased incidence of and improved prognosis for whiplash injury (Cassidy et al., 2000).

Ferrari and Schrader (2001) consider the late whiplash syndrome not as the result of a chronic injury and not merely psychosomatic but as an expression of the patient's cultural expectation. They state that this view "takes away the stigmata of the psychiatric label, while explaining that people's behaviour in response to their injury may generate much of the illness, and therefore the illness is not an incurable injury."

Not all patients with head and neck pain after injury have a psychologic disorder, and not all have their eyes fixed on financial gain. McKinlay, Brooks, and Bond (1983) compared two groups of patients after a blunt head injury, those with and those without a claim for financial compensation. Postconcussion symptoms, intellectual performance, and behavioral changes were similar in the two groups, although claimants did report more symptoms than the control group. No significant difference distinguished the two groups in the time taken to return to work. Radanov et al. (1991) found that psychosocial factors, negative affect, and personality traits were not helpful in predicting the outcome of whiplash injury. Young and Packard (1997) and Saper (2000) summarized the extensive literature on post-traumatic headache, helping to dispel the "myth of nonorganicity."

PROGNOSIS

Settling the legal aspects of the matter does not always lead to disappearance of symptoms and return to work. Balla and Moraitis (1970) followed up 82 patients, 41 of whom suffered from headache, after industrial or traffic accidents. They found that 2 years after financial settlement, 21 patients had not returned to work. Those who did return to work usually did so within a year. Mendelson (1982) reviewed follow-up studies of litigants to ascertain the effect of legal settlement on symptoms attributed to injuries relating to compensation claims. Up to 75% failed to return to gainful employment 2 years after the legal case concluded. Cartlidge and Shaw (1981) distinguished between those patients whose headaches had persisted since discharge from hospital, dropping from about 36% at the time of discharge to about 20% of patients at 1- and 2-year follow-up, and late-acquired headaches that had developed in 20% of cases during the 6 months since the accident. Of the latter group, 83% were pursuing compensation claims, compared with only 20% of the persisting group. Depression was a feature in 44% and 12%, respectively, at the 6-month follow-up. Regarding time from blunt head injury before return to work, McKinlay, Brooks, and Bond (1983) could find no significant difference between those who were claiming compensation and those who were not.

Of 78 patients who suffered a whiplash injury of the neck in Switzerland, 57 had recovered fully within 6 months, whereas 21 had persisting symptoms (Radanov et al., 1991). A poor prognosis related to initial intensity of neck pain, injury-related cognitive impairment, and age. In Lithuania, Greece, and Germany, symptoms of acute whiplash injury usually resolve within 6 weeks (Ferrari & Schrader, 2001), unlike the situation in Norway and North America.

As a late sequel of head injury, a meningioma may develop at the site of a previous skull injury (Walshe, 1961). The evidence is anecdotal, but, as Walshe commented: "the perpetually 'open mind' is not an effective instrument of thought and may too easily become a euphemism for the mind closed to the lessons of experience."

TREATMENT

The early management of head injury may be important in reducing the disability that so often follows. Relander, Troupp, and Bjorkesten (1972) compared the result of an active treatment program with the routine treatment of similar patients in the same hospital. Health care personnel visited the active treatment group daily and explained the nature of the injury to them. Caretakers encouraged patients to get out of bed and start physiotherapy. When patients attended the follow-up clinic, they saw the same doctors who had looked after them in the hospital. The active treatment group returned to work in an average of 18 days, contrasted with 32 days for other patients.

Symptomatic treatment depends on the variety of post-traumatic headache. The vascular forms of headache are best treated with the medications used for managing migraine and cluster headache. Specific forms of treatment for whiplash injury were discussed earlier and are discussed in further detail in Chapter 17. The tension-type headaches may respond to psychologic counseling, relaxation therapy, and tricyclic antidepressant agents.

POSTCRANIOTOMY HEADACHE

The incidence of headache after craniotomy for supratentorial tumors and the surgery of epilepsy is not remarkable. Gee, Ishaq, and Vijayan (2003) reviewed the medical records of 97 patients after such procedures and found that only 11 patients who had not previously experienced headache did so after operation. Most headaches focused on the surgical site.

In contrast, 75% of patients complained of headache after removal of an acoustic neuroma (Vijayan, 1995), with 42% reporting new postoperative pain. Mosek et al. (1999) examined this situation further, finding a headache frequency of 83% after such an operation. They interviewed 48 patients who had undergone resection by a suboccipital craniotomy and found that 58% had postoperative head pain that lasted more than 7 days. These headaches were all in the region of the incision. Within 4 months of operation, 77% of the patients were pain free, but pain persisted in 23%, localized to the incision or the adjacent area. Chronic persistent postoperative pain can develop after either a suboccipital or translabyrinthine approach, but the mechanism remains uncertain.

CONCLUSION

The great difficulty in handling patients with post-traumatic headache lies in differentiating the organic from the psychogenic components. Undeniably, many post-traumatic headaches are of organic origin, in the sense that control of cranial vessels has become more unstable and cranial arteries have become more susceptible to painful dilation since injury. The probability of a head or neck injury causing headache depends on a comparison of the patient's susceptibility to headache before and after head injury, the latent period between injury and the onset of headache or aggravation of any pre-existing symptoms, and the site and nature of the headache.

Ensuring that justice is done to any legal claim and that treatment is appropriate to the variety of headache requires the physician to take an unbiased approach and to carefully assess each patient's personality, cultural background, and his or her headache pattern.

References

Abdel-Dayem, H. M., Abu-Judeh, H., Kumar, M., Atay, S., Naddaf, S., E1-Zeftawy, K., et al. (1998). SPECT brain perfusion abnormalities in mild or moderate traumatic brain injury. *Clin Nucl Med, 23,* 309–317.

Balla, J. I. (1980). Late whiplash syndrome. *Aust N Z J Surg, 50,* 610–614.

Balla, J. I., & Moriatis. S. (1970). Knights in armour. A follow-up study of injuries after legal settlement. *Med J Aust, 2,* 355–361.

Cartlidge, N. E. F., & Shaw, D. A. (1981). *Head injury* (pp. 95–115). London: Saunders.

Cassidy, J. D., Carroll, L. J., Cote, P., Lemstra, M., Berglund, A., & Nygren, A. (2000) Effect of eliminating compensation for pain and suffering on outcome of insurance claims for whiplash injury. *N Engl J Med, 342,* 1179–1186.

Drottning, M., Staff, P. H., & Sjaastad, O. (2002). Cervicogenic headache (CEH) after whiplash injury. *Cephalalgia, 22,* 165–171.

Ellard, J. (1970). Psychological reactions to compensatable injury. *Med J Aust, 2,* 349–355.

Ferrari, R., & Schrader, H. (2001). The late whiplash syndrome: A biopsychosocial approach. *J Neurol Neurosurg Psychiatry, 70,* 722–726.

Gee, J. R., Ishaq, Y., & Vijayan, N. (2003). Postcraniotomy headache. *Headache, 43,* 276–278.

Gilkey, S. J., Ramadan, N. M., Aurora, T. K., & Welch, K. M. A. (1997). Cerebral blood flow in chronic post-traumatic headache. *Headache, 37,* 583–587.

Haas, D. C. (1996). Chronic post-traumatic headaches classified and compared with natural headaches. *Cephalalgia, 16,* 486-493.

Ham, L. P., Andrasik, F., Packard, R. C., & Bundrick, C. M. (1994). Psychopathology in individuals with post-traumatic headaches and other pain types. *Cephalalgia, 14,* 118–126.

Headache Classification Committee of the International Headache Society. (2004). The International Classification of Headache Disorders (2nd ed.). *Cephalalgia, 24*(Suppl. 1), 58–64.

Jacome, D. E. (1986). Basilar artery migraine after uncomplicated whiplash injuries. *Headache, 26,* 515–516.

Keidel, M., & Ramadan, N. M. (2000). Acute posttraumatic headache. In J. Olesen, P. Tfelt-Hansen, & K. M. A. Welch (Eds.), *The headaches* (2nd ed., pp. 765–770). Philadelphia: Lippincott, Williams and Wilkins.

Keidel, M., Rieschke, P., Stude, P., et al.(2001). Antinociceptive reflex alteration in acute posttraumatic headache following whiplash injury. *Pain, 92,* 319–326.

La Rocca, H. (1978). Acceleration injuries of the neck. *Clin Neurosurg, 25,* 209–217.

Lord, S. M., Barnsley, L., Wallis, B. J., & Bogduk, N. (1994). Third occipital nerve headache: A prevalence study. *J Neurol Neurosurg Psychiatry, 57,* 1187–1190.

Lord, S. M., Barnsley, L., Wallis, B. J., McDonald, G. J., & Bogduk, N. (1996). Percutaneous radio-frequency neurotomy for chronic cervical zygapophyseal-joint pain. *N Engl J Med, 335,* 1721–1726.

Magnusson, T., Ragnarsson, T., & Bjornsson, A. (1996). Occipital nerve release in patients with whiplash trauma and occipital neuralgia. *Headache, 36,* 32–36.

McKinlay, W. W., Brooks, D. N., & Bond, M. R. (1983). Post-concussional symptoms, financial compensation and the outcome of severe blunt head injury. *J Neurol Neurosurg Psychiary, 46,* 1084–1091.

Mendelson, G. (1982). Not "cured by a verdict." Effect of legal settlement on compensation claims. *Med J Aust, 2,* 132–134.

Miller, H. (1961). Accident neurosis. *BMJ, 1,* 919–925, 992–998.

Mosek, A. D., Dodick, D. W.,,. Ebersold, M. J., & Swanson, J. R. (1999). Headache after resection of acoustic neuroma. *Headache, 39,* 89–94.

Newman, L. C., Solomon, S., & Lipton, R. B. (1997). Post-traumatic hemicrania continua. *Neurology, 48*(Suppl.), A123.

Nordemar, R., & Thorner, C. (1981). Treatment of acute cervical pain—a comparative group study. *Pain, 10,* 93–101.

Obelieniene, D., Bovim, G., Schrader, H., Surkiene, D., Mickeviàine, B., Miseviàiene, I., et al. (1998). Headache after whiplash: A historical cohort study outside the medico-legal context. *Cephalalgia, 18,* 559–564.

Obelieniene, D., Schrader, H., Bovim, G., Miseviciene, I., & Sand, T. (1999). Pain after whiplash: A prospective controlled inception cohort study. *J Neurol Neurosurg Psychiatry, 66,* 279–283.

Otte, A., Ettlin, T. M., Nitzsche, E. U., Wachter, H., Hoegerle, S., Simon, G. H., et al. (1997). PET and SPECT in whiplash syndrome: A new approach to a forgotten brain. *J Neurol Neurosurg Psychiatry, 63,* 368–372.

Povlishock, J. T., Becker, D. P., Cheng, C. L. Y., & Vaughan, G. W. (1983). Axonal change in minor head injury. *J Neuropath Exp Neurol, 42,* 725–742.

Radanov, B. P., Di Stefano, G., Schnidrig, A., & Ballarini, P. (1991). Role of psychosocial stress in recovery from common whiplash. *Lancet, 338,* 712–715.

Ramadan, N. M., & Keidel, M. (2000). Chronic posttraumatic headache. In J. Olesen, P. Tfelt-Hansen, & K. M. A. Welch (Eds.), *The headaches* (2nd ed., pp.771–780). Philadelphia: Lippincott, Williams and Wilkins.

Ramadan, N. M., Norris, L. L., & Schulz, L. R. (1995). Abnormal cerebral blood flow correlates with disability due to chronic post-traumatic headache. *J Neuroimaging, 5,* 68.

Relander, M., Troupp, H., & Bjorkesten, G. (1972). Controlled trial of treatment for cervical concussion. *BMJ, 2,* 777–779.

Russell, M. D., & Olesen, J. (1996). Migraine associated with head trauma. *Eur J Neurol, 3,* 424–428.

Ryan, G. A., Taylor, G. W., Moore, V. M., & Dolinis, J. (1993). Neck strain in car occupants. The influence of crash-related factors on initial severity. *Med J Aust, 159,* 651–656.

Saper, J. R. (2000). Posttraumatic headache. A neurobehavioural disorder. *Arch Neurol, 57,* 1776–1778.

Simons, D. J., & Wolff, H. G. (1946). Studies on headache: Mechanisms of chronic post-traumatic headache. *Psychosom Med, 8,* 227–242.

Sluijter, M. E., & Koetsveld-Baart, C. C. (1980). Interruption of pain pathways in the treatment of the cervical syndrome. *Anaesthesia, 35,* 302–307.

Tatrow, K., Blanchard, E. B., Hickling, E. J., & Silverman, D. J. (2003). Posttraumatic headache: Biopsychosocial comparisons with multiple control groups. *Headache, 43,* 755–766.

Taylor, J. R., & Kakulas, B. A. (1991). Neck injuries. *Lancet, 338,* 1343.

Tubbs, O. N., & Potter, J. M. (1970). Early post-concussional headache. *Lancet, ii,* 128–129.

Tulyapronchote, R., Selhorst, J. B., Malkoff, M. D., & Gomez, C. R. (1994). Delayed sequelae of vertebral artery dissection and occult cervical fractures. *Neurology, 44,* 1397–1399.

Tyler, G. S., McNeely, H. E., & Dick, M. L. (1980). Treatment of post-traumatic headache with amitriptyline. *Headache, 20,* 213–216.

Vijayan, N. (1995). Postoperative headache in acoustic neuroma. *Headache, 35,* 98–100.

Vijayan, N., & Dreyfus, P. M. (1975). Post-traumatic dysautonomic cephalagia, clinical observations and treatment. *Arch Neurol, 32,* 649–652.

Walshe, F. (1961). Head injuries as a factor in the aetiology of intracranial meningioma. *Lancet, ii*, 993–996.

Warner, J. S. (2000). Posttraumatic headache–a myth? *Arch Neurol, 57*, 1778–1780.

Weiss, H. D., Stern, B. J., & Goldberg, J. (1991). Post-traumatic migraine: Chronic migraine precipitated by minor head or neck trauma. *Headache, 31*, 451–456.

Young, W. B., & Packard, R. D. (1997). Post-traumatic headache and post-traumatic syndrome. In P. J. Goadsby & W. D. Silberstein (Eds.), *Headache* (pp. 253–277). Boston: Butterworth-Heinemann.

Chapter 15
Vascular Disorders

ACUTE ISCHEMIC CEREBROVASCULAR DISEASE

Transient Ischemic Attacks

Fisher (1968) reported that 7 of 20 patients with vertebrobasilar ischemic attacks experienced headache, usually occipital or occipitofrontal in distribution. He described the headache that accompanied transient ischemic attacks (TIAs) in six patients who subsequently developed a complete internal carotid occlusion. The ache was mild, commonly frontal but sometimes radiating to the occiput, and lasted only for the duration of the neurologic deficit. He also questioned 58 patients with transient monocular blindness (amaurosis fugax) but found none who felt pain or discomfort with the attack. This was also the experience of Toole (1984).

Grindal and Toole (1974) reviewed the case histories of 240 patients with TIAs and selected 58 who had a definite, recorded history of headache. They concluded that headache was a prominent symptom in about 25% of patients and was the presenting complaint in nearly one third. Only 50 of the 240 patients had a recorded negative history of headache, so the prevalence of headache in TIAs may have been underestimated. Of 33 patients with carotid insufficiency, the headache was ipsilateral to the diseased carotid in 9, contralateral in 2, and bilateral in the remainder, commonly affecting the frontal region. Headache in vertebrobasilar insufficiency more consistently accompanied the ischemic attacks and affected the occiput or neck in 15 of 23 cases.

Portenoy et al. (1984) found that 10 of 28 patients (36%) had complained of headache before, during, or after their TIAs. Medina, Diamond, and Rubino (1975) commented on late-onset vascular headaches starting in middle age or later in 18 of their 34 patients and recurring independently of their TIAs. These headaches began several years before the onset of TIAs in 13 cases and some months after in 5. The researchers found no association with hypertension or a previous history of migraine.

For 10 years Larsen, Sørensen, and Marquardsen (1990) followed 46 patients aged 18 to 39 years who presented with TIAs. A stroke or myocardial infarction occurred in all 4 patients with cerebrovascular risk factors but in only 2 of the remaining 42 patients. The authors postulate that such episodes in young people may be of migrainous origin, because most of those studies had normal cerebral angiograms. Two thirds were women.

The cause of headaches in transient ischemia remains obscure. Because the site of headache is related to the site of origin of the TIA, some local factor is presumably involved. Edmeads (1979) used cerebral angiography and cortical blood flow studies to investigate 58 patients with TIAs. Frequency of headache in those TIAs with a carotid origin was 26% and for those of vertebrobasilar origin, 17%. No evidence indicated that collateral circulation was any greater in patients with headache than those without. Possibly a transient reflex vascular dilation in response to ischemia or the passage of a platelet embolus may be responsible.

Thromboembolic Stroke

A major cerebral vessel usually occludes without pain. Fisher (1968) recorded some pain or discomfort in 35 of 109 cases (31%) with internal carotid occlusion. Two patients had experienced neck pain. Pain in the neck overlying the carotid artery (carotidynia) may signal the presence of a long intraluminal clot, particularly if it accompanies headache and symptoms of vascular insufficiency (Donnan & Bladin, 1980).

Fisher (1968) determined the incidence of headache with middle cerebral artery occlusion to be 21%, and for the posterior cerebral artery, 50%, whereas nine patients with anterior cerebral artery thrombosis were not aware of headache. Of 94 patients with basal artery occlusion, 41 (44%) had headache or head pain. Pain did not accompany lacunar infarcts. Ferro at al. (1995) found similar figures for headache in vertebrobasilar (57%) and carotid (20%) territory strokes, with a higher frequency in patients who had previously had migraine (odds ratio 6.9). Gorelick et al. (1986) reported a warning ("sentinel") headache days or weeks before stroke in 10% of patients and a headache at onset in 17%.

Size of infarct and attendant edema is usually not enough to account for headache by displacement of intracranial structures. Probably platelet emboli could not release 5-HT or other vasoactive agents in quantities sufficient to cause significant vascular changes. Possibly ischemia of the brain or brainstem may trigger vascular changes or migrainous phenomena. Collateral circulation does not appear to be a factor (Edmeads, 1979).

Episodic headache is one of the main features of the combination of mitochondrial myopathy, encephalopathy, lactic acidosis, and strokelike episodes (MELAS syndrome) (Goto et al., 1992).

In Figure 19.3, vertebral arteriography demonstrates thrombosis of the posterior inferior cerebellar artery.

INTRACRANIAL HEMATOMA

Intracerebral Hematoma

The most important cause of intracerebral hemorrhage is chronic hypertension, and the most common sites are the putamen (60%), thalamus (10%), pons

(10%), and cerebellum (10%). Fisher (1968) reported the frequency of headache as varying from 13% for putaminal hemorrhage to 50% in the case of the cerebellum. Gorelick et al. (1986) found that 55% of patients with intraparenchymal hemorrhage experienced headache, usually unilateral and severe, at the onset. Bleeding into one lobe of the cerebrum is less common than into basal ganglia or thalamus but gives rise to a more localized referral of pain. The patient feels pain around the ipsilateral eye if the hemorrhage is in the occipital lobe, anterior to the ear for the temporal lobe, in the temporal region for the parietal lobe, and in the forehead in the case of the frontal lobe (Ropper & Davis, 1980).

As clinicians would expect, headache is a presenting feature in patients with signs of meningeal irritation or computed tomography (CT) evidence of intraventricular or subarachnoid bleeding, hydrocephalus, transtentorial herniation, or midline shift (Melo, Pinto, & Ferro, 1996). In most patients with cerebral hemorrhage, the headache is overshadowed by the rapid onset of a devastating neurologic deficit, drowsiness, or vomiting. Progressive deterioration or the CT finding of hydrocephalus may dictate urgent evacuation of an intracerebellar hematoma, but contrary to earlier belief, many patients recover well with conservative management (Melamed & Satya-Murti, 1984).

In a follow-up of 90 survivors of intracerebral hemorrhage, Ferro, Melo, and Guerreiro (1998) found that pre-existing headaches remitted in 19%, and headaches, mainly of the tension variety that may accompany depression, developed in 10%.

Subdural and Extradural Hematoma

Extradural (epidural) hematomas are nearly always the result of head injury with a fracture line extending across the middle meningeal artery (Figure 15.1). Headache and impairment of consciousness following head injury should arouse the suspicion of an extradural bleed before dilation of the ipsilateral pupil indicates impending tentorial herniation. Urgent removal of the hematoma is required, because otherwise the patient may die within a matter of hours.

In contrast, subdural hematoma generally runs a slow course, because bleeding takes place from small veins bridging the gap between cortex and venous sinuses. A latent period of weeks or months may separate a minor head injury from the onset of symptoms. Subdural hematomas may present acutely if the bleeding stems from ruptured small arteries on the surface of the cortex. Headache and drowsiness usually antecede neurologic signs.

SUBARACHNOID HEMORRHAGE

Bleeding into the subarachnoid space may take place after head injury, or secondary to an intracerebral hemorrhage or spontaneously in patients with a cerebral aneurysm or angioma (Figure 15.2). Less commonly, bleeding may result from blood dyscrasias, hemorrhage from a cerebral tumor, or some form of arteritis. In different Western series, the ratio of aneurysm to angioma as a cause of subarachnoid hemorrhage varies from 5:1 to 25:1. The pattern is quite different in Asia, where angioma is more common. In about one third of patients, the

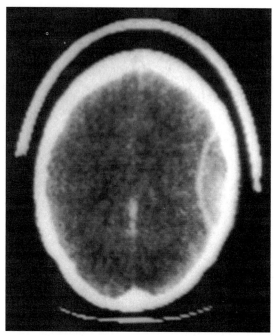

FIGURE 15.1   CT scan of the brain showing a left extradural hematoma. Fresh blood can be seen within the lens-shaped hematoma.

headache of subarachnoid hemorrhage follows exertion. It usually starts suddenly and dramatically, "like a blow on the head." The person may feel a poorly localized sensation of something giving way inside the head, followed by unilateral headache that rapidly becomes generalized and spreads to the back of the head and neck, accompanied by photophobia. The patient may lose consciousness, with or without an epileptic seizure. The neck is usually rigid, and focal neurologic signs appear if the aneurysm has compressed cranial nerves in enlarging or has bled into the brain substance. Pain in the back and legs may follow a subarachnoid hemorrhage after some hours or days, because blood drifting down in the cerebrospinal fluid (CSF) irritates the lumbosacral nerve roots. Hemorrhages may appear in the fundi, spreading out from the optic discs, in approximately 7% of patients, and papilledema appears in 13% (Walton, 1956). Fever, albuminuria, glycosuria, hypertension, and electrocardiographic changes may be present in the acute phase.

One or more brief, severe headaches may precede subarachnoid hemorrhage by several months. Such sentinel headaches have been reported in 31% (Gorelick et al., 1986), 43% (Verweij, Wijdicks, & van Gijn, 1988), and 50% (Òstergaard, 1991) of patients who later developed subarachnoid hemorrhage. The headaches are usually bioccipital, bifrontal, or unilateral and are unlike

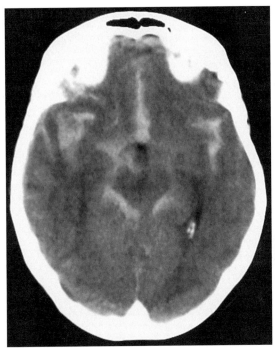

FIGURE 15.2 Subarachnoid hemorrhage. CT scan showing blood in the Sylvian fissures and basal cisterns. (Photograph by courtesy of Professor Mareus Stoodley.)

anything the patient has ever experienced before. They may accompany vomiting, neck stiffness, and blurred or double vision, suggesting that they are caused by a small preliminary leak.

The initial investigation mode for suspected subarachnoid hemorrhage is CT, which is positive in approximately 95% of patients in the first 24 hours (Adams et al., 1983). If the CT scan is negative but the index of suspicion is high, a lumbar puncture should be performed, which usually demonstrates uniformly bloodstained fluid.

After 4 to 12 hours xanthochromia of the cerebrospinal fluid appears, and it disappears 12 to 40 days after the hemorrhage. A lymphocytic cellular reaction and increase in CSF protein to 70 to 130 mg per 100 mL (0.7 to 1.3 g/liter) usually follows subarachnoid hemorrhage (Walton, 1956). Cerebral angiography in patients with proven subarachnoid hemorrhage demonstrates an aneurysm (Figure 15.3) in most cases (Duffy, 1983), and this aneurysm is clipped whenever possible. If the clinician can find no aneurysm or angioma, the patient stays in bed for 4 to 6 weeks and then gradually resumes normal activities.

The recreational use of the drug Ecstasy (3,4-methylenedioxy methamphetamine, MDMA) reportedly caused vasculitis and subarachnoid hemorrhage in two young subjects (Lee et al., 2003).

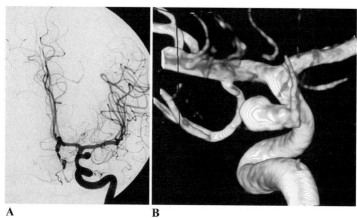

FIGURE 15.3   Posterior communicating aneurysm, demonstrated by cerebral angiography *(A)* and three dimensional angiogram *(B)*.

UNRUPTURED ANEURYSM OR VASCULAR MALFORMATION

Of 220 patients with arteriovenous malformations diagnosed by carotid angiography at the National Hospital for Nervous Diseases in London, 12 (5%) had a history of migraine (Blend & Bull, 1967). Other studies have reported a migraine history in 15% of 110 patients (Paterson & McKissock, 1956) and in 31% of 48 patients (Waltimo, Hokkanen, & Pirskanen, 1975) with arteriovenous malformations. The researchers derived the last figure after carefully questioning all patients about their previous headache pattern.

In Walton's series of 312 cases of subarachnoid hemorrhage, 16 (5%) gave a definite history of migraine. Six of these patients lost their migraine attacks after the episode of hemorrhage. Davis (1967) found that 6% of 431 patients presenting with subarachnoid hemorrhage had a history of migraine. Wolff (1963) found that 7 of 46 patients with subarachnoid hemorrhage had suffered from migraine, and another 12 had periodic recurrent headaches. However, the aneurysm side was not always the headache side, and Wolff considered the headache independent of the presence or absence of aneurysm.

Clearly, unruptured aneurysms are not associated with migraine or other recurrent headaches, but whether arteriovenous malformations appear in migraine patients more than chance would predict is unclear. Bruyn (1984) argues *for* such an association. We remain doubtful, because clinicians undertake cerebral angiography in migraine patients only when the habitual occurrence of neurologic symptoms has alerted them to a possible underlying lesion. More likely, an arteriovenous malformation reduces local cortical perfusion so much that it produces focal neurologic symptoms when cerebral blood flow is further reduced during the aura and is thus responsible for the nature of the aura but not for initiating the migrainous process.

Certainly carotid arteriography is not indicated solely because migraine attacks habitually affect the same side of the head. If the patient also has a loud intracranial bruit, focal fits, or an equivocal CT scan, or has had a subarachnoid hemorrhage, then the likelihood of a positive result from carotid angiography greatly increases. Some patients with cerebral angiomas have repeated small subarachnoid hemorrhages that are confused with migraine attacks or are considered episodes of encephalitis.

VASCULITIS

Savage et al. (2000) summarized various inflammatory diseases of blood vessels, few of which present with headache.

Granulomatous angiitis, as an intracranial manifestation of herpes zoster, causes neurologic deficit that is not usually accompanied by headache (MacKenzie, Forbes, & Karnes, 1981). Systemic lupus erythematosus (SLE) may be associated with headache and papilledema that respond to corticosteroid administration (Silverberg & Laties, 1973). Montalban et al. (1992) found that, of 103 patients with SLE, 32 suffered from migraine headaches. The presence of anticardiolipin antibodies in SLE was 29% but showed no correlation with a tendency to migraine. In the absence of other neurologic symptoms and signs, the presence of headache in this condition does not indicate involvement of the central nervous system (Atkinson & Appenzeller, 1975). By contrast, a related disorder known as *temporal* or *giant-cell arteritis* has headache as its most important presenting symptom.

Giant-Cell Arteritis (Temporal Arteritis)

Temporal or giant-cell arteritis is a rare form of chronic daily headache with clinical importance, because it is a preventable cause of blindness. It usually affects people older than 50 years, but patients as young as 35 years have been reported. The prevalence in the population older than 50 is 133 per 100,000 but rises to 843 per 100,000 in those older than 80 years (Huston et al., 1978). The female-to-male ratio is 2:1.

Headache is the presenting complaint in about half the patients and is a feature in about 85% during the course of the illness. It is commonly bitemporal but may be unilateral or generalized as a constant dull ache. Sudden loss of vision in one eye was the first symptom in 8 of 35 patients examined in our own hospital group (Koorey, 1984). In this series the temporal artery was clinically abnormal in 24 cases, and the examiner found tenderness, thickening, or nodularity of the vessel wall and diminished pulsation (Figure 15.4A). A low-grade fever and other indications of systemic disturbance, such as muscle and joint pain (polymyalgia rheumatica), are a feature in about 25% to 40% of patients. Temporal artery biopsy shows the typical appearance of giant-cell arteritis in about half of the patients with this condition (Murray, 1977) (Figure 15.4B).

Inflammation may spread to arteries other than the temporal and other extracranial vessels. The cause of blindness is involvement of the posterior ciliary artery supplying the optic disc, which produces ischemic papillopathy and

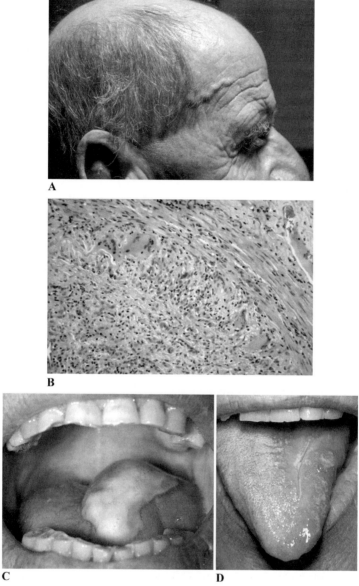

FIGURE 15.4   Temporal arteritis. *A,* A prominent tender temporal artery. *B,* Biopsy appearance of giant-cell arteritis. *C, Gangrene* of one half of the tongue caused by occlusion of the lingual artery. *D,* After resolution of the tongue lesion.

consecutive optic atrophy. Double vision may result from ischemia of the oculo-motor nerve, in which case the pupil is usually spared, or from damage to the extraocular muscles themselves. Approximately 15% of patients report diplopia at some stage of the illness. Pain in the temporal and masseter muscles on chewing (jaw claudication) is virtually pathognomonic of temporal arteritis but occurs in only 25% to 40% of patients in reported series. A rare complication is gangrene of the tongue (Davis & Davis, 1966; Dare, Byrne, & Robertson, 1981). A patient of ours developed this unpleasant condition while on steroid therapy for temporal arteritis (Figure 15.4*C* and *D*). Arteritis may affect the aorta and vertebral, coronary, renal, and iliac arteries. Transient ischemic attacks, vertigo, ischemic neuropathies, and myelopathy have also been reported.

Diagnosis

The erythrocyte sedimentation rate (ESR) ranged from 40 to 140 mm/hour (mean 82 mm/hour) in the case histories Koorey (1984) analyzed. A normal value may be found early in the disease, even when biopsy shows the process is active. If the index of suspicion is high, the clinician should arrange a temporal artery biopsy as a matter of urgency. As soon as the diagnosis is made, steroid therapy should be started on clinical grounds, because blindness can strike suddenly while the patient is awaiting biopsy and subsequent histologic confirmation. Temporal artery biopsy is not always positive, because the disease process may be patchy, with unaffected "skip lesions" (Klein, 1976). Selective extracranial angiography may help identify the affected areas and thus guide the surgeon's hand. Removing a long segment of temporal artery for examination improves the success rate. Even with these precautions, the biopsy may still prove negative. Hall et al. (1983) followed 134 patients who had undergone temporal artery biopsies. Of 46 patients with positive biopsies, polymyalgia rheumatica was a feature in 38%, and jaw claudication occurred in 54%. Temporal arteries were palpable in 67%, and the ESR was 50 mm/hour or more in all cases. The 88 patients with negative biopsies had almost equal frequencies of polymyalgia rheumatica, malaise, fever, and weight loss, but jaw claudication was rare, and the temporal arteries were palpable in only 31%. Only eight of the biopsy-negative patients required long-term steroid therapy. Nonspecific abnormalities in giant-cell arteritis include mild anemia, neutrophil leukocytosis, low serum albumin, increased alpha-2 globulin, and abnormal liver enzyme levels. Hyperthyroidism is an occasional association.

Biopsy demonstrates a thickened arterial wall and intima and often a thrombus in the lumen (see Figure 15.4*B*). The elastic lamellae are disrupted, the media is infiltrated with round cells, and giant cells may be seen. Classification of the condition appears to belong somewhere between acute autoimmune vasculitis and chronic noncaseating granuloma such as sarcoid. Immunoglobins in the arterial wall may represent antibodies to elastin or may be taken up from circulating immune complexes (Liang, Simkin, & Mannik, 1974).

Although the symptoms of temporal arteritis are readily recognizable, their duration before diagnosis in two series was a mean of 5½ months (Dare & Byrne, 1980; Koorey, 1984). The headache may lack distinctive features and may be mistaken for tension headache. Muscle and joint pains are common in the elderly, and clinicians often treat them symptomatically, without investigating.

Early diagnosis is of great importance. A tragic example of a missed opportunity was a patient who became totally blind. She had consulted her medical practitioner 6 months previously for generalized muscular aching, and she had noted pain in the jaws on chewing at that time. A blood count was done, but not an ESR. The practitioner treated her with a series of antirheumatic drugs, without relief, until she went blind in one eye. The hospital admitted her and started steroid treatment immediately, but the next day she lost vision in the other eye. Probably the most common reason for missing the diagnosis is that clinicians mistakenly think that a normal ESR excludes temporal arteritis. Remember, up to 30% of biopsy-confirmed patients may have an ESR of 40 mm/hour or less (Kansu et al., 1977). When the physician suspects the condition on the basis of the clinical history, whether or not the ESR is elevated, it is good policy to have one temporal artery biopsied. Treatment can start immediately, even before the biopsy is taken. Steroid therapy may have to continue for years, and it is reassuring to have a firm histologic diagnosis at the outset.

Prognosis

Temporal arteritis is usually a self-limited inflammatory disease that generally runs a course of 1 to 2 years (Caselli, Hunder, & Whisnant, 1988). The prognosis was worse in those patients Graham et al. (1981) reported from Moorfield's Eye Hospital and neurologic centers in London. Of 90 patients, 44 presented with visual loss, and 32 patients died. Of the surviving patients, the disease "burned out" in a period ranging from 6 months to 7 years in one third, stabilized on low dosage of steroids in one third, and ran a relapsing–remitting course in the remainder. Vision in one or both eyes has been lost in up to 50% of untreated cases, but early introduction of steroid therapy reduces loss to about 13% (Klein et al., 1976). The late incidence of stroke is probably no greater than that of age-matched control patients (Caselli et al., 1988), but Graham et al. (1981) described four patients (of 90 with proven disease) who died in the acute phase of a brainstem stroke, with vertebral arteritis or thrombosis demonstrated in the three autopsied cases. Life expectancy declines in women but not men (Dare, Byrne, & Robertson, 1981; Graham et al., 1981). The outlook is worse if vision has been lost or if the maintenance dosage of prednisone exceeds 10 mg daily.

Treatment

Prednisone 75 mg daily should be started as soon as the condition is diagnosed clinically, pending histologic confirmation. The physician usually reduces dosage in stages every third day down to 30 mg daily. The daily dose can then usually be reduced by 5 mg each week to a maintenance of about 10 mg daily, which is then continued for 3 months. Further reduction depends on the clinical response and the ESR. Most patients can stop steroid therapy after a period of 12 to 14 months.

Side effects of prolonged therapy include Cushingoid features, osteoporosis, and avascular necrosis of the hip. The physician may prescribe intravenous heparin and dextran if there is fluctuating visual impairment.

CAROTID OR VERTEBRAL ARTERY PAIN

Carotid or Vertebral Dissection

West, Davies, and Kelly (1976) reported a distinctive headache syndrome in eight patients with narrowing or occlusion of one internal carotid artery, caused by a dissecting aneurysm of the arterial wall in one operated case. The unilateral pain was associated with a Horner's syndrome on the same side and with contralateral neurologic symptoms or signs in half the patients. The pain involved the head, neck, or face and had a burning or throbbing quality. It subsided over a period of 2 months. Mokri et al. (1986) studied 36 patients with carotid dissection in whom headache, commonly periorbital and frontal, was a presenting symptom in 33, as was neck pain in 7 and focal cerebral ischemic symptoms in 24. An ocular Horner's syndrome was present in 21. Follow-up angiography demonstrated that the stenosis had resolved or diminished in 85% of patients, which was associated with a good clinical recovery. Bogousslavsky, Despland, and Regli (1987) described a similar clinical picture in 30 patients, among whom headache was a feature in 17, associated with monocular blindness in 4 and some other neurologic deficit in 2. Two patients had an isolated neck pain (carotidynia). An ocular Horner's syndrome affected only 20% in this series. Fisher (1982) emphasized that the pain usually occurs in the forequarter of the head but may also involve the cheek, side of the nose, teeth, and jaw. Of his 21 patients with carotid dissection, 12 had neck pain as well.

Dissection of the vertebral arteries causes pain in the upper neck and occiput, associated with a lateral medullary syndrome or cerebellar infarction (Caplan, Zarins, & Hemmati, 1985). One patient of ours developed a severe pain in one side of the occiput and upper neck after the boom of his yacht struck him. The pain became much worse after chiropractic manipulation of his neck, and angiography showed a localized dissection of the vertebral artery at the craniospinal junction (Figure 15.5). Caplan et al. (1985) cite 11 instances in which vertebral artery dissection has followed neck manipulation.

Carotidynia

Carotidynia, a syndrome of neck pain associated with tenderness of the carotid artery, has many causes (Roseman, 1968). One form is of acute onset in young or middle-aged adults, in which the pain persists for an average of 11 days and does not usually recur. The pain radiates to the side of the face in about half of the cases. Tenderness is maximal over the carotid bifurcation. Usually no signs of systemic infection appear, although some patients feel unwell and complain of nasal blockage and lacrimation. The ESR remains normal. The cause is unknown, but the short course of the disorder suggests a viral infection.

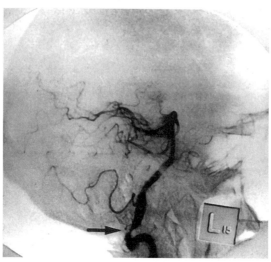

FIGURE 15.5   Dissection of a vertebral artery *(arrow)* caused by a blow to the head followed by manipulation of the neck.

Treatment is symptomatic with analgesics. Prednisolone therapy has not proved helpful.

Another form of carotidynia may appear at any stage of adult life and recurs in attacks lasting minutes to hours, daily or weekly, often in conjunction with throbbing headache (Raskin & Prusiner, 1977). This form responds to ergotamine or substances such as methysergide used to prevent migraine. Tenderness of the carotid artery is not uncommon in migraine, and carotidynia may be an extreme form of this vascular sensitivity (described as "recurrent neck pain" in Chapter 6).

Carotidynia has also been reported with temporal arteritis, fibrosis around the carotid sheath, long intraluminal clots in the internal carotid artery (Donnan & Bladin, 1979), and dissecting aneurysm involving the arterial wall (Chambers et al., 1981). An elongated styloid process has been reported to give rise to pain in the cheek, chin, or neck along the area of distribution of the carotid artery (Eagle's syndrome) (Massey & Massey, 1979).

Postendarterectomy Headache

Some clinicians have reported patients with intense vascular headache, localized to the frontotemporal area of the affected side, following carotid endarterectomy (Leviton, Caplan, & Salzman, 1975; Pearce, 1976; Messert & Black, 1978). The headache comes on after a latent period of 36 to 72 hours and recurs intermittently for 1 to 6 months. Simply restoring normal cerebral perfusion pressure probably could not cause the headache. It is presumably triggered by afferent impulses from the carotid arterial wall.

VENOUS THROMBOSIS

Of 38 patients with thrombosis of cerebral veins or venous sinuses whom Bousser et al. (1985) described, 74% presented with headache, 45% with increased intracranial pressure, 34% with hemiplegia, and 29% with seizures. Of the 38 patients, 9 were eventually found to have Behçet's disease, and 5 had underlying malignant disorders. Four cases followed mild head injury, and four developed after infections of the ear or throat.

The lateral sinus may thrombose after infection of the middle ear and mastoid bone, causing cerebral edema, termed *otitic hydrocephalus* (Figure 15.6). No internal hydrocephalus arises, because the ventricles are normal or small in size. The patient, usually a child, develops headache and papilledema after an ear infection. The sixth nerve may be paralyzed on the side of the lesion, or on both sides, because the expanded brain has stretched the nerves. Radiographs commonly show opacity of the mastoid air cells. Treatment focuses on the infected ear and mastoid (which may include mastoidectomy and removing the clot from the lateral sinus) and on reducing cerebral edema.

Thrombosis of superior sagittal and internal venous sinuses may complicate a low CSF pressure headache following lumbar puncture, particularly if other risk factors are present (Aidi et al., 1999).

Benign idiopathic intracranial hypertension, which may accompany a partial thrombosis of the superior sagittal sinus, is discussed in Chapter 16.

INCREASED VENOUS PRESSURE

Mediastinal obstruction and emphysema can increase venous pressure sufficiently to interfere with cerebral venous drainage and to cause papilledema. Hypoxia associated with these conditions probably increases the tendency for edema of the brain and optic nerve.

A patient of ours experienced a severe headache, at first right-sided and later generalized, that developed on his lying down, flexing his neck, or lifting his arms above his head. On coughing or sneezing, he felt a sharp pain in and behind both eyes, often followed by aching in the right temple (Lance, 1991). He had a

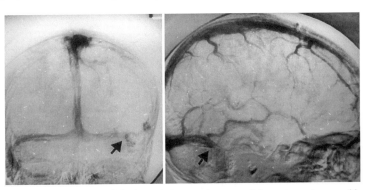

FIGURE 15.6 Thrombosis of the lateral sinus at the apex of the petrous temporal bone.

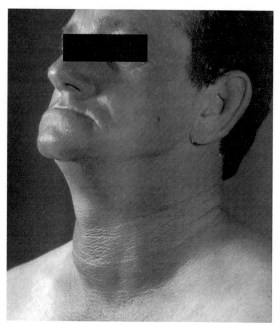

FIGURE 15.7   Increased jugular venous pressure caused by a large goiter. (From Lance, 1991, by permission of the editor of *Headache*.)

large goiter (Figure 15.7), which proved to be Riedel's thyroiditis. Removal of the goiter, which was obstructing his jugular venous flow, completely freed him from headache. A similar increase in jugular venous pressure may be the basis of "weightlifter's headache." The mechanism of headache in thoracic outlet syndrome (Raskin, Howard, & Ehrenfeld, 1985) is unknown but could well relate to venous compression in the neck.

ARTERIAL HYPERTENSION

Clearly, a sudden rise of systemic blood pressure can cause headache. Acute pressor reactions caused by pheochromocytoma and monoamine oxidase (MAO) inhibitors are discussed later. Such headaches are usually bilateral, affecting the occipital or frontal areas, and may involve the whole head. They are commonly severe, bursting or throbbing in quality, and accompany other symptoms of catecholamine release, such as tremor or palpitations. Similar "thunderclap" headaches developing at the climax of sexual intercourse are described in Chapter 13. In acute nephritis or malignant hypertension, blood pressure may also rise rapidly enough to cause headache (Healton et al., 1982).

Whether the insidious onset of hypertension can cause headache is less certain. The typical headache ascribed by various writers over the past 60 years to hypertension is bilateral, usually occipital in site, is present on waking, and eases as the patient rises from bed and begins daily activities. Wolff (1963) pointed out that the headache associated with hypertension may respond to rest and relaxation without any material change in blood pressure. Anxiety is common in hypertensive patients once they know their blood pressure is elevated and may manifest in muscle contraction headache.

A community survey (Waters, 1971) involving 414 people, of whom 36 had a systolic pressure greater than 195 mm Hg and 13 a diastolic pressure higher than 115 mm Hg, disclosed no difference in headache prevalence between the small hypertensive group and the control subjects. However, Bulpitt, Dollery, and Carne (1976) found that 31% of untreated hypertensive patients complained of headaches on waking compared with 15% of normal subjects and treated hypertensive patients, a statistically significant difference. The headache improved more often in those patients whose blood pressure dropped substantially on treatment.

Badran, Weir, and McGuiness (1970) studied a group of 100 patients with a blood pressure of 150/95 mm Hg or more, and 100 matched normotensive controls. Headache was a symptom in 50 hypertensive patients and 39 controls. Headache was significantly more common in hypertensive patients only when the diastolic pressure was 140 mm Hg or more. Eight of twelve patients with papilledema had headache. Of the 11 patients in the grossly hypertensive group, only 2 experienced occipital headache, the remainder being bitemporal or diffuse. Oddly enough, occipital headache was more common in the control group, affecting 20 of the 39 patients. The headache of gross hypertension did indeed occur in the mornings, eased after several hours, and improved in those whose blood pressure responded to treatment. Bauer (1976), in a retrospective survey of 400 patients, could not find any significant correlation between the height of blood pressure and the incidence of headache. A follow-up extending to 15 years showed no difference in mortality between those with headache and those without.

We may tentatively conclude that hypertension by itself is not a common cause of headache but that the association between these disorders may permit control of hypertension to relieve headache.

What of the relationship between hypertension and migraine? Walker (1959) found hypertension significantly more common in patients with migraine older than 50 years. Leviton, Malvea, and Graham (1974) compared frequency of hypertension and vascular disease in parents (with and without migraine) of patients with migraine. High blood pressure was significantly more common in parents with migraine (whether men or women) in a ratio of 1.7:1 ($p < .05$). The incidence of heart attacks under age 70 was almost three times higher in the parents with migraine ($p < .05$), regardless of whether they were hypertensive. Curiously, tendency to stroke did not increase.

Pressor Reactions

Medication with Monoamine Oxidase Inhibitors

Many reports describe patients under treatment with MAO inhibitors who have experienced sudden severe headache, often occipital in site, after taking sympathomimetic agents, drinking red wine, or eating cheeses with a high tyramine content. The headaches accompany a rapid increase in blood pressure and are relieved by the α-noradrenergic blocking agent phentolamine. Some cases of subarachnoid and intracerebral hemorrhage have occurred at the height of the pressor reaction. Patients taking MAO inhibitors must avoid excessive intake of caffeine (in cola-flavored drinks as well as in tea and coffee), any symphathomimetic drugs, and foods that contain large amounts of tyramine. We issue a sheet of instructions to all patients who are prescribed MAO inhibitors, stating they must not eat cheese, meat extracts such as Marmite, red wine, broad beans, chicken liver (pâté), or pickled herring (rich in tyramine). We tell them not to have any injections or take tablets other than those prescribed specifically for headache, such as ergotamine, aspirin, or codeine. They must not use nasal decongestant sprays or tablets for sinusitis containing sympathomimetic agents.

Pheochromocytoma

A rare but interesting cause of acute pressor reactions is pheochromocytoma. Thomas, Rooke, and Kvale (1966) reviewed the clinical histories of 100 patients with proven pheochromocytoma seen at the Mayo Clinic in the preceding 20 years. The attacks in 80% of cases featured episodic headache. It was usually of rapid onset, bilateral, severe, throbbing, and associated with nausea in about half the cases. The headache lasted less than 1 hour in 70% and accompanied other symptoms of catecholamine release in 90%.

Lance and Hinterberger (1976) analyzed the case histories of 27 patients in whom the content of adrenaline and noradrenaline had been assayed in blood, urine, and in the tumor after it had been removed. We were unable to find any distinctive syndrome for tumors producing predominantly one of these amines. Sustained hypertension was more common in the noradrenaline-secreting group, whereas pallor and tremor were more common when the tumor also produced adrenaline. Other symptoms such as palpitations, sweating, and anxiety appeared in both groups. Headaches, apparently related to a rapid increase in blood pressure, were a symptom in 20 of the 27 patients and had the same characteristics as those Thomas, Rooke, and Kvale (1966) had previously described. Blood pressure recorded during a headache ranged from 200/100 mm Hg to 300/160 mm Hg. However, blood pressures as high as 260/100 mm Hg had been recorded in some patients who were not subject to headache. Two patients with bladder pheochromocytoma experienced severe headache starting 15 to 20 seconds after micturition and lasting 1 to 3 minutes. Others described the headache as lasting for a few seconds or minutes only at the onset of their paroxysmal symptoms, but mostly the headache persisted for 5 minutes to 2 hours, subsiding gradually with the other symptoms of the attack. Nausea and vomiting accompanied the headache in seven patients, and two complained of blurred vision. Six patients had collapsed, lost consciousness, or developed focal neurologic signs during the episodes. Attacks followed exertion, straining, emotional upsets, worry, or excitement. High levels of circulating catecholamine causes uptake and storage in other adrenergic tissue, including the adrenal medulla, which releases them on nervous stimulation. This accounts for paroxysmal symptoms being triggered by anxiety and excitement as well as by compression of the tumor.

The diagnosis, which depends on clinical suspicion being aroused when the history is first taken, is confirmed by finding increased excretion of catecholamines in three 24-hour specimens of urine, or elevated blood levels during an attack. Care must be taken that the patient has not taken any sympathomimetic drugs preceding the urine collection, nasal decongestant sprays being the most consistent offender. Blood sugar is usually elevated at the time of the attack, a useful distinction from hypoglycemic attacks, which may simulate pheochromocytoma because of the secondary release of adrenaline in hypoglycemia. The tumor is localized by ultrasound, CT or magnetic resonance imaging (MRI), or aortic angiography if it is present in the characteristic suprarenal site. Bear in mind that pheochromocytomas may arise at any point along the line of development of the sympathetic chain, extending downward from the neck to the pelvis and scrotum. (See also the discussion of thunderclap headache in Chapter 13.)

PITUITARY APOPLEXY

Rapid enlargement of a pituitary tumor is usually caused by hemorrhage and causes sudden headache, vomiting, visual field impairment, and sometimes diplopia. Randeva et al. (1999) reviewed the medical records of 21 male and 14 female patients, ranging from 30 to 74 years of age, of whom 71% had reduced visual fields. Trans-sphenoidal surgery improved visual acuity in 86%.

References

Adams, H. P., Kassell, N. F., Torner, J. C., & Sahs, A. L. (1983). CT and clinical correlations in recent aneurysmal subarachnoid haemorrhage: A preliminary report of the cooperative aneurysm study. *Neurology, 33,* 981–988.

Aidi, S., Chaunu, M.-P., Biousse, V., & Bousser, M.-G. (1999). Changing pattern of headache pointing to cerebral venous thrombosis after lumbar puncture and intravenous high-dose corticosteroids. *Headache, 39,* 559–564.

Atkinson, R. A., & Appenzeller, O. (1975). Headache in small vessel disease of the brain: A study of patients with systemic lupus erythematosus. *Headache, 15,* 198–201.

Badran, R. H. Al., Weir, R. J., & McGuiness, J. B. (1970). Hypertension and headache. *Scott Med J, 15,* 48–51.

Bauer, G. E. (1976). Hypertension and headache. *Aust N Z J Med, 6,* 492–497.

Blend, R., & Bull, J. W. D. (1967). The radiological investigation of migraine. In R. Smith (Ed.), *Background to migraine* (pp. 1–10). London: Heinemann.

Bogousslavsky, J., Despland, P. A., & Regli, F. (1987). Spontaneous carotid dissection with acute stroke. *Arch Neurol, 44,* 137–140.

Bousser, M. G., Chiras, J., Bories, J., & Castaigne, P. (1985). Cerebral venous thrombosis—a review of 35 cases. *Stroke, 16,* 199–213.

Bruyn, G. W. (1984). Intracranial arteriovenous malformation and migraine. *Cephalalgia, 4,* 191–207.

Bulpitt, C. J., Dollery, C. T., & Carne, S. (1976). Change in symptoms of hypertensive patients after referral to hospital clinic. *Br Heart J, 38,* 121–128.

Caplan, L. R., Zarins, C. K., & Hemmati, M. (1985). Spontaneous dissection of the extracranial vertebral arteries. *Stroke, 16,* 1030–1038.

Caselli, R. J., Hunder, G. G., & Whisnant, J. P. (1988). Neurologic disease in biopsy-proven giant cell (temporal) arteritis. *Neurology, 38,* 352–359.

Chambers, S. R., Donnan, G. A., Riddell, R. J., & Sladin, P. F. (1981). Carotidynia: Aetiology, diagnosis and treatment. *Clin Exp Neurol, 17,* 113–123.

Dare, B., & Byrne, E. (1980). Giant cell arteritis. A five-year review of biopsy-proven cases in a teaching hospital. *Med J Aust, 1*, 372–373.

Dare, B., Byrne, E., & Robertson, A. (1981). Acute lingual ischaemia complicating temporal arteritis. *Med J Aust, 1*, 534.

Davis, E. (1967). Subarachnoid haemorrhage. *Med J Aust, 2*, 12–14.

Davis, A. E., & Davis, T. P. (1966). Gangrene of the tongue caused by temporal arteritis. *Med J Aust, 2*, 459–460.

Donnan, G. A., & Bladin, P. F. (1980). The stroke syndrome of long intraluminal clots with incomplete vessel obstruction. *Clin Exp Neurol, 16*, 41–47.

Duffy, G. P. (1983). The warning leak in spontaneous subarachnoid haemorrhage. *Med J Aust, 1*, 514–516.

Edmeads, J. (1979). The headaches of ischemic cerebrovascular disease. *Headache, 19*, 345–349.

Ferro, J. M., Melo, T. P., & Guerreiro, M. (1998). Headaches in intracerebral haemorrhage survivors. *Neurology, 50*, 203–207.

Ferro, J. M., Melo, T. P., Oliveira, V., Salgado, A. V., Crepso, M., Canhão, P., & Pinto, A. N. (1995). A multivariate study of headache associated with ischaemic stroke. *Headache, 35*, 315–319.

Fisher, C. M. (1968). Headaches in cerebrovascular disease. In P. J. Vinken & G. W. Bruyn (Eds.), *Handbook of clinical neurology* (Vol. 5, pp. 124–151). Amsterdam: North Holland.

Fisher, C. M. (1982). The headache and pain of spontaneous carotid dissection. *Headache, 22*, 60–65.

Gorelick, P. B., Hier, D. B., Caplan, L. R., & Langenberg, P. (1986). Headache in acute cerebrovascular disease. *Neurology, 36*, 1445–1450.

Goto, Y., Horai, S., Matsuoka, T., Koga, Y., Nehai, K., Kobayashi, M., et al. (1992). Mitochondrial myopathy, encephalopathy, lactic acidosis, and stroke-like episodes (MELAS): A correlative study of the clinical features and mitochondrial DNA mutation. *Neurology, 42*, 545–550.

Graham, E., Holland, A., Avery, A., & Ross Russell, R. W. (1981). Prognosis in giant-cell arteritis. *BMJ, 282*, 269–271.

Grindal, A. B., & Toole, J. F. (1974). Headache and transient ischemic attacks. *Stroke, 5*, 603–606.

Hall, S., Persellin, S., Lie, J. T., O'Brien, P. C., Kurland, C. T., & Hunder, G. G. (1983). The therapeutic impact of temporal artery biopsy. *Lancet, ii*, 1217–1220.

Healton, E. B., Brust, J. C., Feinfeld, D. A., & Thomson, G. E. (1982). Hypertensive encephalopathy and the neurological manifestations of malignant hypertension. *Neurology, 32*, 127–132.

Huston, K. A., Hunder, G. G., Lie, J. T., Kennedy, R. H., & Elveback, L. R. (1978). Temporal arteritis. A 25 year epidemiologic, clinical and pathologic study. *Ann Intern Med, 88*, 162–167.

Kansu, T., Corbett, J. J., Savino, P., & Schatz, N. J. (1977). Giant cell arteritis with normal sedimentation rate. *Arch Neurol, 34*, 624–625.

Klein, R. G., Campbell, R. J., Hunder, G. G., & Carney, J. A. (1976). Skip lesions in temporal arteritis. *Mayo Clin Proc, 51*, 504–510.

Koorey, D. J. (1984). Cranial arteritis. A twenty year review of cases. *Aust N Z J Med, 14*, 143–147.

Lance, J. W. (1991). Solved and unsolved headache problems. *Headache, 31*, 439–445.

Lance, J. W., & Hinterberger, H. (1976). Symptoms of pheochromocytoma, with particular reference to headache, correlated with catecholamine production. *Arch Neurol, 33*, 281–288.

Larsen, B. H., Sørensen, P. S., & Marquardsen, J. (1990). Transient ischaemic attacks in young patients: A thromboembolic or migrainous manifestation? A 10 year follow up study of 46 patients. *J Neurol Neurosurg Psychiatry, 53*, 1029–1033.

Lee, G. Y. F., Gong, G. W. K., Vrados, N., & Brophy, B. P. (2003). "Ecstasy"-induced subarachnoid haemorrhage: An under-reported neurological complication? *J Clin Neurosci, 10*, 705–707.

Leviton, A., Caplan, L., & Salzman, E. (1975). Severe headache after carotid endarterectomy. *Headache, 15*, 207–210.

Leviton, A., Malvea, B., & Graham, J. R. (1974). Vascular diseases, mortality, and migraine in the parents of migrainous patients. *Neurology, 24*, 669–672.

Liang, C. G., Simkin, P. A., & Mannik, M. (1974). Immunoglobulins in temporal arteries. An immunofluorescent study. *Ann Intern Med, 81*, 19–24.

MacKenzie, R. A., Forbes, G. S., & Karnes, W. E. (1981). Angiographic findings in herpes zoster arteritis. *Ann Neurol, 10*, 458–464.

Massey, E. W., & Massey, J. (1979). Elongated styloid process (Eagle's syndrome) causing hemicrania. *Headache, 19*, 339–344.

Medina, J. L., Diamond, S., & Rubino, R. A. (1975). Headache in patients with transient ischemic attacks. *Headache, 15*, 194–197.

Melamed, N., & Satya-Murti, S. (1984). Cerebellar haemorrhage. A review and reappraisal of benign cases. *Arch Neurol, 41*, 425–428.

Melo, T. P., Pinto, A. N., & Ferro, J. M. (1996). Headache in intracerebral hematoma. *Neurology, 47*, 494–500.

Messert, B., & Black, J. A. (1978). Cluster headache, hemicrania and other head pains: Morbidity of carotid endarterectomy. *Stroke, 9*, 559–562.

Mokri, B., Sundt, T. M., Houser, O. W., & Piepgras, D. G. (1986). Spontaneous dissection of the cervical internal carotid artery. *Ann Neurol, 19*, 126–138.

Montalban, J., Cervera, R., Font, J., Ordi, J., Vianna, J., Haga, H. J., et al. (1992). Lack of association between anticardiolipin antibodies and migraine in systemic lupus erythematosus. *Neurology, 42*, 681–682.

Murray, T. J. (1977). Temporal arteritis. *J Am Geriat Soc, 25*, 450–453.

Òstergaard, J. R. (1991). Headache as a warning symptom of impending aneurysmal subarachnoid haemorrhage. *Cephalalgia, 11*, 53–55.

Paterson, J. H., & McKissock, W. (1956). A clinical survey of intracranial angiomas with special reference to their mode of progression and surgical treatment: A report of 110 cases. *Brain, 79*, 233–266.

Pearce, J. (1976). Headache after carotid endarterectomy. *BMJ, 3*, 85–86.

Portenoy, R. K., Abissi, C. J., Lipton, R. B., Berger, A. R. Mebler, M. F., Baglivo, J., et al. (1984). Headache in cerebrovascular disease. *Stroke, 15*, 1009–1012.

Randeva, H. S., Schoebel, J., Byrne, J., Esiri, M., Adams, C. B., & Wass, J. A. (1999). Classical pituitary apoplexy: Clinical features, management and outcome. *Clin Endocrinol (Oxf), 51*, 181–188.

Raskin, N. H., Howard, M. W., & Ehrenfeld, W. K. (1985). Headache as the leading symptom of the thoracic outlet syndrome. *Headache, 25*, 208–210.

Raskin, N. H., & Prusiner, S. (1977). Carotidynia. *Neurology, 27*, 43–46.

Ropper, A. H., & Davis, K. R. (1980). Lobar cerebral hemorrhages: Acute clinical syndromes in 26 cases. *Ann Neurol, 8*, 141–147.

Roseman, D. M. (1968). Carotidynia. In P. J. Vinken & G. W. Bruyn (Eds), *Handbook of neurology* (Vol. 5, pp. 375–377). Amsterdam: North Holland.

Savage, C. O. S., Harper, L., Cockwell, P., Adu, D., & Howie, A. J. (2000). Vasculitis. *BMJ, 320*, 1325–1328.

Silberberg, D. H., & Laties, A. M. (1973). Increased intracranial pressure in disseminated lupus erythematosus. *Arch Neurol, 29*, 88–90.

Thomas, J. E., Rooke, E. D., & Kvale, W. F. (1966). The neurologist's experience with pheochromocytoma: A review of 100 cases. *JAMA, 197*, 751–758.

Toole, J. (1984). *Cerebrovascular disorders* (3rd ed., p. 342). New York: Raven Press.

Verweij, R. D., Wijdicks, E. F. M., & van Gijn, J. (1988). Warning headache in aneurysmal subarachnoid haemorrhage. *Arch Neurol, 45*, 1019–1020.

Walker, C. H. (1959). Migraine and its relationship to hypertension. *BMJ, 2*, 1430–1433.

Waltimo, O., Hokkanen, E., & Pirskanen, R. (1975). Intracranial arteriovenous malformations and headache. *Headache, 15*, 133–135.

Walton, J. N. (l956). *Subarachnoid haemorrhage*. Edinburgh: Livingstone.

Waters, W. E. (1971). Headache and blood pressure in the community. *BMJ, 1*, 142–143.

West, T. E. T., Davies, R. J., & Kelly, R. E. (1976). Horner's syndrome and headache due to carotid artery disease. *BMJ, i*, 818–821.

Wolff, H. G. (1963). *Headache and other head pain*. London: Oxford University Press.

Chapter 16
Nonvascular Intracranial Disorders

HIGH CEREBROSPINAL FLUID PRESSURE

Internal (Obstructive) Hydrocephalus

Any lesion that obstructs the flow of cerebrospinal fluid (CSF) from the lateral ventricles through the foramen of Monro, third ventricle, aqueduct, and/or fourth ventricle and its exit foramina, or prevents the passage of CSF over the cortex to its absorption site (Figure 16.1), will cause a rapid increase in intracranial pressure so that headache becomes the main presenting symptom. The headache is commonly bilateral and is made worse by coughing, sneezing, or head movement.

A tumor in the vicinity of the third ventricle or within it (such as a colloid cyst) (Figure 16.2) may also interfere intermittently with the function of the midbrain reticular formation so that posture cannot be maintained and the patient thus suffers from "drop attacks," in which he or she slumps heavily to the ground. Severe paroxysmal headaches of recent origin should always arouse suspicion of intermittent obstructive hydrocephalus.

Stenosis of the aqueduct leading from the third ventricle to the fourth may be a congenital malformation that does not produce any symptoms until some systemic infection causes proliferation of its ependymal lining, which then blocks the canal and produces an acute internal hydrocephalus. The aqueduct may also be obstructed by a tumor in the vicinity of the midbrain, such as a pinealoma or glioma (see Figure 19.1), or the aqueduct and fourth ventricle may be displaced or blocked by tumors in the posterior fossa.

Hydrocephalus may progress slowly from conditions in the region of the cisterna magna and foramen magnum. Tumors in this area, cysticercosis, a congenital cystic malformation known as the Dandy-Walker syndrome, platybasia (basilar impression), or Chiari type 1 malformation (see Figure 19.2) may be responsible for obstructing the flow of CSF. Platybasia is a flattening of the floor of the posterior fossa, with anterior parts of the atlas and axis rotated upward. It may be a congenital anomaly, often associated with spina bifida, or may develop

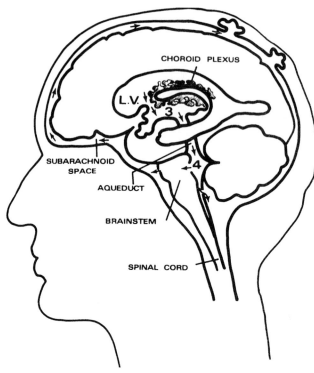

FIGURE 16.1   Cerebrospinal fluid (CSF) circulation. CSF flows from the choroid plexus in the lateral ventricles through the foramen of Monro into the third ventricle (*3*), aqueduct and fourth ventricle (*4*), emerging through the foramina of Magendie and Luschka into the subarachnoid space, to be absorbed mainly by the arachnoid villi in the superior sagittal sinus. (From Lance, 1986, by permission of the publishers, Charles Scribner's Sons, New York.)

through softening of the base of the skull in Paget's disease, osteoporosis, or osteomalacia.

Obstructive hydrocephalus is diagnosed by computed tomography (CT) (see Figure 16.2) or magnetic resonance imaging (MRI; see Figures 19.1 and 19.2). The offending lesion is removed when possible. If not, the pressure in the dilated ventricles can be relieved by a technique using an operating microscope that punches a hole in the thinned floor of the third ventricle (third ventriculostomy), permitting the free flow of CSF into the subarachnoid space (see Figure 19.1). Alternatively, a catheter can be inserted into one lateral ventricle and run subcutaneously to the jugular vein and right atrium (ventriculoatrial shunt) or peritoneal cavity (ventriculoperitoneal shunt).

Communicating Hydrocephalus

The conditions so far considered produce an internal hydrocephalus with dilation of the ventricular system on the central side of the block. Less commonly,

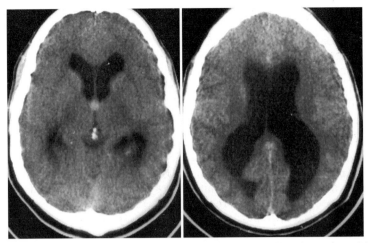

FIGURE 16.2 CT scan showing internal hydrocephalus caused by obstruction of the foramen of Monro. A lesion in this site is commonly a colloid cyst of the third ventricle.

the fluid may emerge freely from the fourth ventricle by the foramina of Magendie and Luschka but be impeded from ascending through the basal cisterns and subarachnoid space because of adhesive arachnoiditis. Researchers have long recognized this as a cause of hydrocephalus in tuberculous or other meningitis, but the condition may also develop quietly in older patients, causing dementia ("normal pressure" hydrocephalus). Progressive arachnoiditis may also follow head injury or subarachnoid hemorrhage.

Cerebral Edema

A sudden elevation of the blood pressure, as in malignant hypertension, may cause headache, presumably by cerebral edema displacing pain-sensitive blood vessels, because the headache is relieved by the intravenous infusion of hypertonic solutions such as 50% glucose but not when CSF pressure is reduced by lumbar puncture (Wolff, 1963). One hemisphere may swell following infarction, as a result of thrombosis of the internal carotid artery, or thrombosis or embolism of one of its main branches. Headache is commonly a symptom of cerebral infarction. Cerebral edema may be sufficiently pronounced to cause papilledema after internal carotid thrombosis, thus simulating an acute presentation of cerebral tumor.

Cerebral edema used to be a major problem after craniotomy but is now largely controlled by high doses of adrenal corticosteroids, such as dexamethasone 16 to 64 mg daily. Potent diuretics, such as furosemide 40 to 120 mg daily, are also valuable in controlling cerebral edema. The oral administration of urea and glycerol has been used with some success at times. The intravenous infusion of mannitol remains a standard procedure. No evidence suggests that steroids are helpful in post-traumatic edema. Decompressive craniectomy or ventricular drainage may become necessary in cases resistant to other measures.

Hypocalcemia may produce cerebral edema, papilledema, and seizures. Prolonged dosage with corticosteroids has been reported to cause headache, vomiting, papilledema, diplopia, and drowsiness. Addison's disease may also cause cerebral edema and papilledema (Jefferson, 1956). Other causes of cerebral edema are considered later, when discussing idiopathic intracranial hypertension.

Idiopathic Intracranial Hypertension (Benign Intracranial Hypertension)

Elevation of CSF pressure without a demonstrable space-occupying lesion or obstruction of the CSF pathways is termed *pseudotumor cerebri, benign intracranial hypertension,* or *idiopathic intracranial hypertension* (IIH). A survey in Iowa and Louisiana in the United States found an annual incidence of 0.9 per 100,000 people (Durcan, Corbett, & Wall, 1988). Among obese people, the incidence increased to 13 per 100,000, and in women aged 20 to 44 years who were more than 20% over ideal weight the incidence reached 19 per 100,000. The female-to-male ratio was 8:1, and the mean weight was 38% above ideal weight for height. The disorder is clearly predominant in overweight women of childbearing age, but no association was found with pregnancy or the use of oral contraceptives (Durcan et al., 1988).

The condition usually presents with generalized headache (92%), transient visual obscuration (72%), and intracranial noises (60%) (Wall & George. 1991). These noises—described as being like "a rushing river," "a waterfall," "water inside a balloon," "a rope twirling," or other buzzing, whistling, or blowing sounds—are presumably caused by turbulent venous flow. Wall and George (1991) preferred the term *idiopathic intracranial hypertension,* because the course is not always benign. Of the 50 patients they studied, 26% initially complained of visual impairment, but on perimetry more than 90% showed some visual loss. Over the follow-up period, averaging 12 months, vision deteriorated in five patients and two became blind. In an earlier study of 57 patients followed for 5 to 41 years (Corbett et al., 1982), 14 developed severe visual loss or became blind, with a much greater risk for patients with high blood pressure, of whom 8 of 13 lost their vision. Rarely, vision may be lost suddenly because of central retinal artery occlusion (Baker & Buncie, 1984).

The insidious onset of headache is usually associated with papilledema, but monitoring of CSF pressure has disclosed some patients in whom pressure was elevated without producing papilledema (Spence, Amacher, & Willis, 1980; Marcelis & Silberstein, 1991). Paresis of one or both sixth cranial nerves develops in 10% to 40% of cases, presumably because cerebral edema displaces and compresses the nerves, and third-nerve palsy has also been reported (Snyder & Frenkel, 1979; McCammon, Kaufman, & Sears, 1981).

Idiopathic intracranial hypertension has been reported as a reaction to certain drugs, such as tetracycline, nitrofurantoin, and nalidixic acid; as the result of excessive intake of vitamin A; and as a sequel to the withdrawal of corticosteroid therapy. The combination of low-dosage tetracycline therapy and vitamin A, used in treating acne, may increase the chances of a patient developing benign intracranial hypertension (Walters & Gubbay, 1981).

The condition must be clearly distinguished from intracranial hypertension caused by venous sinus thrombosis, which it resembles closely. Idiopathic intracranial hypertension appears to be caused by reduced CSF absorption, because CSF production is normal, causing increased total CSF volume. Intracranial pressure builds up in waves, followed by a sudden fall, suggesting that the increased pressure periodically forces fluid through the arachnoid villi. The various causative factors mentioned may all increase resistance to CSF flow across the villi (Johnston & Paterson, 1974). Cerebral blood volume increases in benign intracranial hypertension (Mathew, Meyer, & Ott, 1975), whereas the volume of the lateral and third ventricles is less than in normal controls, indicating that edema or engorgement is causing swelling of the brain (Reid, Matheson, & Teasdale, 1980). Chazal et al. (1979) confirmed a defect in the CSF resorption mechanism, the fault lying in the venous sinuses or in the arachnoid villi. The most plausible hypothesis is a vicious circle of defective CSF absorption, increased CSF pressure, venous engorgement, and cerebral edema, further reducing CSF absorption.

The diagnosis is confirmed by CT demonstration of normal or small ventricles and an elevated CSF pressure (above 250 mm H_2O) with normal CSF constituents.

Medical treatment consists of repeated lumbar puncture, acetazolamide 1000 mg daily to reduce CSF production, and dietary advice to reduce weight. Papilledema and visual field impairment responded more rapidly in patients on a weight reduction program than in a control group (Kupersmith et al., 1998). Weight loss is more important than the use of acetazolamide (Johnson et al., 1998). If visual loss progresses, the clinician often prescribes a short course of corticosteroids and, if there is no improvement, can undertake surgical procedures such as optic nerve sheath fenestration or a lumbar-subarachnoid shunt (Wall & George, 1991). Two thirds of those patients with residual headache improve after the optic nerve sheath is slit (Corbett & Thompson, 1989). Corbett and Thompson emphasized the need for careful follow-up with perimetry, fundus photographs, and measurements of intraocular pressure and cautioned against relying on visual acuity and visual evoked potentials, which are relatively insensitive indices of deterioration.

LOW CEREBROSPINAL FLUID PRESSURE

Postlumbar Puncture Headache

The headache that often follows lumbar puncture is probably caused by continued leakage of CSF from the subarachnoid space after the procedure, which lowers intracranial pressure, withdrawing support for the brain and thus exerting traction on intracranial vessels. Carbaat and van Crevel (1981) showed that the incidence of headache after lumbar puncture was not reduced by having the patient lie flat for 24 hours and was almost 40% whether the patient was kept in bed or allowed to walk about. Hilton-Jones et al. (1982) reported that 38 of their 76 patients developed postlumbar puncture headache, with no significant difference between those lying for 4 hours prone or supine, tilted head up or head down. In a series of 300 patients, headache with nausea was significantly more frequent in those kept at bed rest for 6 hours, affecting 23% compared with 13% who were allowed to get up immediately (Vilming, Schrader, & Monstad, 1988). The total headache incidence was 39% in the recumbent and 35% in the ambulant group. In a series of 203 patients Engelhardt, Oheim, and Neurdorfer (1991) reduced the incidence of postlumbar puncture headache to 2.5% by using an "atraumatic needle" with a conical tip and a side aperture.

Silberstein and Marcelis (1992), in their comprehensive review of CSF dynamics and headache associated with changes in CSF pressure, advocate bed rest, an abdominal binder (to increae venous pressure and thus CSF pressure), and the administration of caffeine as the initial management, followed by a short course of corticosteroids if headache persists. The headache resolves in less than 4 days in 53% of cases and in less than 7 days in 72%. Postlumbar puncture headache may persist for months, with the characteristic postural headache being mistaken for a postviral vascular headache (Lance & Branch, 1994). MRI of the brain usually shows uptake of gadolinium in the thickened meninges, probably caused by diapedesis of red cells inducing a fibrotic reaction (Figure 16.3) (Amor et al., 1996). If headache persists, CSF isotope studies are indicated to determine the site of leakage (Figure 16.4), and the clinician can consider treatment by epidural blood patch, a technique in which 10 to 20 mL of the patient's own blood is injected into the epidural space below the original lumbar

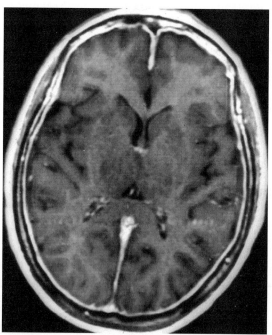

FIGURE 16.3   Thickened meninges enhanced by gadolinium in a low cerebrospinal fluid pressure syndrome. (From Amor et al., 1996, by permission.)

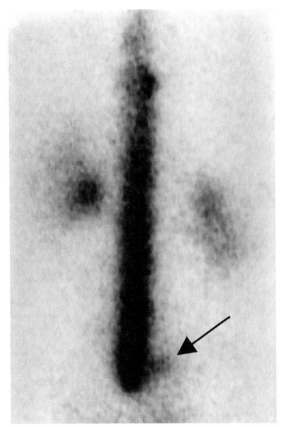

FIGURE 16.4   Isotope study showing leakage of the cerebrospinal fluid from the lumbar sac *(arrow)*.

puncture site. Seebacher et al. (1989) found that five out of six patients treated this way were relieved of headache within 2 hours, whereas none of the six undergoing a sham procedure improved. All the latter lost their headaches after a genuine blood patch.

Other Low-Pressure Syndromes

Intracranial hypotension may be caused by CSF rhinorrhoea as the result of trauma or of bony erosion by a tumor, a spontaneous dural tear, or spinal root avulsion. Patients with connective tissue disorders such as Marfan's syndrome are prone to develop CSF leaks from meningeal diverticula (Ferrante et al., 2003). Trauma may be relatively trivial, such as a sports injury or a roller-coaster ride (Schievink, Ebersold, & Atkinson, 1996). Many start with a minor fall, vigorous exercise, or violent coughing (O'Carroll & Brant-Zawadzki, 1999). Some cases have followed sexual intercourse (see Chapter 13). Silberstein and

Marcelis (1992) also cite systemic medical illnesses, severe dehydration, hyperpnea, meningoencephalitis, uremia, and infusion of hypertonic solutions as causes of low-pressure syndromes.

Intracranial hypotension is classified as "spontaneous" if no obvious source of CSF leakage is found for postural headache and if CSF pressure remains below 60 mm H_2O.

Probably most, if not all, patients with the sudden onset of orthostatic headache have sustained an undetected tear in the dura, causing a slow leak with resulting low CSF pressure. The brain may be displaced downward with incisural or cerebellar herniation, giving the appearance of a Chiari type 1 malformation, which reverses when the low-pressure state resolves. Small bilateral subdural hematomas or hygromas may develop as a secondary phenomenon and may confuse the physician who mistakes it for the source of the headache. Cranial nerves may be stretched. One of O'Carroll and Brant-Zawadzki's patients developed a sixth cranial nerve palsy, and Warner (2002) reported a patient with partial impairment of the third cranial nerve.

Radionucleotide cisternography may detect a CSF leak (see Figure 16.4) and characteristically demonstrates rapid disappearance of the radioactive tracer from the subarachnoid space, with accumulation in the bladder.

Chung, Kim, and Lee (2001) reviewed 30 patients complaining of orthostatic headache, associated in some cases with nausea, dizziness, neck stiffness, blurred vision, tinnitus, hearing difficulties, and radicular pain in the arm. CSF pressure was less than 60 mm H_2O in 82%, cell count rose in 59%, and protein content was elevated in 95%. MRI demonstrated enhancement of the meninges with gadolinium in 83% and showed a subdural hematoma or hygroma in 17%. Radioisotope cisternography identified CSF leakage sites in 52%, most often in the lumbar region. They used epidural blood patches to treat 23 patients, stopping headaches in 70%.

INTRACRANIAL INFECTION

The headache of meningitis or encephalitis is often frontal or retro-orbital, associated with photophobia, nausea, drowsiness, neck stiffness, fever, and general malaise. If the patient has signs of increased intracranial pressure, it is advisable to perform a CT of the brain to exclude subdural empyema, cerebral abscess, or other space-occupying lesions before lumbar puncture. However, this scan should not delay the administration of antibiotics when the clinician suspects a pyogenic infection, because delay can prove fatal.

The clinician makes the diagnosis by clinical assessment and lumbar puncture. In pyogenic infections and in the acute phase of some cases of viral encephalitis, the CSF contains an excess of cells, mostly neutrophils. A purely lymphocytic pleocytosis usually indicates a viral infection but may appear in some cases of tuberculous or cryptococcal meningitis. A low CSF glucose value (in the absence of hypoglycemia) means the infecting organism is metabolizing glucose and indicates a pyogenic, tuberculous, or cryptococcal infection. An exception to this rule is the unusual condition of meningitis carcinomatosis, in which the meninges are infiltrated and sheathed with malignant cells that multiply so rapidly the CSF glucose level drops.

Headache is a common complaint in patients with acquired immunodeficiency syndrome (AIDS), commonly of infectious etiology. Lipton et al. (1991) studied 49 patients infected with human immunodeficiency virus-1 (HIV-1) who presented with headache. They found the cause to be cryptococcal meningitis in 19 patients; toxoplasmosis in 8 patients; progressive multifocal leukoencephalopathy in 1 patient; syphilis in 1 patient; and lymphoma, brain abscess, or undiagnosed mass lesions in 9 patients. No identifiable serious cause of headache was found in the remainder. Ramadan (1997) discusses factors contributing to headache in patients positive for HIV-1.

Headache Associated with Intrathecal Injections

The chemical excitation of nerve endings in the meninges produces a reflex spasm of the neck extensors and sometimes of the lumbar muscles, which is analogous to the contraction of the abdominal wall resulting from peritoneal inflammation and is known as "muscle guarding." Muscle spasm consequent on meningeal irritation causes neck rigidity and Kernig's sign. This is encountered most often in subarachnoid hemorrhage, meningitis, and encephalitis but may also occur after injection of air or chemical agents into the CSF.

CT and MRI are now preferable to the technique of introducing air into the subarachnoid space for diagnostic purposes (pneumoencephalography). This procedure sometimes caused a sterile inflammatory reaction that rivaled meningoencephalitis in its severity and was associated with a CSF pleocytosis. Intrathecal injection of a contrast medium for myelography or antibiotics, baclofen, long-acting steroids, or other agents may sometimes cause a meningitic reaction with headache. The headache usually follows the injection within 5 to 72 hours, is present whether the subject is standing or lying, and clears in a maximum of 14 days. There may be a CSF pleocytosis with negative culture.

INTRACRANIAL GRANULOMA

Sarcoidosis

Approximately 5% of cases of sarcoidosis involve the nervous system. Sarcoid granulomas may obstruct the CSF pathways, resulting in hydrocephalus, or may affect the region of the optic nerves, pituitary, and hypothalamus (Thompson, 1991).

Tolosa-Hunt syndrome is discussed in Chapter 18.

INTRACRANIAL TUMORS

Unless a tumor or other space-occupying lesion affects a strategic position along the line of the drainage pathways of the cerebral ventricles, it can reach a considerable size before causing headache. Because intracranial vessels must be pushed aside before pain is registered, infiltrating tumors, such as the gliomas, may extend throughout one hemisphere without causing headache, because the position of large vessels may remain undisturbed until the last stages of the disease. Tumors that compress the brain from outside, such as meningiomas, are likely to cause seizures, focal cerebral symptoms, progressive impairment of intellectual function, or other neurologic deficit before they produce headache.

Of 163 patients with cerebral tumor that Iversen et al. (1987) reported, 53% suffered from headache, 16% as the first symptom. Headache was twice as common in patients with gliomas and secondary tumors as in patients with meningiomas, and was related to the site rather than to tumor size, occurring more often with occipital, basal, and posterior fossa tumors.

The headache of brain tumor or other space-occupying lesion progressively becomes more severe, aggravated by coughing, sneezing, straining, or bending the head forward. Headache is the initial symptom of patients with posterior fossa tumors, except for those arising in the cerebellopontine angle, and is usually felt in the occipital region. Supratentorial tumors cause frontal headache with extension to the occiput in about one third of cases. A posterior fossa tumor may cause pain by directly compressing the fifth, seventh, ninth, or tenth cranial nerves, which may refer pain to the face, ear, or throat. The person experiences pain in the neck because of irritation of the dura, which is supplied by the upper three cervical nerve roots, and reflex spasm of neck muscles may cause the patient to hold the head to one side. Pain may also be referred to the eye and forehead by convergence of impulses from the upper cervical nerve roots on neurons of the cervical cord, which also serve the trigeminal pathways. Finally, blockage of the CSF flow, increasing intracranial pressure, may cause generalized headache (Forsyth & Posner, 2000).

The headache caused by intracranial tumor is treated surgically by removing the cause whenever possible. Failing that, or as a preliminary to a definitive operation, neurosurgeons may insert a ventricular shunt or prescribe corticosteroids to reduce intracranial pressure.

Pituitary Tumors

Headache is a common symptom of pituitary tumors, particularly in patients with a prolactinoma or acromegaly; headache may affect 85% of the latter. Levy et al. (2002) studied 57 patients with pituitary tumors, among whom 67% complained of headache. Headache did not correlate with pituitary volume or with the extent of cavernous sinus invasion or encasement of the internal carotid artery but was strongly associated with a positive family history of headache. Levy et al. (2003) explored the possibility of the headaches being caused by vasodilator peptides but could not establish a relationship between headache and the presence in the tumor of calcitonin gene–related peptide (CGRP) or substance P.

Prolactin-secreting tumors usually respond to bromocriptine by shrinking and lowering prolactin level. Sumatriptan can be effective in headaches of pituitary origin, and pituitary adenomas respond to the somatostatin analog octreotide (Levy et al., 2003). The headaches of acromegaly improve with long-acting release (LAR) octreotide given once a month intramuscularly, comparable with the response to another somatostatin analog lanreotide (slow release) (McKeage, Cheer, & Wagstaff, 2003).

References

Baker, R. S., & Buncie, J. R. (1984). Sudden visual loss in pseudotumour cerebri due to central retinal artery occlusion. *Arch Neurol, 41,* 1274–1276.

Ben Amor, S., Maeder, P., Gudinchet, F., & Ingvar-Maeder, M. (1996). Syndrome d'hypotension intracranienne spontanee. *Rev Neurol, 152,* 611–614.

Carbaat, P. A., & van Crevel, H. (1981). Lumbar puncture headache: Controlled study on the preventive effect of 24 hours bed rest. *Lancet, ii,* 1133–1135.

Chazal, J., Janny, P., Georget, A. M., & Colnet, G. (1979). Benign intracranial hypertension. A clinical evaluation of the CSF absorption mechanisms. *Acta Neurochir Suppl. (Wien) 28*(2), 505–508.

Chung, S. J., Kim, J. S., & Lee, M. D. (2001). Syndrome of cerebral spinal fluid hypovolemia: Clinical and imaging features and outcome. *Neurology, 56,* 1607–1608.

Corbett, J. J., Savino, S. J., Thompson, H. S., et al. (1982). Visual loss in pseudotumor cerebri: Follow-up of 57 patients from 5 to 41 years and a profile of 14 patients with severe visual loss. *Arch Neurol, 39,* 461–474.

Corbett, J. J., & Thompson, H. S. (1989). The rational management of benign intracranial hypertension. *Arch Neurol, 46,* 1049–1051.

Durcan, F. J., Corbett, J. J., & Wall, M. (1988). The incidence of pseudotumor cerebri: Population studies in Iowa and Louisiana. *Arch Neurol, 45,* 875–877.

Engelhardt, A., Oheim, S., & Neundorfer, B. (1991). Post-lumbar puncture headache: Experiences with an "atraumatic" needle. *Cephalalgia, 11*(Suppl. 11), 356–357.

Ferrante, E., Citterio, A., Savino, A., & Santalucia, A. (2003). Postural headache in a patient with Marfan's syndrome. *Cephalalgia, 23,* 552–555.

Forsyth, P. A., & Posner, J. B. (2000). Intracranial neoplasms. In J. Olesen, P. Tfelt-Hansen, & K. M. A. Welch (Eds.), *The headaches* (2nd ed., pp. 849–859). Philadelphia: Lippincott Williams & Wilkins.

Hilton-Jones, D., Harrad, R. A., Gill. M. W., & Warlow, C. P. (1982). Failure of postural manoeuvres to prevent lumbar puncture headache. *J Neurol Neurosurg Psychiatry, 45,* 743–746.

Iversen, H. K., Strange, P., Sommer, W., & Tjalve, E. (1987). Brain tumour headache related to tumour size, histology and location. *Cephalalgia, 7*(Suppl. 6), 394–395.

Jefferson, A. (1956). A clinical correlation between encephalopathy and papilloedema in Addison's disease. *J Neurol Neurosurg Psychiatry, 19,* 21–27.

Johnson, L. N., Krohel, G. B., Madsen, R. W., & March, G. A., Jr. (1998). The role of weight loss and acetazolamide in the treatment of idiopathic intracranial hypertension (pseudotumor cerebri). *Ophthalmology, 105,* 2313–2317.

Johnston, I., & Paterson, A. (1974). Benign intracranial hypertension. II. CSF pressure and circulation. *Brain, 97,* 301–312.

Kupersmith, M. J., Gamell, L., Turbin, R., et al. (1998). Effects of weight loss on the course of idiopathic intracranial hypertension in women. *Neurology, 50,* 1094–8.

Lance, J. W., & Branch, G. B. (1994). Persistent headache after lumbar puncture. *Lancet, 12,* 414.

Levy, M. J., Classey, J. D., Maneesri, S., et al. (2003). Differential expression of calcitonin gene–related peptide (CGRP) and substance P in pituitary adenomas: In search of a nociceptive peptide. *Cephalalgia, 23,* 687.

Levy, M. J., Jager, H. R., Matharu, M. S., & Goadsby, P. J. (2002). Pituitary tumours and headache: Does size matter? *Cephalalgia, 22,* 592.

Lipton, R. B., Feraru, E. R., & Weiss, G. (1991). Headache in HIV-1–related disorders. *Headache, 31,* 518–522.

Marcelis, J., & Silberstein, S. D. (1991). Idiopathic intracranial hypertension without papilledema. *Arch Neurol, 48,* 392–399.

Mathew, N. T., Meyer, J. S., & Ott, E. O. (1975). Increased cerebral blood volume in benign intracranial hypertension. *Neurology, 25,* 646–649.

McCammon, A., Kaufman, H. H., & Sears, E. S. (1981). Transient oculomotor paralysis in pseudotumor cerebri. *Neurology (NY), 31,* 182–184.

McKeage, K., Cheer, S., & Wagstaff, A. J. (2003). Octreotide long-acting release (LAR): A review of its use in the management of acromegaly. *Drugs, 63,* 2473–2499.

O'Carroll, C. P., & Brant-Zawadzki, M. (1999). The syndrome of spontaneous intracranial hypotension. *Cephalalgia, 19,* 80–87.

Ramadan, N. H. (1997). Unusual causes of headache. *Neurology, 48,* 1494–1499.

Reid, A. C., Matheson, M. S., & Teasdale, G. (1980). Volume of the ventricles in benign intracranial hypertension. *Lancet, ii,* 7–8.

Schievink, W. I., Ebersold, M. J., & Atkinson, J. L. D. (1996). Roller-coaster headache due to spinal cerebrospinal fluid leak. *Lancet, 347,* 1409.

Seebacher, J., Ribeiro, V., Le Guillou, J. L., Lacomblez, L., Henry, M., Thorman, F., et al. (1989). Epidural blood patch as treatment for post-lumbar puncture headache—a double-blind controlled trial. *Cephalalgia, 9*(Suppl. 10), 185–186.

Sechzer, P. H., & Abel, L. (1978). Post-spinal anesthesia headache treated with caffeine. Evaluation with demand method. *Curr Therap Res, 24,* 307–312.

Silberstein, S. D., & Marcelis, J. (1992). Headache associated with changes in intracranial pressure. *Headache, 32,* 84–91.

Snyder, D. A., & Frenkel, M. (1979). An unusual presentation of pseudotumor cerebri. *Ann Ophthalmol, 11,* 1823–1827.

Spence, J. D., Amacher, A. L., & Willis, N. R. (1980). Benign intracranial hypertension without papilledema: Role of 24-hour cerebrospinal fluid pressure monitoring in diagnosis and management. *Neurosurgery, 7,* 326–336.

Thompson, A. J. (1991). Sarcoidosis and the nervous system. In M. Swash & J. Oxbury (Eds.), *Clinical neurology* (pp. 1725–1731). Edinburgh: Churchill-Livingstone.

Vilming, S. T., Schrader, H., & Monstad, I. (1988). Post-lumbar-puncture headache: The significance of body posture. A controlled study of 300 patients. *Cephalalgia, 8,* 75–78.

Wall, M., & George, D. (1991). Idiopathic intracranial hypertension. A prospective study of 50 patients. *Brain, 114,* 155–180.

Walters, B. N. J., & Gubbay, S. S. (1981). Tetracycline and benign intracranial hypertension: Report of five cases. *BMJ, 282,* 19–20.

Warner, G. T. A. (2002). Spontaneous intracranial hypotension causing a partial third cranial nerve palsy: A novel observation. *Cephalalgia, 22,* 822–823.

Wolff, H. G. (1963). *Headache and other head pain* (3rd ed.). New York: Oxford University Press.

Chapter 17
Disorders of the Neck, Cranial, and Extracranial Structures

CRANIUM

It is very rare to find a source of headache within the cranial bones, although we later cite some examples of inflammatory or neoplastic lesions involving the sinuses or petrous temporal bones. Nevertheless the clinician should always run his or her hands over the scalp of any patient complaining of headache. Occasionally a scalp infection or osteomyelitis may give rise to pain that the patient describes as headache. Any expanding lesion of bone that stretches the periosteum may cause local pain. Paget's disease of the skull may be associated with a vascular headache fluctuating in intensity, probably caused by increased cranial blood flow. In Paget's disease the scalp may feel warm because of arteriovenous shunting, which may reach such proportions that cardiac output is substantially increased. The softening of bone in Paget's disease may cause the base of the skull to be invaginated by the atlas and axis, giving rise to "basilar impression" (platybasia). In this condition the posterior fossa is distorted and the flow of cerebrospinal fluid (CSF) may be impaired, with an increase in intracranial pressure, as we described in Chapter 16.

A localized area in the scalp may give rise to constant or stabbing pain (nummular headache) and may be tender to touch (Pareja et al., 2002). Infiltrating the area with local anesthetic or excising the affected area relieves some patients' pain.

NECK

In the fourth of a series of 18 lectures given on "Rest and Pain," between 1860 and 1862, John Hilton (1805–1878) made the following remarks (1950):

> Suppose a person to complain of pain upon the scalp, is it not very essential to know whether that pain is expressed by the fifth nerve or by the great or small occipital? Thus pain in the anterior and lateral part of the head, which are supplied by the fifth nerve, would suggest that the cause must be somewhere in

the area of the distribution of the other portions of the fifth nerve. So if the pain be expressed behind, the cause must assuredly be connected with the great or small occipital nerve, and in all probability depends on disease of the spine between the first and second cervical vertebrae.

Abnormalities of various structures in the neck have been implicated as a source of headache. These structures include the synovial joints, the intervertebral disks, ligaments, muscles, nerve roots, and the vertebral artery (Göbel & Edmeads, 2000). Ample evidence shows that irritation of the upper three cervical roots causes pain in the occiput and may refer pain forward to the orbit on the appropriate side. The most important contributor to the greater occipital nerve and hence to occipital sensation, including pain, is the second cervical root. The C2 dorsal-root ganglion lies dorsal to the atlantoaxial joint (Figure 17.1). Lateral to this point, the C2 dorsal and ventral roots fuse to form a very short spinal nerve, which emerges around the lateral border of the posterior atlantoaxial membrane and then divides into a dorsal and a ventral ramus (Bogduk, 1981a). The ventral ramus gives branches to the lateral atlantoaxial joint on its way to enter the cervical plexus (see Figure 17.1). The C2 dorsal ramus supplies various muscular branches, links with the C1 and C3 dorsal rami, and becomes continu-

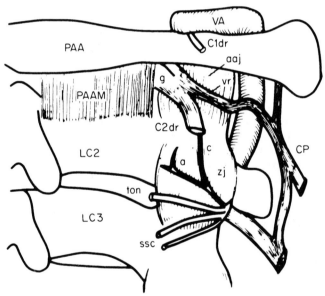

FIGURE 17.1   A diagram of the right C2 ganglion and rami, showing their major relations. *a,* Articular nerve; *aaj,* lateral atlantoaxial joint; *c,* communicating branch C3 to C2; *Cldr,* C1 dorsal ramus; *C2dr,* C2 dorsal ramus (cut proximal to its branching point); *CP,* cervical plexus; *g,* C2 dorsal root ganglions; *LC2,* lamina of C2 vertebra; *LC3,* lamina of C3 vertebra; *PAA,* posterior arch of the atlas; *PAAM,* posterior atlantoaxial membrane; *sc,* nerves to semispinalis capitus; *ton,* third occipital nerve; *VA,* vertebral artery; *vr,* C2 ventral ramus; *zj,* C2–C3 zygapophyseal joint. (From Bogduk, 1981a, by permission of the publishers, Adis Press, Sydney.)

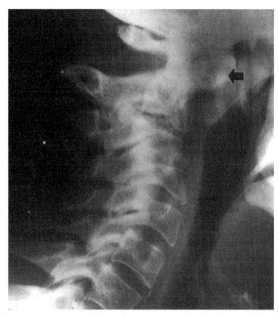

FIGURE 17.2   Rheumatoid arthritis of the upper cervical spine causing dislocation of the odontoid process *(arrow)*.

ous with the greater occipital nerve, which emerges onto the scalp above an aponeurotic sling. For this reason the greater occipital nerve cannot be compressed by spasm of the trapezius, which would draw the aponeurotic sling away from the nerve. Bogduk (1981a) stresses that the C2 nerve is vulnerable to compression only in extreme rotation and extension of the atlas on its axis, with dislocation of the lateral atlantoaxial joints. This is not the type of movement in whiplash injury, which is more likely to damage the lateral atlantoaxial joints and soft tissues than the C2 root itself.

Upper Cervical Syndrome

Disorders of the upper cervical spine affecting the upper three cervical roots can refer pain from the upper neck and occiput forward to the orbital region. Upper cervical instability following trauma, basilar impression (platybasia), and rheumatoid arthritis (see Figure 17.2) are clinical examples. Degenerative changes of the upper cervical zygapophyseal joints accompanying reflex muscle contraction may also cause occipital headache. Examination of the neck may show restricted movement at a joint, a hypomobility lesion, probably caused by intra-articular adhesions, capsular contracture, or local muscle spasm (Bogduk et al., 1985). In contrast, some patients show hypermobility associated with laxity of the ligaments. Neck movement or palpation of the occipital nerves may induce occipital headache as well as local tenderness. Injecting a contrast medium into the cervical facet joints replicated the patients' symptoms in about

50% of cases (Dory, 1983), and after aspirating the contrast medium the researcher then injected triamcinolone 20 to 40 mg into the appropriate joint capsule.

The lateral atlantoaxial (C1–C2) joints may also refer pain to the occiput, as in the neck–tongue syndrome (see Chapter 18). Aprill, Axinn, and Bogduk (2002) found that diagnostic blocks of the atlantoaxial joints relieved 21 of 34 patients with occipital headache.

Treatment of most acute conditions is conservative, immobilizing the neck in a collar and prescribing anti-inflammatory drugs and analgesics, but instability at the craniocervical junction or atlantoaxial joint may require surgical treatment. In the absence of instability, pain arising from the zygapophyseal joints can often be managed by mobilizing the neck. We advise caution for any manipulative procedures. Sudden or forceful chiropractic neck manipulation can dissect the vertebral arteries resulting in brainstem infarction (see Chapter 15). Examination of patients with rheumatoid arthritis, whose upper cervical spine may be severely affected, requires special care.

Injecting local anesthetic agents and steroids into tender areas often helps. Injecting local anesthetic into the suspected joints or block of the second cervical ganglion helps localize the facet joints responsible for pain (Bogduk, 1981b). Rarely, the patient may need surgical treatment by coagulation or section of the nerve supply to facet joints, or section of the second and third dorsal roots, to relieve intractable occipital headaches of cervical origin.

Lesions of the C4/C5 disc space downward may cause "lower cervical syndrome," with referral of pain down the arms, but are not a direct source of headache.

Whiplash Injury

Whiplash injury probably results from injury to structures such as the transverse ligament of the atlas, the capsules of the upper cervical synovial joints, and surrounding soft tissues. A direct blow at the same time may damage the occipital nerves. We consider the condition in Chapter 14 on post-traumatic headache.

Third Occipital Nerve Headache

A subvariety of the upper cervical syndrome is headache arising from the C2–C3 facet joints mediated by the third occipital nerve. The C2–C3 joints are a transition zone between the first and second cervical levels, which enable rotation of the head, and the lower cervical spine, which is responsible for flexion and extension of the neck. Bogduk and Marsland (1986) describe the use of a radiologically controlled block of the nerves supplying the C2–C3 facet joints in diagnosing occipital or suboccipital headache radiating to the forehead. All 10 patients studied had a history of neck injury, precipitation of pain by neck movement, or cervical tenderness. In 7 of 10 patients, the diagnostic nerve block temporarily relieved the headache. Injecting steroids provided relief extending from 2 weeks to 4 months, cryocoagulation for 3 to 6 weeks, radiofrequency coagulation for 3 to 12 months, and open neurectomy for 18 months or more to the time of follow-up.

Cervicogenic Headache

Sjaastad and his colleagues (Fredriksen, Hovdal, & Sjaastad, 1987; Sjaastad, Fredriksen, & Pfaffenrath, 1990) coined the term *cervicogenic headache* to describe episodic unilateral headaches, lasting from 3 hours to a week and recurring at intervals from 2 days to 2 months, that these authors considered to arise from the cervical spine. Although these headaches affected women more than men and were sometimes accompanied by migrainous features such as nausea, vomiting, and photophobia, the authors distinguished them from migraine, because neck movement could precipitate them, they usually started in the upper neck, and pressure over the upper neck or occiput could reproduce the pain. The intimate relationship between trigeminal and upper cervical input to the central nervous system in the genesis of headache is well recognized. It is possible that some "cervicogenic headache" is a variety of migraine triggered from the upper cervical spine in a manner comparable with migraine triggered by other forms of afferent stimulation, such as glare and noise.

In 1998 Sjaastad, Fredriksen, and Pfaffenrath amended the original criteria by stating that a positive response to appropriate local anesthetic blockade was essential for the diagnosis and noting that some cervicogenic headaches could be bilateral. Symptoms and signs referable to the neck, such as reduced range of motion or neck movements precipitating attacks of headache, were obligatory, but no specific radiologic abnormalities need be identified.

Antonaci et al. (2001) selected out of 114 headache patients 62 patients with strictly unilateral pain without side-shift and with pain radiating forward from the neck to the fronto-ocular area. Blockade of the greater occipital nerve with local anesthetic gave relief in only 4 of the 24 patients in whom it was attempted, and these authors found radiologic abnormalities in only 16 of the 62 patients.

The criteria for the diagnosis of cervicogenic headache put forward by the Classification Subcommittee of the International Headache Society (2004) are as follows:

A. Pain, referred from a source in the neck and perceived in one or more regions of the head and/or face, fulfilling criteria C and D.
B. Clinical, laboratory and/or imaging evidence of a disorder or lesion within the cervical spine or soft tissues of the neck known to be, or generally accepted as, a valid source of headache.
C. Evidence that the pain can be attributed to the neck disorder or lesion based on at least one of the following:
   1. Demonstration of clinical signs that implicate a source of pain in the neck
   2. Abolition of headache following diagnostic blockade of a cervical structure or its nerve supply using placebo or other adequate controls
D. Pain resolves within 3 months after successful treatment of the causative disorder or lesion.

"Cervical Migraine"

In the 1920s Barré and Lieou described a form of headache accompanying cervical spondylosis, which they attributed to irritation of the vertebral nerve.

Bartschi-Rochaix (1968) wrote a monograph on the topic in 1949 entitled *Migraine Cervicale.* We doubt whether cervical migraine is an entity separate from vertebrobasilar migraine and whether it bears any relation to changes in the cervical spine. The headaches are described by Bartsch-Rochaix (1968) as bilateral, unilateral, or alternating and are accompanied by giddiness, acoustic symptoms, and blurring of vision or fortification spectra. He considered that the symptoms arise from impaired flow in the vertebral arteries where they are displaced by osteophytes, although headache accompanies only a minority of transient ischemic attacks produced by this mechanism on head rotation.

Bogduk, Lambert, and Duckworth (1981) studied the anatomy and physiology of the vertebral nerve to ascertain whether stimulation of this nerve could reduce blood flow in the vertebrobasilar arterial system. The "vertebral nerve" in humans and monkeys consists of a series of neural arcades formed by communications between gray rami from the sympathetic trunk and ventral rami of the C3–C7 segments. Above C3 direct branches from the C1–C3 ventral rami accompany the vertebral artery. From the C1 ventral ramus nerve, filaments (which have no detectable connection with those from lower levels) follow the vertebral artery across the atlas. Electrical stimulation of the vertebral nerve or cervical sympathetic trunk in the monkey reduced vertebral flow by only 18% in contrast to the 70% reduction in carotid blood flow produced by sympathetic stimulation. The lack of reactivity in the intact vertebrobasilar circulation is surprising in view of the reactivity of isolated segments in vitro. That no single nerve accompanies the vertebral artery along its entire length and the unresponsiveness of the artery to sympathetic stimulation renders untenable any hypothesis linking osteophyte irritation of the "vertebral nerve" with migraine headache. A controlled trial of neck manipulation for treating migraine did not significantly decrease headache frequency (Parker, Tupling, & Pryor, 1978).

Occipital Neuralgia

An aching or paroxysmal jabbing pain in the area of distribution of the greater or lesser occipital nerves characterizes an occipital neuralgia. Diminished sensation or dysesthesias of the affected area usually accompany it (as described in Chapter 18).

Headache with Cervical Spinal Cord Lesions

Spierings, Foo, and Young (1992) examined 20 patients with traumatic transection of the spinal cord between the C2–C3 and C7–C8 levels. Of those patients, 12 had generalized severe throbbing headaches caused by an acute increase in blood pressure associated with urinary obstruction or fecal impaction. These headaches usually accompanied other signs of sympathetic activity such as facial flushing, sweating, and nasal congestion. Sixteen patients had experienced headaches other than bladder and bowel headaches, but none had migrainous features. Only 3 of the 20 patients had never suffered from headache.

EYES

Imbalance of the extraocular muscles (heterophoria), especially convergence weakness, or refractive errors, particularly uncorrected presbyopia, may set up "eye-strain" headache, a form of tension headache that follows visual effort (Lyle, 1968). This condition is much overdiagnosed, and simply correcting a visual disturbance rarely cures headache. Waters (1970) compared visual acuity and ocular muscle balance in groups of patients who were headache prone and headache free. Hyperphoria with near vision was more common in patients with migraine, but no other difference was found. Certain odd ocular pains, which do not seem of any significance, are known as ophthalmodynia (see Chapter 13). These jabbing pains may affect one eyeball and may be repetitive, without obvious cause. Angle closure glaucoma may cause the patient to feel pain deeply in the eye and to feel pain radiate over the forehead in the distribution area of the first division of the trigeminal nerve. The patient may not have mistiness of vision, colored haloes seen around lights, or circumcorneal injection to draw attention to the eye. In the middle-aged or elderly patient, radiation of pain from eye to forehead should arouse suspicion of glaucoma.

Pain in or behind the eye is a common feature of retrobulbar (optic) neuritis and may precede impairment of vision by a few hours or even days (see Chapter 18). Sight becomes blurred and may disappear completely in the affected eye. The most common visual field defect is a central scotoma, because the demyelinating process more often affects the central part of the optic nerve containing fibers from the macula.

Daroff (1998) paraphrased Dr. William Hoyt by stating, "A white eye is not the cause of a monosymptomatic painful eye or headache." The exceptions are optic neuritis and subacute angle-closure glaucoma (SACG). For patients with a headache of recent onset not conforming to a definite headache syndrome, Daroff recommends referral to an ophthalmologist, specifying the need for gonioscopy (measurement of the angle size in the anterior chamber of the eye) to rule out SACG, as well as routine measurement of intraocular tension.

EARS, NOSE, SINUSES, AND THROAT

Vasomotor rhinitis is thought by some to give rise to a midfrontal headache. This statement warrants skepticism, because vasomotor rhinitis is a common disorder and affects many people without causing headache. It does, of course, predispose to sinusitis, which causes headache in the stage of active inflammation or when the ostium of a particular sinus is obstructed. Ryan and Kern (1978) discuss rhinologic causes of headache and facial pain, commenting that chronic sinusitis rarely causes facial pain. Most patients who complain of recurrent "sinus headache" are suffering from one of the varieties of migraine, which may be associated with nasal congestion (Blau, 1988). Headaches resulting from disease of the nose or sinuses usually accompany a feeling of fullness in the affected area and nasal discharge as well as congestion (Close & Aviv, 1997).

Diagnosing sinusitis is usually easy when pain and tenderness are localized to the affected frontal or maxillary sinus or sinuses and percussion over the area increases the pain. Inflammation of the ethmoid or sphenoidal sinuses gives rise to a drilling pain felt deeply in the midline behind the nose. The pain of sinusitis worsens when the patient bends the head forward. If the ostium of the infected sinus is patent, blowing the nose or sneezing usually evokes a throb of pain. If the ostium is obstructed, the patient may awaken with a "vacuum" headache caused by absorbing air from the blocked sinus.

One or both nostrils are usually blocked, and clearing an airway with decongestants lets mucopurulent material discharge from the sinuses, usually relieving pain (Figure 17.3). Using vasoconstrictor nose drops or nasal spray, such as neosynephrine 0.25% every 2 to 3 hours, instilled first with the patient's head bent backward over the end of a bed and then, after some minutes, with the head upright, clears the airway in most patients. When the airway is clear, inhaling steam, followed by applying radiant heat to the affected area, helps clear the ostia. If symptoms of systemic disturbance appear, the patient may need antibiotics, but the first requirement is to ensure that the sinuses are draining freely. If this cannot be accomplished by the simple measures outlined, the patient should be referred to an ear, nose, and throat surgeon. Clinicians often take sinusitis lightly, but it can be treacherous if it persists and can lead to collections of pus in the extradural or subdural spaces, to cerebral abscess, or to spread of infection through the bloodstream. If the ostium of the sinus is obstructed, a mucocele may develop in one frontal sinus and can slowly expand, eroding bone until it projects into the orbit, causing proptosis.

Nasopharyngeal carcinoma invades the cranial nerves more often than does any other malignant growth in the head and neck, because the nasopharynx is close to the foramina of the middle fossa (Figure 17.4). The condition is rare in communities of European origin but is common in China and South-East Asia. The trigeminal nerve or its branches are involved in about half the cases, so pain may be referred to the head. The sixth cranial nerve is also vulnerable and is destroyed in about 70% of patients. In addition the ninth, tenth, and eleventh cranial nerves may be invaded, causing hoarseness and dysphagia. Other symptoms include nasal obstruction, bloody nasal discharge, and enlargement of cervical lymph nodes. About 40% of patients present with headache.

Hippocrates warned that an association of headache with acute pain in the ear is to be dreaded, "for there is danger that the man may become delirious and die"

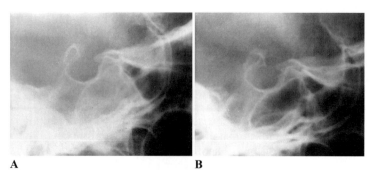

A   **B**

FIGURE 17.3   Sphenoidal sinusitis before *(A)* and after *(B)* treatment.

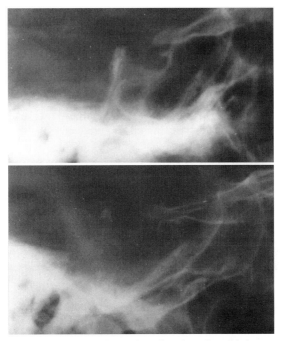

FIGURE 17.4 Nasopharyngeal carcinoma invading the sphenoid sinus and pituitary fossa. Six months separates the x-rays in upper and lower frames.

(Adams, 1948). Otitis media may cause apical petrositis, thrombosis of the lateral sinus, and otitic hydrocephalus (see Figure 15.6). Disease of the petrous temporal bone, whether infectious or neoplastic, can cause pain in the distribution of the first division of the trigeminal nerve and an ipsilateral sixth cranial-nerve palsy (Gradenigo's syndrome). Intracranial abscesses from middle ear disease are uncommon now but may appear in the temporal lobe or cerebellum and present with signs of raised intracranial pressure, focal neurologic disturbance, or meningeal irritation.

A rare clinical syndrome, retropharyngeal tendonitis, presents with severe pains in the back of the neck, aggravated by head movements and swallowing (Fahlgren, 1986). Patients may complain of swelling in the upper pharynx. Body temperature and erythrocyte sedimentation rate (ESR) are often elevated. Radiography demonstrates swollen prevertebral soft tissues and calcification at the level of the atlas and axis. Fahlgren reported 28 patients, but we have never encountered this syndrome.

TEETH

Dental caries or apical root infection can cause a neuralgic pain in the second or third divisions of the trigeminal nerve, with a constant aching component and superadded jabbing pains. The pain is made worse by hot or cold fluids in the mouth. Pains in the lower jaw are almost always of dental origin and warrant careful radiographs of the teeth, because a routine examination may miss apical root infections. Dental malocclusion may trigger pain resembling trigeminal neuralgia (Blair & Gordon, 1973). Heir (1987) summarizes dental causes of pain. Pains in the upper jaw are commonly of dental origin but can readily arise from maxillary sinusitis. The pain of lower-half headache (facial migraine) and cluster headache often includes the upper teeth and gums. Patients may experience atypical facial pain in the nasolabial fold overlying the upper gum (see Chapter 18).

Temporomandibular Joint Disease

A common way for dental disturbance to refer pain to the upper part of the head is through dysfunction of one temporomandibular joint (Cawson, 1986). If the bite is unbalanced by premature contact of one or more teeth or by loss of molar teeth on one side, or if the bite is fixed so that normal lateral or shearing movement of mastication is impossible, the patient adopts the most convenient chewing position, which commonly places an abnormal strain on one temporomandibular joint. This may lead to pain felt in front of or behind the ear on the appropriate side with radiation to the temple, over the face, and down the neck on that side, and is often associated with a blocked sensation in that ear (Costen's syndrome) (Costen, 1934). The condition is made worse if the patient now becomes a chronic "jaw clencher" if he or she was not one already, so that tension symptoms are set up in the temporal and other scalp muscles. Lateral pterygoid-muscle dysfunction and tenomyositis of the masseter muscles may contribute to or be responsible for preauricular pain (Friedman, Agus, & Weisberg, 1983). Ill-fitting dentures or any other source of discomfort in biting or chewing may evoke the same symptoms. In long-standing cases, crepitus may be heard or felt over the affected temporomandibular joint. The clinician can readily palpate the joint by inserting a finger into the external auditory canal and exerting pressure anteriorly on the joint. If this procedure replicates the patient's pain, it confirms the diagnosis. Computed tomography (CT) of the temporomandibular joints did not reveal any correlation between pathologic changes and pain (Tilds & Miller, 1987), but a magnetic resonance study has demonstrated effusion into the painful joint (Schellhas, Wilkes, & Baker, 1989).

The management depends on a dental surgeon carefully adjusting the bite, but advising the patient how to relax the temporal and masseter muscles and administering amitriptyline also help. We discuss the problem in more detail in Chapter 10.

Red Ear Syndrome

Some patients with temporomandibular joint dysfunction, glossopharyngeal neuralgia, or irritation of the third cervical root may suffer from episodic burning pain in one ear lobe, accompanied by obvious reddening of the affected ear (Lance, 1996). In susceptible subjects, the condition may also occur without any apparent structural cause in response to touch or heat.

Raieli et al. (2002) reported eight patients whose red ear episodes were associated with migraine headaches on occasions but recurred independently at other times. These authors postulated that the problem may be a trigeminoautonomic cephalgia mediated by the auriculotemporal nerve, but the ear lobe is innervated by the greater auricular nerve from the third cervical root. We could agree on the term "auriculoautonomic cephalgia." The flushing must be secondary to pain, because facial flushing by itself is not painful. Burning pain is characteristic of small afferent (C fiber) discharge. Whether the ear temperature increases by sympathetic vasodilator activity or antidromic discharge in C fibers releasing vasoactive peptides, described by Ochoa (1993) as the "ABC (Angry Back-firing C-nociceptor) syndrome," remains to be seen. Evans and Lance (in press) discuss the question further.

References

Adams, F. (1948). *The genuine works of Hippocrates* (p. 54). London: Sydenham Society.

Antonaci, F., Ghirmai, S., Bona G., Sandrini, G., & Nappi, G. (2001). Cervicogenic headache: Evaluation of the original diagnostic criteria. *Cephalalgia, 21,* 573–583.

Aprill, C., Axinn, M. J., & Bogduk, N. (2002). Occipital headaches stemming from the lateral atlanto-axial (C1–2) joint. *Cephalalgia, 22,* 15–22.

Bartschi-Rochaix, W. (1968). Headaches of cervical origin. In P. J. Vinken & G. W. Bruyn. (Eds.), *Handbook of neurology* (Vol. 5, pp. 192–203). Amsterdam: North Holland.

Blair, G. A. S., & Gordon, D. S. (1973). Trigeminal neuralgia and dental malocclusions. *BMJ, 4,* 38–40.

Blau, J. N. (1988). A note on migraine and the nose. *Headache, 28,* 495.

Bogduk, N. (1981a). The anatomy of occipital neurolgia. *Clin Exp Neurol, 17,* 167–184.

Bogduk, N. (1981b). Local anaesthetic blocks of the second cervical ganglion: A technique with application in occipital headache. *Cephalalgia, 1,* 41–50.

Bogduk, N., Corrigan, B., Kelly, P., Schneider, G., & Farr, R. (1985). Cervical headache. *Med J Aust, 143,* 202, 206–207.

Bogduk, N., Lambert, G. A., & Duckworth, J. W. (1981). The anatomy and physiology of the vertebral nerve in relation to cervical migraine. *Cephalalgia, 1,* 11–24.

Bogduk, N., & Marsland, A. (1986). On the concept of third occipital headache. *J Neurol Neurosurg Psychiatry, 49,* 775–780.

Cawson, R. A. (1986). Temporomandibular cephalalgia. In F. Clifford Rose (Ed.), *Handbook of clinical neurology* (Vol. 4[48], pp. 413–416). Amsterdam: Elsevier.

Classification Subcommittee of the International Headache Society. (2004). The International Classification of Headache Disorders, 2nd ed. *Cephalalgia, 24*(Suppl. 1), 114–120.

Close, L. G., & Aviv, J. (1997). Headaches and disease of the nose and paranasal sinuses. *Semin Neurol, 17,* 351–4.

Costen, J. B. (1934). A syndrome of ear and sinus symptoms dependent upon disturbed function of the temporomandibular joint. *Ann Otol Rhinol Laryngol, 43,* 1–15.

Daroff, R. B. (1998). Ocular causes of headache. *Headache, 38,* 661.

Dory, M. A. (1983). Arthrography of the cervical facet joints. *Radiology, 148,* 379–382.

Evans, R. W., & Lance, J. W. (in press). The red ear syndrome: An auriculo-autonomic cephalgia. *Headache, 44.*

Fahlgren, H. (1986). Retropharyngeal tendinitis. *Cephalalgia, 6,* 169–174.

Fredrikson, T. A., Hovdal, H., & Sjaastad, O. (1987). "Cervicogenic headache": Clinical manifestations. *Cephalalgia, 7,* 147–160.

Friedman, M. H., Agus, B., & Weisberg, J. (1983). Neglected conditions producing preauricular and referred pain. *J Neurol Neurosurg Psychiatry, 46,* 1067–1072.

Göbel, H., & Edmeads, J. G. (2000). Disorders of the skull and cervical spine. In J. Olesen, P. Tfelt-Hansen, & K. M. A. Welch (Eds.), *The headaches* (2nd ed., pp. 891–898). Philadelphia: Lippincott, Williams & Wilkins.

Heir, G. M. (1987). Facial pain of dental origin—a review for physicians. *Headache, 27,* 540–547.

Hilton, J. (1950). *Rest and pain* (p. 77). E. W. Walls & E. E. Philipp (Eds.). London: Bell.

Lance, J. W. (1996). The red ear syndrome. *Neurology, 47,* 617–620.

Lyle, T. K. (1968). Ophthalmological headaches. In P. J. Vinken & G. W. Bruyn (Eds.), *Handbook of clinical neurology* (Vol. 5, pp. 204–207). Amsterdam: North Holland.

Ochoa, J. L. (1993). The human sensory unit and pain: New concepts, syndromes and tests. *Muscle Nerve, 16,* 1009–1016.

Pareja, J. A., Caminero, A. B., Serra, J., Barriga, F. J., Baron, M., Dabato, J. L., et al. (2002). Nummular headache: A coin-shaped cephalgia. *Neurology, 548,* 1678–1679.

Parker, G. B., Tupling, H., & Pryor, D. S. (1978). A controlled trial of cervical manipulation for migraine. *Aust N Z J Med, 89,* 589–593.

Raieli, V., Monastero, R., Santangelo, G., Eliseo, G. L., Eliseo, M., & Camarda, R. (2002). Red ear syndrome and migraine: Report of eight cases. *Headache, 42,* 147–151.

Ryan, E. R., Jr., & Kern, E. B. (1978). Rhinological causes of facial pain and headache. *Headache, 18,* 44–50.

Schellhas, K. P., Wilkes, C. H., & Baker, C. C. (1989). Facial pain, headache, and temporomandibular joint inflammation. *Headache, 29,* 228–231.

Sjaastad, O., Fredriksen, T. A., & Pfaffenrath, V. (1990). Cervicogenic headache: Diagnostic criteria. *Headache, 30,* 725–726.

Sjaastad, O., Fredriksen, T. A., & Pfaffenrath, V. (1998). Cervicogenic headache: Diagnostic criteria. *Headache, 38,* 442–445.

Spierings, E. L. H., Foo, D. K., & Young, R. R. (1992). Headaches in patients with traumatic lesions of the cervical spinal cord. *Headache, 32,* 45–49.

Tilds, B. N., & Miller, P. R. (1987). Radiographic pathology of the temporomandibular joints, and head pain. *Headache, 27,* 427–430.

Waters, W. E. (1970). Headache and the eye. A community study. *Lancet, ii,* 1–4.

Chapter 18
Cranial Neuralgias and Central Causes of Facial Pain

Pain in the head is mediated by afferent fibers in the trigeminal nerve, nervus intermedius, glossopharyngeal and vagus nerves, and the upper cervical roots via the occipital nerves. Impulses giving rise to the sensation of pain may be generated by compression or distortion of these nerves, exposure to excessive heat or cold, or other sources of irritation. Lesions of the central connections of sensory fibers can also cause pain referred to the distribution of the appropriate nerves.

Neural pain is neuralgia that may be constant or intermittent and aching or stabbing in quality. Sometimes its origin can be determined from the case history, physical signs, or imaging, but in other cases no cause may be apparent.

Clinicians encounter some difficulty in classifying trigeminal or glossopharyngeal neuralgia as primary or secondary, because many, perhaps most, patients have an aberrant blood vessel impinging on the nerve and presumably causing their symptoms. For this reason The Classification Subcommittee of The International Headache Society (2004) prefers the term *classical* for patients in whom imaging has not shown a neuroma or similar identifiable cause. If a patient has such a lesion, the Subcommittee classifies the neuralgia as symptomatic.

TRIGEMINAL NEURALGIA

The lifetime prevalence of trigeminal neuralgia has been calculated as 700 per million of the population (Macdonald et al., 2000). It affects women more than men, in a ratio of 1.6:1. Its alternative name, *tic douloureux,* should be pronounced in the French manner, because Anglicization to "tic doloroo" pains the Francophone scarcely less than the condition itself. The disorder usually begins after age 40, with a mean varying from 50 to 58 years of age in different reported series. Familial occurrence is rare.

Clinical Features

The pain is strictly limited to some part of the distribution of the trigeminal nerve, involving the right side more than the left, in the ratio 3:2. It usually starts in the second or third divisions, affecting the cheek or chin. Less than 5% start in the first division. All three divisions have been involved in 10% to 15% of reported cases, and the pain has become bilateral in 3% to 5%.

The pain is sudden, intense, and stabbing in quality, lasting only momentarily but often recurring in repeated paroxysms. A dull background pain sometimes persists. The patient can always identify trigger factors such as talking, chewing, swallowing, or touching the face or gums as in shaving or cleaning the teeth. The pain may also have many trigger points, areas around the nose or lips that are particularly liable to evoke a paroxysm if touched, the pain commonly being in the same division as the trigger point. In some cases the pain may be precipitated by sensory stimuli outside the trigeminal area or even by other modalities such as bright lights or noise. The pain may recur daily for weeks or months and then remit for a period of time, even for years, before returning. This periodicity sometimes leads to confusion between trigeminal neuralgia and cluster headache. Indeed, some authors have reported (rare) associations of the two conditions, but the characteristic lancinating pain of trigeminal neuralgia bears little resemblance to the sustained pain of cluster headache, which lasts for 10 minutes or more each time. Clinicians have not yet fully defined the overlap with the SUNCT syndrome (see Chapter 12). Trigeminal neuralgia may occasionally occur with glossopharyngeal neuralgia, so that pain is referred to the ear and throat as well as to the area of trigeminal distribution. Trigeminal neuralgia tends to become progressively worse in frequency and severity of episodes.

Classical trigeminal neuralgia usually does not produce a clinically detectable sensory loss. Thus, if sensation is impaired, the clinician must consider other conditions, such as neuroma or multiple sclerosis. In this case the condition is termed *symptomatic* or *secondary trigeminal neuralgia.*

After repeated jabs of neuralgia, facial flushing sometimes occurs, probably caused by release of vasodilator peptides. Drummond, Gonski, and Lance (1983) found face flushing in the cutaneous distribution area of the appropriate division after the Gasserian ganglion was thermocoagulated to relieve trigeminal neuralgia (Figure 18.1), while the levels of calcitonin gene–related peptide (CGRP) and substance P rose in external jugular venous blood (Goadsby, Edvinsson, & Ekman, 1988). The distribution of flushing is similar to that during cluster headache (see Figure 12.1).

Fromm et al. (1990) have described prodromal symptoms of pain resembling sinusitis or toothache that may precede by some days the onset of typical trigeminal neuralgia. Such pains may last for several hours and be triggered by jaw movements or by hot or cold fluids; the resulting confusion of symptoms may lead to unnecessary dental procedures.

Etiology

The most common cause of trigeminal neuralgia is probably an aberrant vessel compressing the trigeminal root where it enters the pons. In the past, clinicians have proposed compression of the divisions, mainly second and third, by the internal carotid artery and the possibility of degenerative changes or herpes simplex infection of the Gasserian ganglion as causes, but these theories have little to support them.

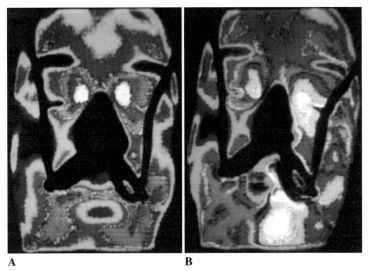

A   **B**

FIGURE 18.1 *A* and *B*, Thermogram taken before and after coagulation of the trigeminal ganglion. The white area *(B)* shows that the eye, nostril, cheek, and chin are warmer on the operated side. Note the similarity with cluster headache in the distribution of the facial flush (see Figure 12.1). The dark lines converging on the patient's nose are oxygen tubes.

Dandy (1934) recorded his personal observations in 215 operated cases. He found a gross lesion distorting the trigeminal nerve in 60% of patients, the most common being the impingement on the nerve of a hardened superior cerebellar artery (66 cases) or a branch of the petrosal vein (30 cases). Other causes included acoustic neuromas, cholesteatomas, an osteoma, basilar artery aneurysms, angiomas, and adhesion of the sensory root to the brainstem.

Jannetta (1976) refined the posterior fossa approach to the trigeminal nerve, using microsurgical techniques, and concluded that *all* tic douloureux is "symptomatic tic douloureux." The trigeminal root entry zone was compressed or distorted by a branch of the anterior inferior cerebellar artery in the 4% of patients in whom the first division was primarily affected, whereas the superior cerebellar artery was responsible when the second and third divisions were affected. In 100 consecutive patients with trigeminal neuralgia, Jannetta found tumors in 6%, plaques of multiple sclerosis in 4%, atrophic areas of nerve in 2%, and vascular compression of the trigeminal nerve in the remaining 88%. Richards, Shawdon, and Illingworth (1983) explored the posterior fossa in 52 patients. Arterial loops compressed the trigeminal root in 37 (71%), and clinically unsuspected tumors did so in 3 cases. Progressive elongation and tortuosity of arterial loops seems to account for the condition becoming more common with advancing age. Haines, Jannetta, and Zorub (1980) examined the trigeminal nerves in 20 cadavers of patients known to have been free of trigeminal neuralgia. Of the 40 nerves, 11 were in contact with an artery, but it distorted only 4.

Veins compressed an additional four nerves. In contrast, of 40 trigeminal nerves surgeons exposed in treating trigeminal neuralgia, adjacent arteries compressed 31, and veins compressed 8. The painful jabs of pain probably result from demyelination of the trigeminal root, which favors the theory that the pain stems from generation of spontaneous afferent volleys (Love & Coakham, 2001).

Neurophysiology

Stohr, Petruch, and Scheglmann (1981) obtained somatosensory evoked potentials by stimulating the lipsin 17 patients with unoperated trigeminal neuralgia. The latency of the response was delayed about 2 msec on the affected side in 7 patients, confirming compression of the trigeminal nerve or ganglion on that side. A comparison of responses evoked from the lower lip in 10 patients treated by retro-Gasserian glycerol injection, with 20 normal controls, showed diminished amplitude and prolonged latency of responses on the operated side (Dalessio et al., 1990). Trigeminal evoked potentials can therefore serve either as an indication for posterior fossa operation or as a check on the success of any destructive procedure.

Experimental demyelination of the trigeminal root in cats and monkeys follows about 3 weeks after inserting sutures through the root, and at this time the nerve is hyperexcitable (Burchiel, 1980). A single stimulus evoked multiple discharges, and afferent volleys evoked an after-discharge. Action potentials were generated at the site of the lesion and were enhanced by hyperventilation and suppressed by diphenylhydantoin. In the peripheral or central trigeminal pathways of humans, vascular or other compression or primary demyelination, as in multiple sclerosis, could cause such lesions. Thus, using anticonvulsants to damp down neural hyperexcitability has logical application for controlling trigeminal neuralgia in humans.

Treatment

Clinicians once used diphenylhydantoin in medically managing trigeminal neuralgia, but now commonly use carbamazepine 200 mg, the dose being increased slowly from half a tablet to up to two tablets three times daily or the equivalent in slow-release form, to reach a blood level that will control the pain without inducing giddiness and ataxia. Carbamazepine nearly always causes some degree of leukopenia. For this reason, a blood count should be obtained on patients who develop any infection. The blood may be checked every 3 months as a routine, but it is doubtful whether regular blood counts really fulfill any useful function, because clinically significant leukopenia is rare and may appear quite suddenly. Tomson et al. (1980) found the optimum blood level for control of pain to lie between 24 and 43 μmol/liter (5.7 to 10.1 μg/mL). It is best to administer carbamazepine in divided doses three times daily, because trigeminal neuralgia tends to recur 6 to 9 hours after each dose, or in the controlled-release form 400 mg twice daily.

The second choice of medication for those patients not responding to carbamazepine is baclofen. Baclofen proved superior to placebo in a crossover trial

(Fromm, Terrence, & Chattha, 1984) and relieved 74% of patients in an open trial with a dosage of 40 to 80 mg daily. Of 50 patients, 37 were free of pain after 2 weeks. Six patients were unable to tolerate baclofen because of drowsiness and nausea. Eighteen patients remained controlled on baclofen for a mean duration of 3 years, although twelve of these required the addition of carbamazepine or phenytoin.

Clonazepam 0.5 to 2.0 mg three times daily is also effective in suppressing trigeminal neuralgia, but drowsiness and mood changes limit its use. Intravenous infusion of lignocaine (lidocaine) can temporarily control the painful paroxysms of trigeminal neuralgia, but mexiletine, a lidocaine derivative taken orally in doses of 10 mg/kg body weight daily, has not proved beneficial (Pascual & Berciano, 1989).

If the condition persists despite medical treatment, a surgical approach becomes necessary. Surgeons devised operations to decompress the Gasserian ganglion or sensory root, giving temporary relief, or to compress these structures, for more lasting relief, but injecting alcohol or glycerol became preferred. More recently, balloon compression or controlled thermocoagulation of the Gasserian ganglion has relieved pain with less impairment. The technique offers hope of sparing the corneal reflex and thus preventing ocular complications and is effective in 90% of cases, but 17% still have troublesome dysesthesias, and 3% have "anesthesia dolorosa" (Illingworth, 1986). A follow-up of 1200 patients claimed that 99% of patients achieved immediate relief, with a recurrence rate of 20% in 7 to 9 years (Taha & Tew, 1997). Postoperative dysesthesia varied from 7% of patients with mild hypalgesia to 36% of patients with analgesia.

Jannetta (1976) advocated posterior fossa exploration, using a binocular microscope to examine the nerve at the point of entry into the pons. Dissecting any compressing artery or vein away from the trigeminal root and placing a small piece of polyvinyl chloride sponge between the nerve and the offending vessel suddenly or gradually abated pain in all but four of Jannetta's patients followed for periods of up to 94 months. A report from this team on 1155 patients followed for a median of 6.2 years found that 30% had recurrences of tic, some requiring reoperation (Barker et al., 1996). McLaughlin et al. (1999) presented a review of 4415 operations performed over 29 years. Complications were few, with cerebellar and hearing loss each less than 1% and declining with improving techniques. This procedure is usually the treatment of choice in younger patients, because it spares facial sensation, but thermocoagulation of the Gasserian ganglion (radiofrequency trigeminal rhizotomy or gangliolysis) or glycerol injection around the ganglion are less invasive (Illingworth, 1986) for the older patient who is not responding to medication.

More recently still, researchers have advocated fine-beam radiotherapy (gamma knife radiosurgery) for relieving trigeminal neuralgia (Young et al., 1997). Of 51 patients treated, 38 became free of pain and 7 substantially improved. Eight of another nine patients in whom the pain stemmed from a tumor also found relief. Brisman (2000) reported the best results when radiosurgery was the first option, but 33 of 42 patients still had relief at 12 months follow-up, even when previous surgical procedures had failed.

GLOSSOPHARYNGEAL NEURALGIA

Glossopharyngeal neuralgia, which is about 100 times less common than trigeminal neuralgia, causes a similar type of lancinating pain in the ear, base of the tongue, tonsillar fossa, or beneath the angle of the jaw. The distribution is not only in the sensory area of the glossopharyngeal nerve but also in those of the auricular and pharyngeal branches of the vagus nerve. Swallowing, talking, or coughing provoke it. Of 217 cases Rushton, Stevens, and Miller (1981) reported, 25 also had trigeminal neuralgia. Pain may predominate in the pharynx or in the ear, presenting as pharyngeal or otalgic forms of neuralgia (Bruyn, 1986b). Glossopharyngeal neuralgia may follow compression of the nerve by neoplasms, infections, or blood vessels. Minagar and Sheremata (2000) have also reported it as a symptom of multiple sclerosis. Cardiovascular disturbances such as bradycardia, hypotension, and even transient asystole have been reported to accompany glossopharyngeal neuralgia on occasions (Bruyn, 1986b). The ear on the affected side occasionally becomes red and painful (Lance, 1996).

If the pain does not respond to carbamazepine, phenytoin, or baclofen, microvascular decompression or intracranial section of the glossopharyngeal nerve and the upper two rootlets of the vagus nerve is usually necessary.

NERVUS INTERMEDIUS NEURALGIA

The nervus intermedius, part of the facial nerve, mediates sensation from the external auditory canal and part of the external ear. A patient with geniculate herpes may experience pain in the associated area of distribution (Ramsay-Hunt syndrome). It remains doubtful as to whether stabbing pains in the ear ever stem from the nervus intermedius or whether they represent the otalgic variation of glossopharyngeal neuralgia (Bruyn, 1986c).

SUPERIOR LARYNGEAL NEURALGIA

The superior laryngeal is a terminal branch of the vagus nerve. It can give rise to a rare disorder characterized by severe pain in the lateral aspect of the throat, submandibular region, and under the ear, brought on by swallowing, shouting, or turning the head. The pain may be constant or lancinating, triggered by pressure on the side of the throat. It may occasionally follow respiratory infections, tonsillectomy, or carotid endarterectomy (Bruyn, 1986e). Local anesthetic block of the superior laryngeal nerve confirms the diagnosis, and neurectomy relieves the condition.

NEURALGIAS OF TERMINAL BRANCHES OF THE TRIGEMINAL NERVE

Figure 18.2 shows terminal branches of the trigeminal nerve.

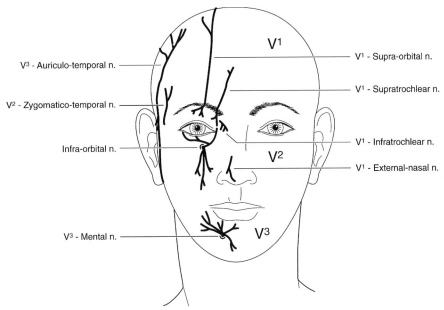

FIGURE 18.2   Terminal branches of the trigeminal nerve.

Supraorbital Neuralgia

In supraorbital neuralgia, the patient feels a constant or jabbing pain in the inner canthus of the eye and forehead, in the distribution of the first division of the trigeminal nerve (Sjaastad et al., 1999). The nerve is characteristically tender to touch in the supraorbital notch, and local anesthetic blockade and subsequent ablation of the nerve by a radiofrequency probe or surgical section relieves the pain. Pain was accompanied by diminished sensitivity to touch or pin prick in a frontal strip above the eyebrow in 4 of the 18 patients reported by Caminero and Pareja (2001).

Nasociliary Neuralgia

Nasociliary neuralgia is a rare condition that may arise from a blow to the face or may occur spontaneously. Touching the outer surface of the nose provokes a stabbing pain that radiates upward to the midfrontal region. Applying local anesthetic to the nerve or into the nostril on the affected side stops the pain (Bruyn, 1986a).

Other Terminal Branch Neuralgias

Injury or entrapment of other peripheral branches of the trigeminal nerve may cause constant or lancinating pain in the areas that nerve innervates. Examples are neuralgias of the infraorbital, lingual, alveolar, and mental nerves (De Vries & Smelt, 1990).

Nummular Headache

Pareja et al. (2002) described a distinctive localized pain, the shape of a coin 2 to 6 cm in diameter, felt in the scalp as a continuous sensation that sometimes develops into a severe or stabbing pain. Research has not established the underlying cause, but nummular headache is presumably a neuralgia of a terminal twig of a trigeminal nerve branch. The condition is benign and may remit. The term *nummular* means "coin-shaped."

OCCIPITAL NEURALGIA

In occipital neuralgia the patient characteristically feels an aching or paroxysmal jabbing pain in the distribution area of the greater or lesser occipital nerves, and usually with diminished sensation or dysesthesias in the affected area (Hammond & Danta, 1978). The patient may also feel tenderness over the point where the nerve crosses midway between the mastoid process and the occipital protuberance, whereas the lesser occipital nerve crosses it about 4 cm behind the ear (Figure 18.3).

If the occipital pain is continuous and there is no impairment of sensation, it may be a referred pain from the atlantoaxial or C2–C3 facet joints, from the posterior

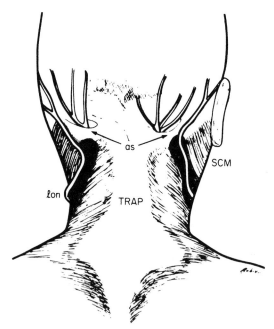

FIGURE 18.3   Occipital nerves. The greater occipital nerve emerges from an aponeurotic sling (as), and the lesser occipital nerve (lon) lies lateral to it. Muscles labeled are trapezius (TRAP) and sternocleidomastoid (SCM). (From Bogduk, N. [1981b]. The anatomy of occipital neuralgia. *Clin Exper Neurol, 17*, 167–184, by permission of Adis Press, Sydney.)

fossa, or even from the first division of the trigeminal nerve, the descending spinal tract of which converges with the C2–C3 afferent fibers on second-order neurons in the upper three segments of the spinal cord. The distinction can often be made by assessing the response to infiltration of the tender area by a local anesthetic agent or blockade of the second cervical ganglion (Bogduk, 1981c). Proceed with caution, because inadvertently injecting local anesthetic into the cerebrospinal fluid via an underlying long-nerve root sleeve may lead to respiratory arrest.

This condition overlaps with the upper cervical and third occipital nerve syndromes described in Chapter 17.

The patients with occipital neuralgic pain whom Hammond and Danta (1978) reported illustrate the difficulty in differential diagnosis. Of these patients, nine had migrainous features, two suffered from rheumatoid arthritis, and three had cervical spondylosis. Of the remainder, four had a history of direct trauma to the occipital region and eight of whiplash or other injury to the cervical spine.

Carbamazepine may relieve the pain if it is paroxysmal in nature. Transcutaneous nerve stimulation provides short-term relief, and immobilization in a collar may ease the pain partially or completely. Neurectomy of the appropriate nerve may stop the pain completely, but pain may later recur with neuroma formation. Bogduk (1985) prefers nerve and facet joint blocks to detect the precise origin of occipital pain, with a goal of then treating with intra-articular injection of steroids or selective thermocoagulation of the appropriate nerve.

NECK–TONGUE SYNDROME

Lance and Anthony (1980) described an unusual syndrome affecting mainly children and young adults on sudden rotation of the neck. The patient experiences a sharp pain in the upper neck or occiput, which may be accompanied by numbness or tingling in these areas. At the same time, the ipsilateral half of the tongue becomes numb or feels as though it were twisting in the mouth. The explanation is that proprioceptive fibers from the tongue travel via links from the lingual nerve to the hypoglossal nerve and then to the second cervical root (Figure 18.4). Bogduk (1981a) has pointed out that during rotation of the neck the C2 central ramus is drawn over the atlantoaxial joint, which it innervates. Transient subluxation of the atlantoaxial joint produces local pain by stretching the joint capsule and numbness of the tongue by stretching the C2 ventral ramus, which contains proprioceptive fibers from the tongue.

Other cases have been described in normal subjects and in patients with degenerative spondylosis, ankylosing spondylitis, and psoriatic arthritis. Bertoft and Westerberg (1985) reported that five of their seven nonrheumatic cases had a similarly affected parent or sibling, suggesting a genetically determined laxity of ligaments or joint capsules.

Cervical manipulation has improved some patients. In one patient with upper cervical disease, fusion at the C2–C3 level abolished symptoms (Bertoft & Westerbeg, 1985), and sectioning the second cervical spinal nerve reduced the more extensive symptoms of another patient (Elisevich et al., 1984). Our own patients have not been sufficiently incapacitated by their symptoms to warrant any intervention.

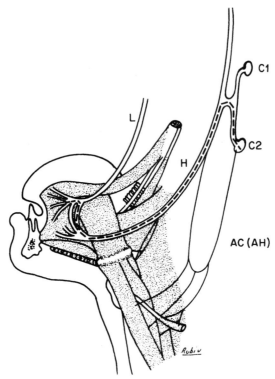

FIGURE 18.4   The anatomic basis for the neck–tongue syndrome. Proprioceptive fibers from the tongue (dashed line) travel from the lingual nerve (L) to the hypoglossal nerve (H) and then to the second cervical root (C2). AC (AH), Ansa cervicalis (ansa hypoglossi). (From Lance & Anthony, 1980, by permission of the editor of the *J Neurol, Neurosurg Psychiatry*).

EXTERNAL COMPRESSION

Wearing a tight hat, a band around the head, a protective construction hard hat, or tight swimming goggles (Pestronk & Pestronk, 1983) may induce headache by external compression.

EXPOSURE TO COLD

Exposing the bare head to subzero temperatures or diving into cold water can cause headache, presumably from excessive stimulation of temperature-sensitive receptors in the face and scalp. Pain induced by dipping the top of the head into cold water (<18°C) reaches a peak in 60 seconds and spreads from the vertex to temples and occiput (Wolf & Hardy, 1941). The only areas of the body from which these authors could not provoke pain by exposure to cold were the ear lobes and the glans penis.

Ice-Cream Headache

Drake (1850) commented on the possible injurious effects of eating ice cream: "first, swallowing it before the ice has dissolved in the mouth, when it sometimes raises an acute pain in the pharynx, and gives a sense of coldness and sinking in the stomach; second, eating it when the stomach is torpid and inactive from dyspepsia, and the individual is inclined, at the time, to sick headache."

Holding ice or ice cream in the mouth, or swallowing a cold food or drink as a bolus, may cause discomfort in the palate and throat. It may also refer pain to the forehead or temple via the trigeminal nerve and to the ears via the glossopharyngeal nerve. Raskin and Knittle (1976) found that 15 of 49 subjects not normally prone to headache had experienced infrequent mild ice-cream headaches at some time of their lives. In contrast, 55 of 59 migraine patients were subject to such headaches, which were frequent and severe in 46. Most patients felt the pain in the midfrontal region, but eight reported pain in the temporal and maxillary regions and two in the occiput.

Drummond and Lance (1984) reported that 189 (36.7%) of 530 patients attending a headache clinic had experienced ice-cream headache. The prevalence of such headaches increased in direct proportion to the number of migrainous symptoms associated with the patient's customary headache (Figure 18.5).

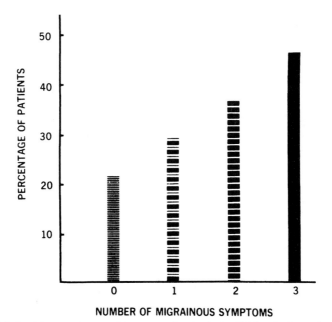

FIGURE 18.5   The prevalence of ice-cream headache in 530 headache patients grouped according to the number of migraine characteristics (unilateral headache, focal neurologic symptoms, and gastrointestinal disturbance) experienced by each. The prevalence increases progressively from 20% in tension-type headache (no migraine symptoms) to almost 50% in typical migraine headache (all three groups of migraine symptoms). (From Drummond & Lance, 1984, by permission of the publishers, Adis Press, Sydney.)

Although the headache was usually midline or bilateral, the pain affected only one side of the head for 18 of the 90 patients for whom the site had been documented. In 13 of these 18, and in 17 of the 72 patients with bilateral headache, the site of ice-cream headache coincided with the area their other headaches habitually affected. Fuh et al. (2003) reported that 40.6% of 8359 adolescents in Taiwan were prone to ice-cream headache, more common in migrainous subjects. Of 1084 students who were also subject to other headaches, 53.2% described the same location for both.

Wolff (1963) found that applying ice to the palate referred pain to the frontal region, and cooling in the posterior pharynx caused pain behind the ears.

That ice-cream headache is more common in migraine patients and often affects the part of the head afflicted by the customary headache suggests migraine patients may have a segmental disinhibition of central pain pathways that causes undue susceptibility to an afferent volley of impulses from excitation of cold receptors in the oropharynx.

STRUCTURAL LESIONS COMPRESSING, IRRITATING, OR DISTORTING CRANIAL NERVES OR UPPER CERVICAL ROOTS

The first division of the trigeminal nerve may be compressed in the orbit, in the superior orbital fissure, in the cavernous sinus, or near the apex of the petrous temporal bone. Tumors such as a meningioma growing from the sphenoid wing or a pituitary tumor may refer pain to the forehead, accompanying diminished sensibility over the area supplied by the first division of the trigeminal nerve. The sudden onset of severe pain behind and above one eye may indicate enlargement of an aneurysm of the internal carotid or posterior communicating artery. Meningioma may also compress the Gasserian ganglion. A neuroma may arise from the fifth nerve. Trigeminal nerve compression is often painless. When pain is present, it may be constant or stabbing in quality, often accompanying sensory impairment in the appropriate distribution area.

Involvement of the nervus intermedius refers pain to the external auditory canal; involvement of the glossopharyngeal nerve refers pain to the base of the tongue and tonsillar fossa; and involvement of the vagus nerve refers pain to a region in or behind the ear.

Raeder's Paratrigeminal Neuralgia

The term *Raeder's syndrome* is applied to pain of trigeminal distribution, usually the ophthalmic division, in association with an ocular (postganglionic) sympathetic deficit comprising ptosis, miosis, and impairment of sweating over the medial aspect of the forehead but not elsewhere on the face. Because this combination may have many different causes, the syndrome simply serves to draw attention to the region of the carotid siphon as the site of disturbance, but the nature of the disturbance must be determined by the history and special investigations.

Two of the five patients Raeder described in 1924 did not have pain as a presenting symptom. One had a parasellar tumor, two cases resulted from trauma, and in two cases the cause was unknown (Mokri, 1982). Mokri (1982) and

Sjaastad et al. (1994) have since then summarized the many descriptions in the literature. They fall into two groups: those with episodic pain that we now recognize as cluster headache and those with aneurysms, neoplasms, inflammation, or trauma involving the internal carotid artery and impinging on the first division of the trigeminal nerve. Sjaastad et al. (1994) distinguish the features of Raeder's syndrome from the supraorbital fissure syndrome of Tolosa-Hunt and the posterior cavernous sinus syndrome of Gradenigo. The concept of Raeder's syndrome has some localizing value but no more than that.

Gradenigo's Syndrome

Lesions of the apex of the petrous temporal bone cause pain referred to the frontotemporal region and ear in conjunction with a paralysis of the sixth cranial nerve, which runs across the bone at that point. Gradenigo's syndrome was originally described as a complication of middle ear infection but may also appear with tumors arising from or invading this area.

OPTIC NEURITIS

Pain in or behind the eye usually precedes impairment of vision by some hours or days in optic (retrobulbar) neuritis. The eyeball is usually tender to pressure and aches on eye movement. The characteristic visual field defect is a central scotoma. The optic fundi are usually normal on examination, but if demyelination involves the nerve head, the optic disc swells (papillitis).

In a prospective survey of patients followed for 5 years, 10% of patients with a normal brain magnetic resonance imaging (MRI) scan had developed clinically definite multiple sclerosis, whereas 51% of those with three or more lesions visible on their MRI scan had signs of multiple sclerosis (Optic Neuritis Study Group, 1997). The pain and visual disturbance of optic neuritis usually responds rapidly to corticosteroids.

OCULAR DIABETIC NEUROPATHY

In diabetes mellitus, one or more of the ocular motor cranial nerves may become paralyzed, accompanied or preceded by pain in or around the affected eye. Pain may precede diplopia by up to 7 days. The third cranial nerve is most commonly involved, often with sparing of pupillary function, but the fourth and sixth cranial nerves are also susceptible.

POSTHERPETIC NEURALGIA

Herpes zoster is caused by reactivation of the varicella-zoster virus, which researchers think lies dormant in the trigeminal, geniculate, and dorsal root ganglia after chickenpox infection in early life. The incidence of postherpetic neuralgia is about 10% when all age groups are considered but increases with age, reaching 50% by 60 years. The distribution of the rash and subsequent pain follows trigeminal distribution in about 23% of cases (Watson, 1990), mostly affecting the ophthalmic division. The rash may also involve the external auditory meatus, the soft palate, or the area supplied by the upper cervical roots. Paralysis of the third, fourth, or sixth cranial nerves or a facial palsy may accompany the herpetic eruption. The combination of a herpetic rash in the external auditory canal and a facial palsy, which results from invasion of the geniculate ganglion, is known as Ramsay-Hunt syndrome. An unpleasant burning pain often precedes the skin eruption by 2 to 4 days. Pain in the distribution area of the first division of the trigeminal nerve may cause diagnostic difficulties when it appears several days before the rash or, on rare occasions, without any rash at all.

Postherpetic neuralgia has been defined as pain persisting 3 months or more after onset of the rash. The pain is characteristically burning, with occasional stabbing pains, and the lightest touch over the affected area may be felt as painful (allodynia). Nurmikko and Bowsher (1990) found lowered sensory threshold for warmth, cold, tough, pin prick, and vibration over the affected areas in patients whose rash was followed by neuralgic pain but not in those who escaped postherpetic neuralgia. Allodynia was present in 87% of the patients with postherpetic neuralgia and extended to the maxillary division in half the patients after ophthalmic herpes. All modalities of sensation were affected, contradicting the view that neuralgic pain depends on the selective destruction of large afferent fibers.

In reviewing the gate-control theory of pain, Nathan (1976) summarized the conflicting views in various reports of the pathologic changes herpes zoster causes, concluding that selective destruction of a certain range of nerve fibers cannot explain the condition. Fibrous tissue involves skin and nerves, with the degeneration of large fibers being followed by destruction of smaller fibers. The pain presumably arises from a disturbed pattern of afferent impulses and removal of some central inhibitory influence, because pain usually persists after section of the trigeminal nerve or medullary tractotomy. The descending (spinal) tract of the trigeminal nerve is the direct rostral continuation of the tract of Lissauer in the spinal cord. Like the tract of Lissauer, the ventrolateral portion of the descending trigeminal tract acts to suppress sensory transmission in its neighboring segments, and the dorsomedial portion facilitates transmission (Denny-Brown &Yanagisawa, 1973). Fibers from the ophthalmic division of the trigeminal nerve lie in the ventrolateral segment, so perhaps the virus of herpes zoster selectively damages this inhibitory area, permitting unrestrained outflow of afferent impulses producing postherpetic neuralgia.

Whether administering corticosteroids or acyclovir at the onset of herpes zoster can prevent postherpetic neuralgia remains controversial (Portenoy, Duma, & Foley, 1986; Watson, 1990; Editorial, 1990). The usual practice is to prescribe a course of steroids at the onset in any patient who is not immunosuppressed. Watson (1990) recommends prednisone 60 mg daily with gradual reduction in dosage over 2 weeks. When the rash is extensive or ophthalmic herpes threatens sight, acyclovir should be prescribed instead. Some reports indicate that 800 mg five times daily for 7 to 10 days reduces the incidence of postherpetic neuralgia (Editorial, 1990). Whereas some publications claim steroids alone or acyclovir alone help prevent postherpetic neuralgia, administering both agents together clearly does not confer any additional advantage (Esmann et al., 1987). Time and further trials may reveal the best method of preventing this unpleasant condition.

Once postherpetic neuralgia has established itself, what then? Blockade of peripheral nerves, roots, or the sympathetic nervous system and various surgical procedures are of no proven benefit (Portenoy et al., 1986). Amitriptyline has proved useful in managing persistent pain since its effectiveness was demonstrated for chronic tension headache (Lance & Curran, 1964). Watson et al. (1982) demonstrated its benefit in postherpetic neuralgia in a double-blind crossover study in which 16 of 24 patients obtained relief by a (median) dose of 75 mg daily. The tablets are best taken at night, to minimize daytime drowsiness, and the dosage should be increased gradually. For patients unable to tolerate amitriptyline, imipramine can be useful. Carbamazepine helps control the stabbing component of postherpetic pains but not the constant burning pain. We have recently found gabapentin useful in some patients.

Topical application of a cream containing capsaicin (usually starting with 0.025%) has been successful in open trials but not in one double-blind trial (Editorial, 1990). The theoretical basis for its use is that it discharges substance P from nerve terminals, desensitizing them.

Shanbrom (1961) reported that an intravenous drip of 500 mg of 0.1 to 0.2% procaine, repeated up to 10 times if necessary, relieved 13 of 16 patients. We have used a lignocaine (lidocaine) drip, 1 g of lignocaine being added to 500 mL of 5% glucose in N/5 saline and administered at the rate of 2 mg/minute (1 mL/minute). This drip may be repeated daily for 3 days or more. Diminution of postherpetic pain often outlasts the duration of the infusion and is sometimes permanent.

Bates and Nathan (1980) used transcutaneous electrical nerve stimulation in 74 patients with postherpetic neuralgia resistant to other forms of therapy, placing the electrodes above and below the scarred area. One third of the patients derived continuing benefit for 1 year, and one quarter for 2 years or more.

TOLOSA-HUNT SYNDROME

Involvement of the superior orbital fissure by granuloma causes recurrent painful ophthalmoplegia (Tolosa-Hunt syndrome) that may be mistaken for ophthalmoplegic migraine and must be distinguished from other retro-orbital lesions such as intracranial aneurysms and sphenoid wing meningioma. It is probably identical with pseudotumor of the orbit. Tolosa (1954) described the condition in a patient who died after surgical exploration for left retro-orbital pain associated with ophthalmoplegia and who was found at autopsy to have granulomatous tissue surrounding the intracavernous portion of the internal carotid artery. Hunt et al. (1961) noted the responsiveness of the syndrome to steroid therapy. Although more than 200 cases have been reported since then, few have had histologic confirmation.

One of our own patients came in with severe left-sided headache, retro-orbital pain, nausea, and diplopia (Goadsby & Lance, 1989; see Figure 5.3). After a 6-year history of recurrence of such episodes, sometimes with proptosis and paralysis of the left third and sixth cranial nerves, and repeated investigations, we at last obtained a positive computed tomography (CT) scan. Biopsy disclosed a granuloma with some multinucleated giant cells. Kline and Hoyt (2001) reviewed the condition. Painful ophthalmoplegia may accompany Horner's syndrome and sensory impairment in the distribution of the first or second divisions of the trigeminal nerve. Paresis may occur with the onset of pain or within 2 weeks; it resolves within 72 hours when treated with corticosteroids but persists for 8 weeks or so if untreated. Orbital phlebography in Tolosa-Hunt syndrome shows narrowing of the third segment of the superior ophthalmic vein, often combined with partial occlusion of the cavernous sinus (Hannerz, Ericson, & Bergstrand, 1986). These authors examined 13 patients with Tolosa-Hunt syndrome and 83 other patients with the same sort of orbital pain characteristics. Of 50 patients who had abnormal orbital phlebograms, 17 had orbital pain without neurologic deficit, 20 had associated visual impairment, and the remaining 13 had involvement of extraocular muscle innervation, 1 with additional optic nerve signs. The authors considered that retroorbital vasculitis and granulomatous disease of presumably immunologic origin is more common than reported cases of Tolosa-Hunt syndrome would suggest. Of 41 patients treated with steroids, 39 lost their characteristic pain, supporting this view. A study by Hannerz (1992) emphasized that about one third of patients with Tolosa-Hunt syndrome had episodes of periorbital pain without ophthalmoplegia and that chronic fatigue and other systemic symptoms were not uncommon.

Diagnosis may be made by MRI (de Arcaya et al., 1999). It is important to exclude other causes of similar symptoms, which Kline and Hoyt (2001) delineate. The major categories are vascular lesions such as aneurysms, tumors of various sorts, mucoceles, sarcoid and Wegener's granulomatosis.

OPHTHALMOPLEGIC MIGRAINE

Recurrent attacks of migrainelike headache accompanied or followed by paresis of the third, fourth, or sixth cranial nerves have traditionally been considered a variation of migraine. That ophthalmoplegia may develop as long as 4 days after headache begins, and that MRI often shows gadolinium uptake in the cisternal part of the affected cranial nerves (Figure 18.6), has prompted suggestions that the condition is a recurrent demyelinating neuropathy (Mark et al., 1998; Lance & Zagami, 2001). The relationship between headache and neural involvement is unclear. The older concept, that the ophthalmoplegia results from an ischemic neuropathy triggered by migrainous vasospasm, has not been disproved. As with Tolosa-Hunt syndrome, it is important to exclude compression of the cranial nerves caused by aneurysm or other space-occupying lesions.

CENTRAL CAUSES OF FACIAL PAIN

Anesthesia Dolorosa

In the unpleasant and intractable condition of anesthesia dolorosa, the patient feels pain or other disagreeable sensations in a body area that is numb from some deafferenting disease or procedure, comparable with a phantom limb (Bowsher,

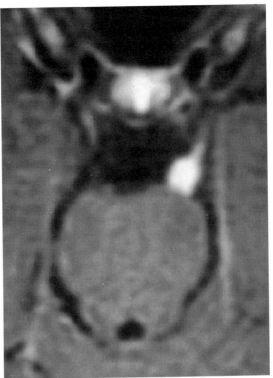

FIGURE 18.6 Ophthalmoplegic "migraine." Magnetic resonance image with gadolinium showing enhancement of the intracisternal portion of the oculomotor nerve. (From Lance and Zagami, 2001, by permission of the editor of *Cephalalgia*).

1996; Boivie & Casey, 2000). It is as if central pain pathways, deprived of their normal afferent input, discharged spontaneously to convey a false message of perceived pain to higher centers. After radiofrequency lesions of the Gasserian ganglion, anesthesia dolorosa has affected up to 3% of patients, and other disturbing sensations were reported in another 17% (Illingworth, 1986). Dysesthesia varied from 7% to 36% in the series Taha and Tew (1997) reported, depending on the extent of postoperative sensory impairment.

Central Poststroke Pain

Pain and burning sensations in the face and scalp may be caused by central lesions involving the second-order trigeminal neurons, the quintothalamic tract, the ventrobasal nuclei of the thalamus, or, less often, of the thalamocortical pathway. These pathways or nuclei may be damaged by vascular disease or multiple sclerosis and, less commonly, by syringomyelia or glioma. The pain often extends to the limbs and trunk on the affected side, and the clinician can usually detect diminished sensibility to pin prick and temperature over the painful half of the face or body. Touching the hypesthetic area may evoke pain (allodynia).

Facial pain following a thalamic lesion is part of a hemisyndrome. Poststroke pain has been reported to follow hemorrhages into the posterior limb of the internal capsule, but the face was involved in only 4 of 20 patients (Kim, 2003). With lateral medullary infarction (Wallenberg syndrome), the patient may feel pain only in one side of the face but commonly also feels pain in the opposite side of the body (Bowsher, Leijon, & Thuomas, 1998).

The condition is notoriously difficult to control. Tricyclic antidepressants such as amitriptyline and anticonvulsants such as carbamazepine, clonazepam, and sodium valproate may be helpful (Miles & Bowsher, 1991).

Multiple Sclerosis

Trigeminal neuralgia has been a symptom of multiple sclerosis in 1% to 8% of cases in reported series (Selby, 1975). However, 2% to 3% of patients with trigeminal neuralgia have multiple sclerosis (Jensen, Rasmussen, & Reske-Nielsen, 1982). In 80% to 90% of the documented cases, other symptoms of multiple sclerosis preceded the onset of trigeminal neuralgia by 1 to 29 years. In the remainder, facial pain was the presenting symptom, and other signs of multiple sclerosis followed 1 month to 6 years later. Of patients with multiple sclerosis and trigeminal neuralgia, the pain becomes bilateral in 11% to 14%, compared with 3% to 4% of patients with the idiopathic form. The pain arises from a plaque of multiple sclerosis in the pons at the entry zone of the trigeminal nerve. Jannetta (1976) observed such plaques in 4% of patients subjected to posterior fossa exploration for trigeminal neuralgia. Less commonly, a plaque of multiple sclerosis can cause glossopharyngeal neuralgia (Minager & Sheremata, 2000). Watkins and Espir (1969) reported that migrainous headache was more common in patients with multiple sclerosis, affecting 27% of patients compared with 12% of a control group. This supports the concept that migraine has a central origin.

Persistent Idiopathic Facial Pain

By definition, the term *persistent idiopathic facial pain* (previously known as *atypical facial pain*) embraces all those patients whose symptoms do not fit in with a recognized pattern of headache or neuralgic symptoms. In practice, a distinctive group of patients has what might be called *typical atypical facial pain,* so the term *persistent idiopathic facial pain* is preferable. This pain commonly affects patients in their 30s or 40s, women more often than men (Clough, 1991). The most common sites are in the nasolabial fold or on the chin overlying the lower gum. The pain is usually constant, fluctuating in intensity, and aching or drilling in quality. We could say it bears the same relationship to "lower-half headache" that tension headache does to migraine. It often starts after some apparently innocuous dental procedure or minor facial trauma.

In the past, this condition has been perceived as a hysterical conversion phenomenon or symptom of depression. Lascelles (1966) could find no justification for the former view in his study of 93 patients but considered that the majority had depressive symptoms with fatigue, agitation, and sleep disorders. It is important to note that most of the patients had good premorbid personalities, so their psychologic symptoms may well be a reaction to their depressing illness. Kerr (1979) considered that a small neuroma at the site of trauma could initiate atypical facial pain, which then became a self-perpetuating pain phenomenon.

We regard the condition as an organic syndrome of central origin for the following reasons:

1. The pain is remarkably similar in site and quality from patient to patient and is consistent with hyperexcitability of the trigeminal nerve, commonly the second division, or its central connections.
2. The most common sites of pain coincide with trigger points for trigeminal neuralgia.
3. The pain often starts after dental procedures, indicating the possibility that some infection could be introduced at that time or that herpes simplex virus, a permanent resident in the second and third trigeminal divisions of many people, might be activated to involve central pain pathways and to initiate a reaction akin to the neuralgia following herpes zoster.
4. Thermographic assessment of the facial circulation in nine of our patients with unilateral atypical facial pain demonstrated increased heat loss from the cheek of the affected side in six patients and from the orbit in four (Drummond, 1988). This suggests a reflex vasodilator response to activity in the trigeminal system and supports the concept of an organic basis for this disorder.

Jaegher, Singer, and Kroening (1986) reported two patients, one with intense unilateral facial pain following extraction of an upper molar tooth and the other with pain following sinus operations, who improved after stellate ganglion block. These authors described this syndrome as "reflex sympathetic dystrophy of the face."

Facial pain around the ear or temple may precede the detection of an ipsilateral lung carcinoma causing referred pain by invading the vagus nerve. Eross et al. (2003) warn that the clinical triad of a smoker suffering periauricular pain who has a high erythrocyte sedimentation rate (ESR) should have a lung CT scan. Previously refractory facial pain responds to effective treatment of the lung lesion.

Surgical measures do not usually relieve atypical facial pain and may make it worse. Regular administration of imipramine, amitriptyline, and dothiepin often eases the pain. We have also found baclofen useful in some instances. Electroconvulsive therapy has helped some patients who were severely depressed (Lascelles, 1966).

Burning Mouth Syndrome

A burning sensation in the mouth or tongue can be a symptom of a local or systemic disorder that responds to treatment of the underlying condition. When no medical, mucosal, or dental cause can be found, the condition is termed *burning mouth syndrome*. It may be associated with subjective dryness, paresthesia, and altered taste (Zakrzewska, 2002). The pain may be confined to the tongue (glossodynia).

The syndrome affects predominantly women, increasing in prevalence with age, particularly following menopause. Many patients have symptoms of anxiety, depression, and personality disorders. The cause of the syndrome is unknown. One third to one half of patients improve spontaneously.

Treatment is unsatisfactory. Antidepressants and low-dose clonazepam (mean 1 mg daily) have been employed, but evidence of their effect is lacking.

NEURALGIAS OF UNCERTAIN VALIDITY

Sluder's Sphenopalatine Neuralgia

Sluder (1910) reported 60 patients in whom symptoms and signs indicated disturbance of the sphenopalatine ganglion. He described pain at the root of the nose, also involving the eye, jaws, teeth, and ear. On the affected side he noticed diminished sensibility of the soft palate, a higher arch of the palate, and diminished taste sensation. Applying cocaine 20% to the mucosa overlying the sphenopalatine ganglion relieved pain.

Sluder cited examples of a 27-year-old woman with episodes of such pain recurring from three times weekly to once every 3 months (which may have been facial migraine), patients with pain accompanying respiratory infections, and one patient whose pain extended down the arm and leg. The International Headache Society Classification Subcommittee considered this condition the same as cluster headache, but it is more likely a collection of facial pains of differing etiology. Bruyn (1986d) reviewed the literature on the syndrome.

Vail's Vidian Neuralgia

Vail (1932) considered that many of the cases Sluder described had pain arising from the vidian nerve rather than the sphenopalatine ganglion and ascribed the cause to inflammation of the sphenoid sinus. He described 31 cases, 28 of whom were female, between 24 and 59 years of age. The attacks often came on between 2 and 3 AM, suggesting that many of these patients may have had migraine or cluster headache. The diagnosis, like that of Sluder's neuralgia, is of historical interest only.

Eagle's Syndrome

In 1937 W. Eagle reported that pain in the upper pharynx radiating to the ipsilateral ear, and made worse by swallowing, was related to an elongated styloid process (Montalbetti et al., 1995). He later reported 200 cases, claiming that approximately 4% of people with a long styloid process suffer from facial/pharyngeal pain. We remain skeptical, because we have not seen a convincing example.

References

Barker, F. G., II, Jannetta, P. J., Bissonette, P. A.-C., Larkins, M. V., & Jho, H. D. (1996). The long-term outcome of microvascular decompression for trigeminal neuralgia. *N Engl J Med, 334,* 1077–83.

Bates, J. A. V., & Nathan, P. W. (1980). Transcutaneous nerve stimulation for chronic pain. *Anaesthesia, 35*, 817–823.

Bertoft, E. S., & Westerberg, C. E. (1985). Further observations on the neck–tongue syndrome. *Cephalalgia, 5*(Suppl. 3), 312–313.

Bogduk, N. (1981a). An anatomical basis for the neck–tongue syndrome. *J Neurol Neurosurg Psychiatry, 44*, 202–208.

Bogduk, N. (1981b). The anatomy of occipital neuralgia. *Clin Exper Neurol, 17*, 167–184.

Bogduk, N. (1981c). Local anaesthetic blocks of the second cervical ganglion: A technique with application in occipital headache. *Cephalalgia, 1*, 41–50.

Bogduk, N. (1985). Greater occipital neuralgia. In D. M. Long. (Ed.), *Current therapy in neurological surgery* (pp. 175–180). Toronto: Decker; St. Louis: Mosby.

Boivie, J., & Casey, K. L. (2000). Central pain in the face and head. In J. Olesen, P. Tfelt-Hansen, & K. M. A. Welch (Eds.), *The headaches* (2nd ed., pp. 939–945). Philadelphia: Lippincott, Williams & Wilkins.

Bowsher, D. (1996). Central pain: Clinical and physiological characteristics. *J Neurol Neurosurg Psychiatry, 61*, 62–9.

Bowsher, D., Leijon, G., & Thuomas, K. A. (1998). Central poststroke pain. Correlation of MRI with clinical pain characteristics and sensory abnormalities. *Neurology, 51*, 1352–1358.

Brisman, R. (2000). Gamma knife radiosurgery for primary management for trigeminal neuralgia. *J Neurosurg, 93*(Suppl. 3), 159–161.

Bruyn, G. W. (1986a). Charlin's neuralgia. In P. J. Vinken, G. W. Bruyn, & H. L. Klawans (Eds.), *Handbook of clinical neurology*. Vol. 4(48). *Headache,* ed. F. Clifford Rose (pp. 483–386). Amsterdam: Elsevier.

Bruyn, G. W. (1986b). Glossopharyngeal neuralgia. In P. J. Vinken, G. W. Bruyn, & H. L. Klawans (Eds.), *Handbook of clinical neurology*. Vol. 4(48). *Headache,* ed. F. Clifford Rose (pp. 459–473). Amsterdam: Elsevier.

Bruyn, G. W. (1986c). Nervus intermedius neuralgia (Hunt). In P. J. Vinken, G. W. Bruyn, & H. L. Klawans (Eds.), *Handbook of clinical neurology*. Vol. 4(48). *Headache,* ed., F. Clifford Rose (pp. 487–494). Amsterdam: Elsevier.

Bruyn, G. W. (1986d). Sphenopalatine neuralgia (Sluder). In P. J. Vinken, G. W. Bruyn, & H. L. Klawans (Eds.), *Handbook of clinical neurology*. Vol. 4(48): *Headache,* ed. F. Clifford Rose (pp. 475–487). Amsterdam: Elsevier.

Bruyn, G. W. (1986e). Superior laryngeal neuralgia. In P. J. Vinken, G. W. Bruyn, & H. L. Klawans (Eds.), *Handbook of clinical neurology*. Vol.4(48). *Headache,* ed. F. Clifford Rose (pp. 495–500). Amsterdam: Elsevier.

Burchiel, K. J. (1980). Abnormal impulse generation in focally demyelinated trigeminal roots. *J Neurosurg, 53*, 674–683.

Caminero, A. B., & Pareja, J. A. (2001). Supraorbital neuralgia: a clinical study. *Cephalalgia, 21*, 216-223.

Classification Subcommittee of the International Headache Society (2004). *The International Classification of Headache Disorders* (2nd ed.), (Suppl.1), 126–136.

Clough, C. G. (1991). Atypical facial pain. In M. Swash & J. Oxbury (Eds.), *Clinical neurology* (pp. 370–372). Edinburgh: Churchill Livingstone.

Dalessio, D. J., McIsaac, H., Aung, M., & Polich, J. (1990). Non-invasive trigeminal evoked potentials: Normative data and application to neuralgia patients. *Headache, 30*, 696–700.

Dandy, W. E. (1934). Concerning the cause of trigeminal neuralgia. *Am J Surg, 24*, 447–455.

de Arcaya, A. A., Cerezal, L., Canga, A., Polo, J. M., Berciano, J., & Pascual, J. (1999). Neuroimaging diagnosis of Tolosa-Hunt syndrome. MRI contribution. *Headache, 39*, 321–325.

Denny-Brown, D., & Yanagisawa, N. (1973). The function of the descending root of the fifth nerve. *Brain, 96*, 783–814.

De Vries, N., & Smelt, W. L. (1990). Local anaesthetic block of posttraumatic neuralgia of the infraorbital nerve. *Rhinology, 28*, 103–106.

Drake, D. (1850). *A systematic treatise, historical, epidemiological and practical, on the principal diseases of the interior valley of North America, as may appear in the Caucasian, African and Indian and Esquimaux varieties of its population*. Cincinnati: W. B. Smith.

Drummond, P. D. (1988). Vascular changes in atypical facial pain. *Headache, 28*, 121–123.

Drummond, P. D., Gonski, A. G., & Lance, J. W. (1983). Facial flushing after thermocoagulation of the Gasserian ganglion. *J Neurol Neurosurg Psychiatry, 46*, 611–616.

Drummond, P. D., & Lance, J. W. (1984). Neurovascular disturbances in headache patients. *Clin Exp Neurol, 20,* 93–99.

Editorial. (1990). Postherpetic neuralgia. *Lancet, 336,* 537–538.

Elisevich, K., Stratford, J., Bray, G., & Finlayson, M. (1984). Neck–tongue syndrome: Operative management. *J Neurol Neurosurg Psychiatry, 47,* 407–409.

Esmann, V., Geil, J. P., Kroon, W., Fogh, H., Peterslund, N. A., Petersen, C. S., et al. (1987). Prednisolone does not prevent post-herpetic neuralgia. *Lancet, ii,* 126–129.

Eross, E. J., Dodick, D. W., Swanson, J. W., & Capobianco, D. J. (2003). A review of intractable facial pain secondary to underlying lung neoplasms. *Cephalalgia, 23,* 2–5.

Fitzek, S., Baumgartner, U., Fitzek, C., Magerl, W. L., Urban, P., Thomke, F., et al. (2001). Mechanisms and predictors of chronic facial pain in lateral medullary infarction. *Ann Neurol, 49,* 493–500.

Fromm, G. H., Graff-Radford, S. B., Terrence, C. F., & Sweet, W. H. (1990). Pre-trigeminal neuralgia. *Neurology, 40,* 1493–1495.

Fromm, G. H., Terrence, T. F., & Chattha, A. S. (1984). Baclofen in the treatment of trigeminal neuralgia: Double-blind study and long-term follow-up. *Ann Neurol, 15,* 240–244.

Fuh, J. L., Wang, S. J., Lu, S. R., & Juang, K. D. (2003). Ice-cream headache–a large survey of 8359 adolescents. *Cephalalgia 23,* 977–981.

Goadsby, P. J., Edvinsson, L., & Ekman, R. (1988). Release of vasoactive peptides in the extracerebral circulation of man and the cat during activation of the trigeminovascular system. *Ann Neurol, 23,* 193–196.

Goadsby, P. J., & Lance, J. W. (1989). Clinicopathological correlation in a case of painful ophthalmoplegia: Tolosa-Hunt syndrome. *J Neurol Neurosurg Psychiatry, 52,* 1290–1293.

Haines, S. J., Jannetta, P. J., & Zorub, D. S. (1980). Microvascular relations of the trigeminal nerve. An anatomical study with clinical correlation. *J Neurosurg, 52,* 381–386.

Hammond, S. R., & Danta, G. (1978). Occipital neuralgia. *Clin Exp Neurol, 15,* 258–270.

Hannerz, J. (1992). Recurrent Tolosa-Hunt syndrome. *Cephalalgia, 12,* 45–51.

Hannerz, J., Ericson, K., & Bergstrand, G. (1986). A new aetiology for visual impairment and chronic headache. The Tolosa-Hunt syndrome may be only one manifestation of venous vasculitis. *Cephalalgia, 6,* 59–63.

Hunt, W. E., Meagher, J. N., Lefever, H. E., & Zeman, W. (1961). Painful ophthalmoplegia. Its relation to indolent inflammation of the cavernous sinus, *Neurology 11,* 56–62.

Illingworth, R. (1986). Trigeminal neuralgia: Surgical aspects. In P. J. Vinken, G. W. Bruyn, & H. L. Klawans (Eds.), *Handbook of clinical neurology.* Vol. 4 (48). *Headache,* ed. F. Clifford Rose (pp. 449–458). Amsterdam: Elsevier.

Jaeger, B., Singer, E., & Kroening, R. (1986). Reflex sympathetic dystrophy of the face. Report of two cases and a review of the literature. *Arch Neurol, 43,* 693–695.

Jannetta, P. J. (1976). Microsurgical approach to the trigeminal nerve for tic douloureux. *Progr Neurol Surg, 7,* 180–200.

Jensen, T. S., Rasmussen, P., & Reske-Nielsen E. (1982). Association of trigeminal neuralgia with multiple sclerosis: Clinical pathological features. *Acta Neurol Scand, 65,* 182–189.

Kaufman, D. I., Trobe, J. D., Eggenberger, E. R., & Whitaker, J. N. (2000). Practice parameter: The role of corticosteroids in the management of acute monosymptomatic optic neuritis. *Neurology, 54,* 2039–2044.

Kerr, F. W. L. (1979). Craniofacial neuralgia. In J. J. Bonica, J. C. Liebeskind, & D. G. Albe-Fessard (Eds.), *Advances in pain research and therapy* (pp. 283–295). New York: Raven Press.

Kim, J. S. (2003). Central post-stroke pain or paresthesia in lenticulocapsular haemorrhages. *Neurology, 61,* 679–682.

Kline, L. B., & Hoyt, W. F. (2001). The Tolosa-Hunt syndrome. *J Neurol Neurosurg Psychiatry, 71,* 577–582.

Lance, J. W. (1996). The red ear syndrome. *Neurology, 47,* 617–620.

Lance, J. W., & Anthony, M. (1985). Neck–tongue syndrome on sudden turning of the head. *J Neurol Neurosurg Psychiatry, 43,* 97–101.

Lance, J. W., & Curran, D. A. (1964). Treatment of chronic tension headache. *Lancet, i,* 1236–1239.

Lance, J. W., & Zagami, A. S. (2001). Ophthalmoplegic migraine: A recurrent demyelinating neuropathy? *Cephalalgia, 21,* 84–85.

Lascelles, R. G. (1966). Atypical facial pain and depression. *Br J Psychiatry, 112,* 651–659.

Love, S., & Coakham, H. B. (2001). Trigeminal neuralgia: Pathology and pathogenesis. *Brain, 124,* 2347–2360.

Macdonald, B. K., Cockerell, O. C., Sander, J. W., & Shorvon, S. D. (2000). The incidence and lifetime prevalence of neurological disorders in a prospective community-based study in the U.K. *Brain, 123,* 665–676.

Mark, A. S., Casselman, J., Brown, D., Sanchez, J., Kolsky, M., Larsen, T. C. 3rd, et al. (1998). Ophthalmoplegic migraine: Reversible enhancement and thickening of the cisternal segment of the oculomotor nerve on contrast-enhanced MR images. *AJNR, Am J Neuroradiol, 19,* 1887–1891.

McLaughlin, M. R., Jannetta, P. J., Clyde, B. L., Subach, B. R., Comey, C. H., & Resnick, D. K. (1999). Microvascular decompression of cranial nerves: Lessons learned after 440 operations. *J Neurosurg, 90,* 1–8.

Miles, J. B., & Bowsher, D. (1991). Chronic pain syndromes. In M. Swash & J. Oxbury (Eds.), *Clinical neurology* (pp. 649–657). Edinburgh: Churchill Livingstone.

Minager, A., & Sheremata, W. A. (2000). Glossopharyngeal neuralgia and MS. *Neurology, 54,* 1368–1370.

Mokri, B. (1982). Raeder's paratrigeminal syndrome. Original concept and subsequent deviations. *Arch Neurol, 39,* 395–399.

Montalbetti, L., Ferrandi, D., Pergami, P., & Savoldi, F. (1995). Elongated styloid process and Eagle's syndrome. *Cephalalgia, 15,* 80–93.

Nathan, P. W. (1976). The gate-control theory of pain. A critical review. *Brain, 99,* 123–158.

Nurmikko, T., & Bowsher, D. (1990). Somatosensory findings in postherpetic neuralgia. *J Neurol Neurosurg Psychiatry, 53,* 135–141.

Optic Neuritis Study Group. (1997). The five-year risk of MS after optic neuritis. *Neurology, 49,* 1404–1413.

Pareja, J. A., Caminero, A. B., Serra, J., Barriga, F. J., Baron, M., Dobato, J. L., et al. (2002). Nummular headache: A coin-shaped cephalgia. *Neurology, 58,* 1678–1679.

Pascual, J., & Berciano, J. (1989). Failure of mexiletine to control trigeminal neuralgia. *Headache, 29,* 517–518.

Pestronk, A., & Pestronk, S. (1983). Goggle migraine. *N Engl J Med, 308,* 226.

Portenoy, R. K., Duma, C., & Foley, K. M. (1986). Acute herpetic and postherpetic neuralgia: Clinical review and current management. *Ann Neurol, 20,* 651–661.

Ragozzino, M. W., Melton, L. J., Kerland, L. T., Chu, C. P., & Perry, H. O. (1982). Population-based study of herpes zoster and its sequelae. *Medicine, 61,* 310–316.

Raskin, N. H., & Knittle, S. C. (1976). Ice cream headache and orthostatic symptoms in patients with migraine. *Headache, 16,* 222–225.

Richards, P., Shawdon, H., & Illingworth, R. (1983). Operative findings on microsurgical exploration of the cerebello-pontine angle in trigeminal neuralgia. *J Neurol Neurosurg Psychiatry, 46,* 1098–1101.

Rushton, J. G., Stevens, J.C., & Miller, R. H. (1981). Glossopharyngeal (vagoglossopharyngeal) neuralgia. A study of 217 cases. *Arch Neurol, 38,* 201–205.

Selby, G. (1975). Diseases of the fifth cranial nerve. In P J. Dyck, P. K. Thomas, & E. H. Lambert (Eds.), *Peripheral neuropathy* (pp. 533–569). Philadelphia: Saunders.

Shanbrom, E. (1961). Treatment of herpetic pain and postherpetic neuralgia with intravenous procaine. *JAMA, 176,* 1041–1043.

Sjaastad, O., Elsas, T., Shen, J.-M., Joubert, J., & Fredriksen, T. A. (1994). Raeder's syndrome: "anhidrosis," headache and a proposal for a new classification. *Funct Neurol, 9,* 215–234.

Sjaastad, O., Stolt-Neilsen, A., Pareja, J. A., & Vincent, M. (1999). Supraorbital neuralgia. The clinical manifestation and a possible therapeutic approach. *Headache, 39,* 204–212.

Sluder, G. (1910). The syndrome of sphenopalatine-ganglion neurosis. *Am J Med Sci, 140,* 868–878.

Stohr, M., Petruch, F., & Scheglmann, K. (1981). Somatosensory evoked potentials following trigeminal nerve stimulation in trigeminal neuralgia. *Ann Neurol, 9,* 63–66.

Taha, J. M., & Tew, J. M. (1997). Treatment of trigeminal neuralgia by percutaneous radiofrequency rhizotomy. *Neurosurg Clin N Amer, 8,* 31–39.

Tolosa, E. (1954). Periarteritic lesions of the carotid siphon with the clinical features of a carotid infraclinoidal aneurysm. *J Neurol Neurosurg Psychiatry, 17,* 300–303.

Tomson, T., Tybring, G., Bertilsson, L., Ekbom, K., & Rane, E. (1980). Carbamazepine therapy in trigeminal neuralgia. Clinical effects in relation to plasma concentration. *Arch Neurol, 37,* 699–730.

Vail, H. H. (1932). Vidian neuralgia. *Ann Otol Rhinol Laryngol, 41,* 837–856.

Watkins, S. M., & Espir, M. (1969). Migraine and multiple sclerosis. *J Neurol Neurosurg Psychiatry, 32,* 35–37.

Watson, C. P. N. (1990). Postherpetic neuralgia: Clinical features and treatment. In H. L. Fields (Ed.), *Pain syndromes in neurology* (pp. 223–238). London: Butterworths.

Watson, C. P., Evans, R. J., Reed, K., Merskey, H., Goldsmith, L., & Warsh, J. (1982). Amitriptyline versus placebo in postherpetic neuralgia. *Neurology, 32,* 671–673.

Wolf, S., & Hardy, J. D. (1941). Studies on pain. Observations on pain due to local cooling and on factors involved in the "cold pressor" effect. *J Clin Invest, 20,* 521–533.

Wolff, H. G. (1963). *Headache and other head pain* (pp. 36–37). New York: Oxford University Press.

Young, R. F., Vermeulen, S. S., Grimm, P., Blasko, J., & Posewitz, A. (1997). Gamma knife radiosurgery for treatment of trigeminal neuralgia: Idiopathic and tumour related. *Neurology, 48,* 608–614.

Zakrzewska, J. M. (2002). Burning mouth. In J. M. Zakrzewska & S. O. Harrison (Eds.), *Pain research and clinical management* (Vol. 14, pp. 263–366). Amsterdam, Elsevier Science.

Chapter 19
The Investigation and General Management of Headache

A systematic case history (Chapter 2) and its interpretation (Chapter 4) are usually sufficient for the diagnosis of migraine, cluster, and tension-type headache. When headaches are of recent onset, of uncertain pattern, or if they accompany progressive neurologic signs or systemic disturbance, investigation becomes obligatory. The clinical approach depends on the length of the headache history and the mode of presentation.

DIFFERENTIAL DIAGNOSIS

The Acute Severe Headache

The abrupt onset of a severe headache (thunderclap headache) usually requires immediate investigation (Day & Raskin, 1986; Wijdicks, Kerkhoff, & van Gijn, 1988). The following possibilities must be considered:

With Neck Rigidity

Subarachnoid hemorrhage
Meningitis, encephalitis
Systemic infections (meningism)

Without Neck Rigidity

Pressor responses (such as pheochromocytoma, reaction while on monoamine oxidase [MAO] inhibitors, "benign sex headache" at orgasm)
Acute obstructive hydrocephalus (such as colloid cyst of the third ventricle)
Expanding intracranial aneurysm
Carotid or vertebral artery dissection
Migraine
Segmental vascular constriction (Call-Fleming syndrome)

Wijdicks et al. (1988) followed 71 patients with such headaches and concluded that angiography was not indicated if computed tomography (CT) scan and cerebrospinal fluid (CSF) study were normal. See Chapter 13 for a discussion of thunderclap headache.

The Subacute Onset of Headache

The recent development of headache may indicate a sinister etiology. The following are possible causes:
- An expanding intracranial lesion (such as hematoma, tumor, abscess)
- Progressive hydrocephalus
- Temporal arteritis in patients older than 55 years
- Idiopathic (benign) intracranial hypertension
- Intracranial hypotension

Recurrent Discrete Episodes of Headache or Facial Pain

Recurrent discrete episodes of headache or facial pain may be differentiated into the following categories:
- Migraine, including "lower-half" headache (facial migraine)
- Cluster headache
- Trigeminal and other cranial neuralgias
- Transient ischemic attacks
- Intermittent obstructive hydrocephalus
- Paroxysmal hypertension (such as pheochromocytoma)
- Tolosa-Hunt syndrome
- Cough, exertional, and sex headaches
- Hypnic headaches
- Ice cream headache
- Ice-pick pains
- Sinusitis (rarely a cause of episodic headache)

Chronic Headache or Facial Pain (More Than 1 Year Duration)

Chronic headache or facial pain (lasting more than 1 year) may be classified as follows:
- Tension-type headache
- Migraine
- New daily persistent headache
- Post-traumatic headache
- Persistent idiopathic (atypical) facial pain
- Postherpetic neuralgia

It is unlikely that headache caused by intracranial lesions or temporal arteritis would persist for more than 1 year without diagnosis.

INVESTIGATION

Only a few headache patients require investigation beyond a careful history and physical examination. Clinical judgment determines which of the following tests are necessary.

Blood Count and Erythrocyte Sedimentation Rate

A blood count and a measurement of erythrocyte sedimentation rate (ESR) are routine tests for patients admitted to the hospital. General practitioners should also perform them when the patient has symptoms of systemic disorder, infection, or meningeal reaction, or when dealing with a patient older than 55 years in whom the possibility of temporal arteritis must be ruled out. Polycythemia may accompany hemangioblastoma of the cerebellum. Leukemia may present with intracranial deposits. Anemia may indicate neoplasia or other systemic disease and may accentuate any tendency to headache. A high ESR also can direct attention to some locus of infection, hidden malignancy, multiple myeloma, one of the collagen diseases, or subacute bacterial endocarditis, any of which may produce intracranial manifestations. *Note: It is sound practice always to request an ESR with a full blood count.*

Plain X-rays

Investigating headache rarely requires simple radiography of the skull unless the clinician is seeking evidence of sinusitis, mastoiditis, a skull fracture, or platybasia.

Opinions differ about the significance of certain findings. Some European authors regard hyperostosis frontalis interna as an inflammatory condition producing headache. It is a common variation of the normal from middle age onward, particularly in female patients. "Thumbing," a beaten-copper appearance of the cranial vault, may be a normal variation, although it alerts the observer to the possibility of long-standing raised intracranial pressure. In the young child, the sutures should be carefully observed, because they separate when intracranial pressure increases.

In most patients with headache, the skull radiograph will appear normal. If an intracranial lesion is suspected, a chest x-ray should also be obtained to exclude primary or secondary carcinoma, tuberculosis, sarcoid, bronchiectasis, or other relevant conditions.

Computed Tomography

In developed countries, it is difficult to dissuade anybody with any sort of headache from having a CT scan of the brain. However, injecting a contrast agent carries the risk of an allergic reaction, although with nonionic contrast media the risk is small. Always ask about a patient's response to injected contrast media on any previous occasion and about a history of allergic reactions of any kind in the past.

CT has become the initial investigative tool for patients with suspected sub-arachnoid hemorrhage, intracranial space-occupying lesions, or hydrocephalus. Interpretation of particular CT appearances may vary from country to country. For example, an enhancing lesion diagnosed as a glioma in Western countries would more likely be diagnosed as a tuberculoma in India. Cysticercosis is diagnosed as a possible cause of obstructive hydrocephalus in some South American, Mediterranean, or Asian countries.

Compared to conventional radiology, CT can give greater resolution of temporomandibular joint degeneration, sinus pathology, and fractures of the temporal and facial bones, which may be of particular value in managing post-traumatic headache and facial pain.

Abnormalities shown by CT of patients with migraine are discussed in Chapter 7. The CT appearance of a third ventricular tumor is illustrated in Chapter 16 (Figure 16.2).

Magnetic Resonance Imaging

Magnetic resonance imaging (MRI) complements CT in defining the outline and determining the nature of intracranial lesions. It is particularly helpful for finding the site of obstruction in CSF pathways (Figure 19.1) and in detecting Chiari type 1 malformation (Figure 19.2). It is useful in assessing whether an arteriovenous malformation has bled previously, by showing the presence or absence of hemosiderin surrounding the defect and in depicting posterior fossa tumors and white matter lesions.

MRI can demonstrate thrombosis of the superior sagittal or other venous sinuses (Donohoe, Waldman, & Resor, 1987; Salvati, 1990). It clearly displays dissection of the internal carotid artery, because it shows the bright signal that a

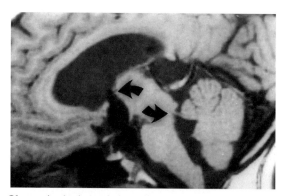

FIGURE 19.1   Obstructive hydrocephalus relieved by third ventriculostomy. MRI showing obliteration of the aqueduct (caudal end indicated with *lower arrow*) by a glioma of the midbrain tectum. Surgery has reduced pressure in the dilated lateral and third ventricles by making a communication between the posterior part of the distended floor of the third ventricle and the subarachnoid space. A flow void indicates passage of cerebrospinal fluid through the foramen of Monro and the ventriculostomy *(upper arrow)*. (Photograph courtesy of the Departments of Neurosurgery and Radiology, Prince of Wales Hospital, Sydney.)

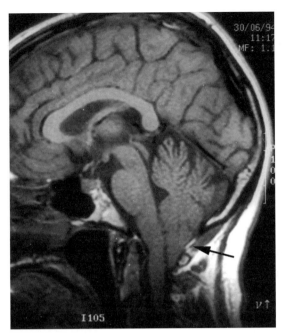

FIGURE 19.2   MRI of the brain shwoing a Chiari type 1 malformation. A tongue of cerebellum extends down to the C2 level *(arrow)*.

subintimal clot causes, surrounded by a dark flow void (Cox, Bertorini, & Laster, 1991).

MRI of patients with basilar artery migraine (Jacome & Leborgne, 1990) and those with cluster headache (Sjaastad & Rinck, 1990) has not shown any specific abnormality. Small lesions have appeared in the white matter of patients who have migraine more often than in control subjects (Igasashi et al., 1991). Magnetic resonance angiography has substantially reduced the need for conventional arteriograms.

Carotid and Vertebral Angiography

For investigating transient ischemic attacks, angiography demonstrates arterial dissection (see Figure 15.5) and stenosis or occlusion (Figure 19.3) of the major arteries. Cerebral angiography shows the site of origin of aneurysms (see Figure 15.3), the feeding vessels of arteriovenous malformations, and the vascular supply of brain tumors. It can sometimes show bilateral subdural hematomas that CT may miss when they are in their isodense phase. MRI can often show clots in the superior sagittal sinus better than angiography can.

Electroencephalography

Electroencephalography (EEG) is rarely required for diagnosis of headache, unless there are accompanying epileptic features. The association of migraine

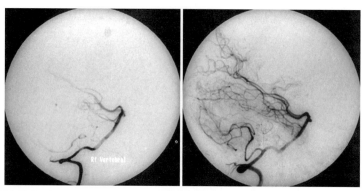

FIGURE 19.3   Posterior inferior cerebellar artery (PICA) thrombosis. The sparse filling of the vertebrobasilar circulation and the absence of the PICA on the left contrasts with the normal circulation on the right.

with epilepsy is discussed in Chapters 6 and 7, and the rare occurrence of headache as an ictal phenomenon is mentioned in Chapter 12. Occasionally EEG may prove helpful in a suspected case of herpes simplex encephalitis in which the CT scan is normal by showing a temporal slow-wave focus.

Lumbar Puncture

Lumbar puncture is performed when clinical suspicion of subarachnoid hemorrhage is high but CT scan of the brain is normal. It is also used to diagnose meningitis and encephalitis and to measure CSF pressure (e. g. in idiopathic intracranial hypertension).

It is always advisable to perform a CT scan of the brain before performing lumbar puncture if the clinician sees any indication of raised intracranial pressure or possibility of an intracranial space-occupying lesion. When a CT scanner is readily available, the clinician can start patients with suspected meningitis on antibiotic therapy immediately, transfer them to the CT scan unit, and obtain the CSF sample once the CT scan is available. Administering antibiotics for such a short period will not affect identification and culture of the infecting organism, but delay in starting antibiotics can prove fatal in fulminating meningitis. If the clinician must do a lumbar puncture urgently in a patient with raised intracranial pressure, for example, one with papilledema and possible meningitis in a hospital without ready access to CT, it is a worthwhile precaution to have at hand a 20-mL syringe filled with normal saline. If signs of coning develop after lumbar puncture, the clinician can inject saline intrathecally and elevate the foot of the patient's bed.

A small point concerning the technique of lumbar puncture that one of the authors has found useful is to infiltrate the skin with local anesthetic 1 to 2 cm laterally to the midline at the selected intervertebral disc space and, as it is inserted from this point, to angle the lumbar puncture needle toward the midline. The suggested track passes through soft tissues until the needle touches the spine. A gentle tapping movement of the needle will indicate to the examiner whether the needle is in contact with bone or with the elastic interlaminar ligament. If the latter, the clinician can insert the needle through the ligament with confidence that CSF will emerge when the stilette is removed. The advantages of this oblique approach are that it is usually painless and permits tactile sensing of the needle point position. In contrast, the firm pressure required to penetrate the interspinous ligament in the midline approach makes it difficult to perceive when the needle has entered the lumbar sac.

Cerebrospinal Fluid Isotope Studies

Inserting a radionuclide tracer into the CSF to locate the site of leakage in low pressure syndromes is discussed in Chapter 16 (Figure 16.4).

GENERAL PRINCIPLES OF MANAGEMENT

What do patients with headache expect from their doctors? Will they leave the consulting room content or with their expectations unfulfilled? Fitzpatrick and Hopkins (1981) found that dissatisfaction was more common in patients with migraine than in those with tension headache, headache duration of longer than 1 year, or significant psychiatric symptoms. Common criticisms were that clinicians did not tell patients what their diagnosis meant and did not discuss causes of their disorder or ways to avoid or alleviate episodes.

After taking the history and completing the examination, the doctor must take enough time with the patient to ensure that he or she understands the problem and to explain why investigations are or are not necessary for that particular patient. If the history is typical of migraine, cluster, or tension headache, explain this to the patient to dispel fears of cerebral tumor at the outset. Sometimes the clinician must yield to pressure and order CT of the brain to complete the process of reassurance.

Some patients hope to find a simple cause for their headaches and a simple cure. For patients with no discernible structural basis for their headaches, it may help to explain they have been born with a sensitive nervous system that responds to various stimuli by pain in blood vessels of the brain and scalp. They can also be told they can reduce the frequency and severity of attacks by physical and mental relaxation and by avoiding trigger factors, and that most patients also benefit from pharmacologic agents other than analgesics. Because some people are reluctant to use any medication, it is worthwhile taking the trouble to explain that preventive treatment is designed to build up the body's own pain control pathway to prevent recurring attacks and that acute therapy is aimed at constricting blood vessels and turning off nerves to stop the painful process.

After prescribing treatment and clarifying the rationale for it, warn the patient about any common side effect, advise him or her to start with small doses, and ask that he or she make an appointment to come in again and report progress. The patient should understand that no medication benefits everyone who takes it and that the endeavor to control headaches depends on the continuing collaboration between patient and doctor. As the efficacy of our management improves, so will the cooperation and satisfaction of the patients.

References

Cox, L. K., Bertorini, T., & Laster, R. E. (1991). Headache due to spontaneous internal carotid artery dissection. Magnetic resonance imaging evaluation and follow up. *Headache, 31,* 12–16.

Day, J. W., & Raskin, N. H. (1986). Thunderclap headache: Symptom of unruptured cerebral aneurysm. *Lancet, ii,* 1247–1248.

Donohoe, C. D., Waldman, S. D., & Resor, L. D. (1987). Magnetic resonance imaging in cerebral venous thrombosis. *Headache, 27,* 155–157.

Fitzpatrick, R., & Hopkins, A. (1981). Referrals to neurologists for headaches not due to structural disease. *J Neurol Neurosurg Psychiatry, 44,* 1061–1067.

Igarashi, H., Sakai, F., Kan, S., Okada, J., & Tazaki, Y. (1991). Magnetic resonance imaging of the brain in patients with migraine. *Cephalalgia, 11,* 69–74.

Jacome, D. D., & Leborgne, J. (1990). MRI studies in basilar artery migraine. *Headache, 30,* 88–90.

Salvati, C. A. (1990). Cerebral venous thrombosis shown by MRI. *Headache, 30,* 650–651.

Sjaastad. O., & Rinck, P. (1990). Cluster headache: MRI studies of the cavernous sinus and the base of the brain. *Headache, 30,* 350–351.

Wijdicks, E. F. M., Kerkhoff, H., & van Gijn, J. (1988). Long-term follow-up of 71 patients with thunderclap headache mimicking subarachnoid haemorrhage. *Lancet, ii,* 68–70.

APPENDIX A: AN EXPLANATION FOR PATIENTS OF HYPERVENTILATION AND ANXIETY ATTACKS

Anxiety attacks with hyperventilation (overbreathing) are commonly associated with headache. They can be overcome by recognizing the cause and obeying a few simple rules.

What Are the Symptoms?

- Light-headedness, dizziness, faintness, "giddiness"
- Tightness or pain in the chest
- Dry mouth
- Heart beating faster
- Blurring of vision
- Sweating
- Trembling of hands and legs
- Weakness ("jelly legs")
- Pins and needles in hands, feet, and around mouth
- Headache
- Anxiety, fear, or panic
- Sensation of being unable to breathe
- A feeling of having a heart attack, passing out, losing control, or of being about to die
- Spasms of hands and feet (in prolonged episodes)

When you overbreathe you may swallow air, causing:

- Distension of the stomach
- Burping
- Passing wind

What Do You Mean by Overbreathing?

- Taking deep sighing breaths
- Yawning often
- Rapid, shallow breathing
- Deep breathing

When Is This Most Likely to Happen?

- When you are tense, bored, or depressed
- In crowds, at a party, or in a supermarket

How Does This Cause Symptoms?

Normally nature takes care of the rate and depth of breathing. The carbon dioxide (CO_2) in your blood makes you breathe enough to eliminate it and get sufficient oxygen.

If you override nature and breathe too much, you wash out too much CO_2. This reduces the blood flow to your brain and makes you feel dizzy. It also reduces the available calcium in the blood, which can cause "pins and needles" and make the hands and feet spasm. Adrenaline increases in the bloodstream, causing a feeling of anxiety, sweating, and trembling, and makes the heart beat faster. Contraction of muscles causes pain and tightness in the chest and headache.

How Can You Stop It?

Look for the first signs of sighing or yawning. Do not do the following:

- Open the windows.
- Run outside.
- Take deep breaths.

  Instead,

- Sit down.
- Hold your breath and count to i0.
- Breathe out slowly and say "relax" to yourself.
- Then breathe in and out slowly every 6 seconds (10 breaths per minute).
- As soon as possible, forget about your breathing and let nature do it for you.

General Principles

- Take it easy. It is not a disaster if you forget someone's name, burn the dinner, or don't have time to mow the lawn. Talk more slowly. Walk more slowly. You have plenty of time.
- Think positively. You can handle a problem as well as the next person. All the people you meet in the street or around a conference table have their problems, too. Spread out your workload throughout the day. Give yourself enough time for each task.
- Remain calm.
- Don't bottle up your feelings—discuss any worries or things that make you angry or upset.
- Eat regular meals and don't hurry them.
- Limit yourself to five cups of tea or coffee each day.
- Cut out smoking or have fewer than 10 cigarettes per day.

- Learn to recognize any tendency to overbreathe.
- Learn to relax your muscles—no frowning or jaw clenching.
- Get regular exercise.
- Take time out for social activities and holidays.

You can control your attacks completely by following these rules.

APPENDIX B: RELAXATION EXERCISES: INSTRUCTIONS FOR PATIENTS WITH MIGRAINE OR TENSION-TYPE HEADACHES

What Does Muscle Contraction Have to Do with Headache?

The blood vessels and nerve fibers of your scalp lie in muscle. Place your fingers on each temple and clench your jaw. You will feel the muscle belly of your temporal muscle swell as it contracts. Let your jaw go loose, and the muscle becomes flat again. Many people contract these muscles all day without realizing it, so they are working continuously, which may set up a constant dull ache in the temples. The vessels that run through the muscles often constrict while the muscle is contracting. During sleep the muscles may relax and the vessels dilate, so that a person may wake in the middle of the night or the early morning with a throbbing headache in the temples. Others may grind their teeth at night during sleep and may therefore wake up with aching jaws and a raw, tender spot on their upper gum caused by sideways movement of the jaw during sleep. Overcontracting the jaw muscles is very common in tense or anxious people, who often do not realize their muscles are not relaxed.

Do you feel your jaw muscles aching at the end of your day, after an unpleasant or difficult conversation, or after an argument? Do you feel an ache in one or both temples at these times or wake up with a headache in this area? If your headache is in one temple only, check your bite to see if you chew equally and evenly on both sides and can move your jaw freely from side to side. If you have back teeth missing on one side or the other, the strain of chewing is shifted to the other side, which causes an ache in the hinge joint of your jaw and in your temple. If this is the case, see your dentist about balancing your bite, as this factor can be very important in excessive jaw clenching.

Just as chronic jaw clenching is a common cause of aching in the temples, chronic frowning is a common cause of pain in the forehead. Do others say to you that you frown a lot or look worried most of the time? This can indicate that you are using your scalp muscles without being aware of doing so.

Pain in your neck can also result from muscle contraction. Some people walk about holding their neck stiffly as though it were a solid block of wood.

This may be an attempt to protect your neck, because when you move it you feel a sensation of grating in your neck, or because you have found out that an x-ray shows some of the disks in your neck, have degenerated. Disk degeneration is quite common even in young people and is almost universal in older age groups. If you have had a whiplash injury to the neck or your attention drawn to your neck in any way, your muscles may contract to splint your neck. This sets up a vicious cycle of pain leading to muscle spasm, which leads to more pain.

Muscle contraction or tension headache is usually a constant tight, pressing feeling in your forehead, temples, or back of your head and may spread all around your head "like a tight band." Because your scalp muscles are linked together by a sheet of strong tissue that passes over your skull, muscle contraction may also cause the feeling of pressure on top of your head. Sharp jabbing pains may also be felt, because muscle contraction compresses scalp nerves.

Overcontraction of muscle is a habit that develops over the years and often starts in childhood. About one in seven patients with tension headache can remember having similar headaches even when younger than age 10. This habit may be associated with mental tension and anxiety but may have become an automatic reaction that continues even when there are no obvious problems of any sort.

Are You Able to Relax?

The most natural form of treatment is to train the muscles of your body to relax, and the first step is to realize that you are not as relaxed as you thought you were. Try these simple tests.

1. Sit in a chair and lean back. Ask someone to lift your arm in the air in a comfortable position as though it were resting on the side of an armchair. Take your time, and relax completely. Then ask your friend to take away his or her hands, which have been supporting your arm. When the supporting hands are taken away, what does your arm do? If it flops lifelessly downward, you are indeed relaxed. If it stays in the air, or you move it slowly downward, you are not relaxed. Your muscles are contracting continuously without you realizing it.
2. Lie on a bed or couch with your head on a pillow, and try to relax completely. When you consider that you have achieved this, ask your helper to pull the pillow away from under your head. Does your head drop limply onto the bed? Or does it stay poised in midair as though the pillow were still there? If you are still holding your head in the air above an invisible pillow, your muscles must be contracting without you realizing it.

Once you have acknowledged that excessive muscle contraction is playing a part in the aching of your head or neck, and that you do not really know whether the muscles are contracting or not, you are ready to start relaxation exercises.

Paradoxically, you cannot relax about relaxing. It is not a passive process. It is no use saying to someone "relax" and imagining that he or she can do so without further thought. You cannot say to yourself "relax" and then do it unless you have carefully practiced the art of "switching off" the nerve supply to your muscles. This is a voluntary action as deliberate as turning off a light switch and must be practiced until it can be done at will and done rapidly.

At first it is necessary to set aside at least 10 minutes each night and morning for your exercises. It is a great help to have someone with you in the early stages to ensure that you are completely relaxed when you think you are. We will call this person your "helper." It is obviously a great advantage if your helper can be a trained physiotherapist or occupational therapist, but this is not always possible, and a well-motivated husband or wife, relative, or friend can be very valuable in ensuring that your exercises are done thoroughly and that relaxation is practiced until it becomes complete.

The Sequence of Relaxation Exercises

Lie down on a firm surface such as a carpeted floor. A bed with an inner-spring mattress will do, but not one with a soft, sagging mattress. A pillow can be used to support your head at first but can be discarded later as relaxation becomes easier. For the first few sessions wear only a short-sleeved shirt and shorts so that muscle contraction can be seen as well as felt. Lie on your back with legs slightly separated and arms comfortably flexed at your elbow so that your elbows are by your sides with hands resting on your body. Now you will contract and relax various muscles in turn.

Legs

Contract your leg muscles so that your legs become rigid pillars. The muscle bellies stand out as your muscles contract. Concentrate on the sensation set up by your muscles contracting, and the feeling of tension in them. Then, suddenly and deliberately, "switch off the power supply" so that your muscles go limp. Concentrate on whether any sensation is coming from your muscles now. Are they completely relaxed? At this point it is helpful for your helper to put his or her hand behind your knees and lift them up sharply to see if your leg is completely floppy and that your muscles do not contract again as soon as your limb is moved passively. If they are not completely relaxed, or if they contract again when your limb is touched or moved, repeat the sequence.

On the first few attempts, many people only relax halfway. This can be detected by watching the muscles closely. After the first relaxation, the muscle bellies are not as prominent as they were, but some contraction may remain. Try again to switch off, and this second attempt may be rewarded by seeing the muscle become completely flaccid. Your helper can then bend your legs at the knee, move them about, or roll them backward and forward with your feet flopping like a rag doll. This sequence can be completed by lifting one leg, letting it drop downward like an inanimate object, then doing the same with the other.

Arms

Brace your arms so that your elbows are forced downward on the couch (or on the helper's hand if he or she is checking degree of relaxation). Hold your arms rigidly and stop the muscle contraction suddenly so arms become limp and lifeless. Your helper should then be able to bounce your elbow up and down without any resistance being offered. Repeat this sequence until you are aware of the sensation of muscle contraction and the contrast with the feeling of relaxation, and your helper is satisfied that your arm can become truly flaccid.

Neck

Lift your head from the pillow and then let it *drop* backward. Your helper may provide resistance by pressing on your forehead until you feel the contraction of the muscles in the front of your neck. When your head is dropped backward, your helper can rock it gently to and fro to make certain that there is no residual activity in your muscles. Now *push* your head backward into the pillow and register the sensation of contraction of the muscles in the back of your neck. Stop the contraction suddenly, so that your helper can rotate your head freely on your neck. Repeat this until relaxation is satisfactory.

Forehead

Frown upward so that your brow is furrowed. If you have difficulty doing this, look upward as far as your eyes will move, and the skin on your forehead will crease. Again, feel the sensation of tension in your muscles, then close your eyes and let your forehead muscles relax. Your helper can detect the presence or absence of contraction by seeing whether the skin of your forehead moves freely with his or her hand.

Eyes

Screw your eyes up tightly and become aware of the sensation of tension; then relax your muscles and lie with your eyes lightly closed. Make sure that there is no trembling or flickering of your closed eyelids and that your eye muscles feel entirely relaxed.

Jaws

Clench your jaw firmly and concentrate on feeling the sense of tightness in your temples as well as in your jaw itself. Then switch off and let your jaw fall open. Push your jaw open, perhaps against the pressure of your helper's hand, then relax completely. Move your jaw sideways to the right as far as it will go, and experience the sensation this gives to your jaw and temple before relaxing. Then do the same to the left. Complete the sequence by clenching your jaw firmly again, and let your jaw drop open loosely. Your helper should then be able to hold the tip of your jaw with his or her fingers and waggle your jaw up and down rapidly without any opposition from your jaw muscles.

This is the hardest of all relaxation procedures to achieve, so do not be disappointed if you don't succeed on the first occasion. You may need repeated practice to enable your jaw muscles to cease all activity so that your helper can easily move your jaw. It is very important to persevere until you accomplish this, because overcontraction of jaw muscles is a common factor in tension headache, and the switching-off process must be thoroughly learned.

Whole Body Relaxation

Once you can relax your legs, arms, neck, forehead, eye, and jaw muscles in order, lie for 5 minutes with all muscles relaxed. Once you have achieved total relaxation, the process becomes negative rather than positive. In other words, you permit natural relaxation to continue rather than willing yourself to relax actively. At this stage, it helps to think of some beautiful and tranquil scene, to imagine yourself lying on a grassy bank on a warm summer's day with the drowsy sounds of summer in the background. Everyone has some particular sound he or she associates with peace and tranquility. It may be the rippling of a trout stream, the humming of bees, the song of birds, the soughing of wind in the trees, or distant music. Choose your own theme and your own mental picture and live in that scene for a few minutes. As you do, feel the sensation of heaviness creep over your legs, trunk, and arms, then spread to your neck and head, eyes, and face. Lie completely inert, with all muscles relaxed, a feeling of heaviness throughout your body, and a pleasant scene pictured in your mind. Feel the sensation of freedom in your mind and in your head. This can become a permanent freedom if your muscles obey you all the time as well as they do at that moment.

After Relaxation Exercises Are Finished

The final and most important step is to carry the art of relaxation into your everyday life. Watch the way you stand, sit, speak on the telephone, talk to people, write, type, or perform any other activity of a typical day. Check that all your muscles not essential to your task of the moment are in a state of relaxation. You can handle any situation, irrespective of the degree of mental stress, without physical tension once you become accustomed to the idea. You actually perform more efficiently if you tackle any problem in an orderly fashion without excessive and useless muscle contraction. If you notice any warning sensations of tension in your scalp, jaw, or neck muscles, you must pause a moment to ensure that these muscles are switched off in the manner you have practiced. In this way you will finish your day feeling much fresher and with much less chance of headache making your day a misery.

Keep Practicing

There is no point in performing the exercise routine religiously for a week and then forgetting the whole thing. If you do, unless you are a very exceptional person the old habits of muscle contraction will assert themselves again. Keep practicing, stay relaxed, and free yourself from headache.

Index